Intuitive Eating

HOHM PRESS

HUMBART "SMOKEY" SANTILLO, N.D.

Printed in the United States of America
ISBN: 0-934252-27-0

Library of Congress Card Number: 93-077511
Published by Hohm Press P.O. Box 2501 Prescott, Arizona 86302
602-778-9189

Design and Typesetting:
Kim Johansen
Pièce de Résistance Ltée.

To my children, Nicholas and Jessica:

I have felt what this world could be like through the eyes of my children.

TABLE OF CONTENTS

PART III: ACTION STEPS

PART IV: APPENDICES

FOREWORD

by Victor P. Kulvinskis

IT is a teacher's great pleasure to be exceeded by a student. I have known Smokey Santillo for twenty-five years. We started out as teacher and student and evolved into friends and colleagues. I was just one of many teachers who played a role in Smokey's development. In whatever field he entered, and there were many, he always expanded the borders, created structure where there was none, and innovated creative models and systems for healing the body.

Smokey Santillo is a holistic person, and the quality of his life has made him an inspiration and role model for others. He has healed himself of many chronic health problems and rejuvenated and maintained his body into his current youthful form. Smokey is an accomplished jazz musician, an outstanding athlete, a great family man, a respected researcher and teacher, and a compassionate and effective counselor.

In the 80s, after working with over ten thousand clients, Smokey guided the growing field of herb usage into a model of holistic healing rather than just more therapy. His now classic work, *Natural Healing With Herbs*, stands as a witness to his contribution to this field.

Motivated by personal tragedy, we worked together on creating the nutritional support for the self-healing of his father from liver cancer. He was both excited and surprised by how quickly the body was able to recover with the assistance of *aspergillus* enzymes plus herbs in conjunction with a low-protein, predigested, mucus-lean diet oriented towards live foods. This initiated his research into the field of enzymes. He fused this knowledge with his oriental studies and understanding of magnetism and this resulted in his pioneering a new system for enzyme formula development and application. His studies were articulated in his book *Food Enzymes* and the marketplace was revitalized with his many new enzyme-based formulas for balancing the acupuncture meridians, the chakras, and the glandular system.

As Smokey became more involved with the use of fresh fruit and vegetable juices he redefined a bio-chemical foundation for juicing. Using elements of Oriental medicine, saliva and urinary testing, and particular juices for particular organs of the body, the new science of "Juiceology" was born. At the same time he evolved a system for preserving the essence of the juices by the removal of water. This makes it possible to reconstitute juice at any time.

This new book, *Intuitive Eating*, is a perfect continuation in Smokey's ongoing service to the needs of the public. More folks would be vegetarians if they were guided in their transition in ways that were tasty, appealing, and safe—offering them the benefits of long-term health. As the title implies, *Intuitive Eating* is a text to develop your intuition so that you will know at all times what to eat, how, when and where, as well as why. All the answers are within. The book will act as a key to open you to your true nature.

Intuitive Eating will teach you how to cleanse your internal system, rebuild it with upgraded nutrition, and help you to eventually evolve into a live-food-oriented system that will take into account your unique balance. I have used many of the methods recommended here and have found them to be extremely beneficial.

Smokey provides us with a system that the public is already gravitating towards. According to Brain Reserve, a leading New York consulting firm that boasts a 95% success rate in forecasting future markets for Fortune 500 companies such as American Express, Eastman Kodak, and the Hearst Corporation, vegetarianism in the 1990s will be more than just a passing trend. It will be a permanent lifestyle shift. The transitional system of *Intuitive Eating* is a invaluable resource for anyone wishing to make that shift.

Examples of this movement to vegetarianism are observable in many areas. In the summer of 1992, the American Dietetics Association held the Second International Congress on Vegetarian Nutrition. It was attended by leading experts such as Dr. Campbell from Cornell University and Dr. Dean Ornish. Furthermore, the Cornell-China-Oxford Project on Nutrition, Health and Environment which was conducted by Dr. Chen Junshi (Deputy Director, Institute of Nutrition and Food Hygiene, Chinese Academy of Preventive Medicine) and Dr. T. C. Campbell (Cornell University) in their preliminary findings of the study involving 6,500 people in China in 1983 showed that a diet of mostly plant foods is "associated with reduced risk of the kinds of diseases that tend to kill...Humans evolved as a 'vegetarian species' and have not adjusted to the risk of eating animal products." (USA Today, 5-9-90). This project represented the movement of vegetarianism into the mainstream.

Previously, doctors, nutritionists, and dietitians have looked at vegetarianism as a counter-culture phenomenon and simply hoped that no harm would come to those who practiced such non-traditional eating habits. Now it is more widely accepted that a vegetarian diet is actually safer and healthier than the standard American diet. For most health professionals this represents a radical change in thinking. It will be only a matter of time before *Intuitive Eating* will be the book used for training many health professionals because it teaches that vegetarianism, when properly applied, can be the main healing agent and preventive method of handling disease and the key to assured longevity.

In a 1977 report of the U.S. Department of Health, Education and Welfare, the Secretary of H.E.W. stressed that: "You, the individual can do more for your own health and well being than any doctor, any hospital, any drug, and exotic medical device." The report went on: "Indeed, a wealth of scientific research reveals that the key to whether a person will be healthy or sick, live a long life or die prematurely, can be found in several simple personal habits: one's habit with regard to smoking, one's habit of diet, sleep and exercise, as well as attitude."

I feel that Smokey's Santillo's book is the natural answer to our major health dilemmas as Americans. It stands on the foundation of self-responsibility as expressed by the H.E.W. Report. *Intuitive Eating* has the keys to open the doors to inner understanding and wisdom. It makes it possible and practical to understand your body and apply the Hippocratic principle of "Let food by your medicine and medicine be your food" in a balanced way to assure a life of health, joy, success, and longevity. The body is self-healing, but first it needs to have the toxins reduced and be introduced to the food of intuition which will help it rebuild itself every year in a healthier and more beautiful expression.

Everyone can be an intuitive eater. Age is no limit! The natural state of health is our birthright and we can free ourselves of degenerative diseases. But, unless we use a system like the one found in *Intuitive Eating,* Americans will continue to search for the potion of health and the evasive fountain of youth without success.

I fully endorse this book, *Intuitive Eating,* as the most practical and scientifically based system for self healing.

Victor Kulvinskas, M.S.
Author: *Survival Into the 21st Century*; *Vegetarian Lifestyle Directory and Travel Guide*, and others.
Survival Foundation
Royal, AR 71958

PREFACE

by Jay Kordich

TO begin with, let me express how honored I am that Smokey Santillo asked me to say a few words on behalf of his new book.

Although I did not meet Smokey until late 1989, our relationship goes back a few years before that. In 1987 I picked up a copy of Smokey's book *Food Enzymes:The Missing Link To Radiant Health.* I read it over and over because I was amazed at how closely this young doctor's views on enzymology correlated to mine. I was excited to have a book that so accurately put into written form what I had been teaching to people over the past thirty-five years.

I proceeded to carry Smokey's book with me in the pocket of my juicer bag, using it as my own private handbook. I took the book with me to juicing lectures and seminars, employing it often as a reminder and reference on the subject of enzymes. In late 1989, after conducting a lecture in Buffalo, New York, a pleasant-looking young man approached me and introduced himself as Dr. Santillo. As you can imagine, I was absolutely astounded. Here I had been packing his book around—I even had it with me at that moment—and here he was introducing himself as one of my greatest fans. Little did he know at the time that I had been closely following his career, too.

Happily, Smokey joined our company and conducted juicing lectures and seminars himself. With great pride I have watched him grow into a true expert on our subject of enzymology. Once a protege of mine, I now consider him to be a colleague in the field. He is helping to perpetuate this subject which is of utmost importance for our healthy existence on this planet.

I am very happy to see Smokey's new book, *Intuitive Eating*, become a reality. It is filled with timely information that is worth seriously considering. Although both Smokey and I are vegetarians and therefore do not endorse the consumption of meat, I note that Smokey's Transition Diet does provide a way for non-vegetarians to take advantage of his program as well. Following the stages he sets forth, moreover, anyone wishing to leave meat-eating behind will be encouraged and supported by his gradual and practical approach.

Of course I am particularly pleased to see that his book contains an entire chapter on juicing; juicing is my life. But, more than that, *Intuitive Eating* goes beyond the ideal of "conscious" or purposeful eating. It challenges us to re-evaluate what we thought was out of our control. In his poignant chapter, "Nutrition Against Disease," Smokey convincingly shows that in fact our destinies are ours to determine. In addition, *Intuitive Eating* is conveniently divided into sections to help us easily learn how to nutritionally care for our bodies.

I know I speak for Smokey when I invite you to read *Intuitive Eating* and employ his methods to increase your overall health.

Best Wishes,

Jay Kordich
author, The Juiceman's Power of Juicing
(New York: William Morrow and Co., 1992)

INTRODUCTION

Why I Wrote This Book

WHEN I was a child the atmosphere around my family dinner table was like a war zone. Since my parents grew up during the Depression and knew what it was like to go without food, the fear of food scarcity was indelibly instilled in our minds. We had to use survival tactics, eating all we could as fast as possible. We talked little and stuffed ourselves with heavy proteins and starches at each meal.

Going to bed on a full stomach was common. It was nothing for me to eat three sticks of pepperoni, half a quart of milk, and a quarter of a pound of cheese as a bedtime snack. There were hardly any raw fruits or vegetables in my diet, and absolutely no freshly made juices. For me the results were allergies, constipation, and swollen joints at an early age.

I went to college on a track and football scholarship and continued my heavy diet of cooked foods. By the age of 21 my perverted eating habits began to take their heaviest toll. My weight increased from 190 to 230 pounds, and my allergies and joint pains were so severe that I needed to get allergy shots once a week. When my prescribed medication wasn't working any longer, my regular doctor started sending me to different specialists. But they played a guessing game about how to treat my condition and indiscriminately used a wide range of drugs, some of which even caused me to pass out for short periods of time. I was actually allergic to them. It didn't take me long to realize that this method of treatment was a road leading nowhere.

Inquisitive, and blessed with an interest in health, I went to a health food store one day to search for an answer. The owner of the store suggested a book called *The Mucousless Diet Healing System* by Professor Arnold Ehret, (Beaumont, CA: Ehret Literature Publishing Co., 1972). Here Ehret explained that meat, dairy, eggs, and too much cooked food were the cause of most physical disease. He asserted that fruits, vegetables, seeds and nuts (most of them to be eaten raw) were the perfect foods for human beings. It sounded good to me. So, without preparation or guidance I started this strict regime with vigor.

Immediately my body began to eliminate poisons from all excretory organs, including bowels, sinuses, kidneys, the complete urinary tract, and the lungs. But, instead of eliminating my congestion, it actually increased it, and this went on painfully for months. I had a fever for 101 days and became so weak that walking half a mile was a monumental task. Something had to be wrong.

So I re-read Ehret's book, and there it was. Somehow I had overlooked the three chapters in which he explained how to make a dietary change. He warned that the body can become extremely weak trying to eliminate toxins that have been retained for years in the cells, the bowels, and the organs. Using two or three *transitional diets* was therefore absolutely necessary.

I had changed too dramatically without giving my body a chance to clean out at each stage and to adapt to each transitional step. No wonder I was congested! During each step the organs needed time to adjust, and time and energy to eliminate excess toxins, mucous, etc. Overburdening the eliminatory organs was also causing enzyme deficiencies and immune deficiency problems.

I remedied this by establishing a 60% raw food diet and cooking 40% of my foods. In this first step I also left out meat, dairy, and eggs. I started fasting periodically — 1 day a week, 2 days at the end of every month, 7-10 days at the end of every four months. It took me two years and several more transitional steps to evolve the diet I am living on now, even though my arthritis and allergies were gone after the first six months of my dietary regime. It was that dramatic!

Today I eat 90% raw food and 10% cooked food with one quart of freshly made raw fruit and vegetable juice daily. When I feel the need for extra carbohydrates I cook some rice or potatoes. At the age of 42 I am still able to play the same sports I played when I was in high school and college. As a matter of fact I have tied my fastest high school 40-yard dash time this year — which is 25 years later. I did this on a diet that most athletes feel they would shrivel up and die on. (Being an athlete I have trained with professional football players doing the same exercise routines they were doing. They felt they needed 3500 to 5000 calories per day. My intake, however, was only 1500 calories per day. And I have been eating this way for over twenty years.)

All of this is an example of knowing how much food is really necessary, as well as the proper kind of food to eat. I know exactly when my body needs protein, and how much. I know when I need carbohydrates, juices, or water. I essentially eat only what is necessary and get maximum output from the food I eat. And I haven't had a symptom of either arthritis or allergies for over twenty years either!

Over the sixteen years of my practice, working with thousands of people, I have used acupuncture, kinesiology, herbs, homeopathy, and mental therapeutics. While each therapy and philosophy was valuable in itself, no one approach was the answer for everybody. Even though ten people may have had the same symptoms, no two people needed the same therapy. Some fevers were caused by congestion, for example, while others were the result of fatigue, adrenal exhaustion, or infections. The one common element was that each person was unique. Consequently, different therapies were needed to bring each person back into balance.

There were a few other factors common to every case. Those who got well were those who took responsibility for their health. That meant the development of a greater self-awareness, including their relationship with food and nutrition. Because of individual differences it was clearly imperative for people to get to know themselves and their nutritional needs.

All my experience, my research, and the five books that I have written, were guides which led me to the creation of this book, *Intuitive Eating*. Too much material has been written telling people what they should eat instead of what they can do to learn to trust their body's innate wisdom, and to find out what their individual needs really are. *Intuitive Eating* not only explains what foods lead to regeneration and what foods lead to degeneration, but now to travel a safe, long-term, transitional dietary path so that you can reclaim what your body knows and needs.

• • •

> If you're going to be a doctor, you have to be able to get sick people well. That's what it's all about not just collecting their money. The important thing is to get sick people well, and when you can prove you can do that, first of all to yourself, and then to your patients, and it's predictable and reliable and dependable, well there isn't anything like it!"
>
> \- *Dr. D.J. Scott*

I am dedicated to helping people help themselves to get well, and this book, *Intuitive Eating,* is part of that dedication. You are invited to actively participate with me in this process. What a wonderful feeling it will be to get to know yourself again and to learn what you need for your optimum health.

ACKNOWLEDGEMENTS

I have been blessed with many wonderful friends.
I would like to thank the following people for their love
and continuous support.

Dawn Santillo, my wife, and Cindy Grogan, for their many hours of work helping with the recipe sections; Regina Sara Ryan, my editor; John Blair from NSA; Dr. D.J. Scott, D.C.; Paul and Dawn St. John; Dr. Richard Gerow, D.C.; Diane and Dr. Frank Torelli, D.C.; Dino and Debby Ruse, Charley Fox, Dan McCue. Special thanks to Jay and Linda Kordich, Victoras Kulvinskas, Rob and Kathy Palano, Teri Oles, N.D., Uri Le Baron and his family, Joe and Robin Miano, Dave Schiavone, my saxophone teacher; Lou Piccone, Terrie South, Jack Lee, Sal Andolina, Fred Gelotte, Pat Kane, Kevin Delapenta, Joe and Edie Clouse, Bobby Maguire, Tony Collier, Melissa and Melanie, Donna Portale, Jim Sullivan, Traci and Dave Bissonette, Mom Bedell, Chris and Patty Best, Dr. Mike Marfino, D.D.S., Barb and Bob Metz, Mike Starr, Dave Alan, Ellin Larsin, Mike Barnhart, Sue Martin, Ben Habberman, Bob Gosch, Kay Ranno, Lucy Beatty, Hank Paolucci, Jim Piotrowski, Ray Stapell, Gary Heuck, Diane Parnagian, Sam and Kathy Mameli, Rick Utt, Frank Berrafato, Bobby Romano, Michael and Christopher DellaPenna, and Hoagy and the Blues Bombers.

PART I

OVERVIEW

CHAPTER 1

Intuitive Eating

IMAGINE what it would be like to be so attuned to your body that you knew exactly what it needed — when the system could profit from some additional protein; what vegetables or fruits would immediately remedy an acid or alkaline imbalance; what foods would help you through a period of emotional turmoil. Now take this a step further. See yourself eating very little on some days, yet feeling light and strong. See yourself on other days eating 2000 calories and feeling good. Imagine being so sensitized to your body's genuine needs that you naturally gravitate towards the foods and the eating style that will work best for your system.

This is no fantasy. It is a very real possibility for you, one that I have lived and shared with thousands of clients. This is *Intuitive Eating*.

THE DEFINITION

Intuitive Eating is a personalized relationship to food and nutrition that is characterized by self-awareness and environmental sensitivity. It is based on an energy-efficiency model of human health — the understanding that disease and health are primarily functions of optimal nutrition, and that with better diet human beings can maximize their use of energy and capacity for regeneration in all aspects of their lives.

Intuitive Eating is incorporated into one's lifestyle only through a gradual process of education, coupled with a series of transitional dietary changes and detoxification methods as necessary. With this foundation, *Intuitive Eating* becomes the guiding principle whereby each individual comes to know what to eat, how much to eat, when to eat, and what foods to use to bring about a balance and harmony of mind and body.

WHY WE NEED INTUITIVE EATING

A. Everyone Is Different.

There have been so many books written about nutrition that many people are discouraged before they start. Whether you read the advocates of the "meat and potato" diet, the Macrobiotic, the Lacto-vegetarian, the High Protein diet, or whatever, you find that each proclaims it is the only diet the human race should eat. How can this be true when human beings are so metabolically different? It can't be!

When you consider that some people start off on their nutritional journey because of being seriously overweight, while others are lacking weight, you get an idea of why the same program cannot work for everybody. Some people exercise more than others, some have jobs that require hard labor while their next door neighbor sits all day in front of a computer terminal. Certainly their needs for proteins or carbohydrates will differ. Then there is the realistic subject of convenience. Some of us are away from home for most of the day so we can't always eat the way we may want to. Even our organs are different sizes and weights. Genetics definitely plays a role in what is required for adequate nutrition.

Consider further that elderly people or those suffering from chronic disease conditions may be unable to digest certain foods. They will need a diet that takes this into account. For the past three or four generations, however, our educational programs about nutrition have failed us. What is being taught in most of our school systems about proper eating is outdated. For example, the recommendation of a high-protein diet for everyone is not scientifically verifiable.

So, we need education, and not only education about what foods are healthy and what foods are not. We need some basic environmental education which places nutritional needs within a broader context and inspires us to appreciate our place in the planetary ecological system. We need education about the miraculous nature of the human body — the ongoing miracles of digestion and utilization of food. We need education about what regenerates and what degenerates the human organism, and we need some guidance to implement these new understandings for ourselves and our families.

Only by honoring ourselves and our similarities to others, and celebrating our differences, will we find a way through this confusing jungle of nutritional data.

B. We Are Out of Touch With Our Own Nature.

Ideally we should know our own body better than any physician, but how many people will even offer their doctor an opinion about what they think is going wrong? How many doctors will even ask what we think about our own condition? What will it take to learn to trust ourselves, to "listen" to the body and feel confident that we are "reading" its messages accurately?

In the realm of nutrition, most people are immune to their natural inclinations. Because of eating junk foods, fast foods, overcooked, highly processed and overly spiced diets, our natural cravings have been changed. The literal poisons that we have put into our systems have either over-stimulated or depressed our glandular secretions, resulting in either depressed or overly excited emotional states. Our life energy is being controlled and drained by over-eating (a national habit) and by eating deficient foods. And the more deficient the food, the greater the number of false cravings we will experience. We get entangled then in a cycle of false desires which only lead us farther and farther from our specific needs. Where that leads is obvious. Who can dispute that we in the U.S. at least, have become a nation of addicts?

This loss of intuitive sensitivity to our bodies' needs has resulted in a variety of new diseases and numerous types of physical malfunctioning. It seems that every five years or so we see another epidemic in the U.S. Not long ago it was hypoglycemia and herpes; now it is AIDS; all caused by our sophisticated and cultured lifestyle. We are leading an abnormal existance, like domesticated animals who develop diseases unknown to their wild cousins. A 1988 Surgeon General's Report stated that 68% of all the deaths in the United States are diet-related.[1]

The natural world would exist perfectly without our help or interference. Observe how the seasons come and go, how plants arise producing food, how wild animals acquire their food and eat it in its natural state. How perfect the plan of nature is, and how desparately we need to get back in closer alignment with that.

C. Food is Energy

Food is the body's prime source of energy — the energy that we need internally for the maintenance of life, as well as the energy we put out into the world in the form of work or play. Our choice of food, then, together with all other aspects of our relationship to food, will determine the quantity and quality of our life energy.

When a diet is "heavy," i.e. requiring a lot of internal energy to break it down into usable form, that taxes the body's internal energy reserves. Since the body is always using food nutrients for healing, rebuilding, and detoxification, the ideal foods are those which will assist in this process rather than rob energy from it. This is especially true when there is a state of illness or imbalance, like the common cold. Energy conversation is the key in treating illness. Most of the energy in the body should be used for healing, not depleted unnecessarily. How different that is from the "normal" diets of most people. Few understand this principle of energy conservation, and even fewer practice it.

This balance of energy is especially important to maintain

whenever we decide to "clean up our act," nutritionally speaking. Any program of nutritional change, including any "cleansing" or detoxification methods, must include an understanding of these principles. Tremendous deficienies in enzymes and other nutrients can develop even in a healthy person, which is why a good percentage of vegetarians may look weak and malnourished at times. Without a program that supplies these nutrients during illness or transitions, it will be extremely difficult to regain the strength needed for overall metabolic functioning.

We need a diet that is energy efficient, that supplies the necessary enzymes and nutrients for proper digestion. We need a diet that is adaptable to everyone — no matter what their age or physical condition. We need a diet that honors the environment, and restores us to a place of nutritional self-awareness. No one diet will do this for everyone. But, everyone can establish a new relationship to food and eating that does it for them. *Intuitive Eating* is that relationship.

COMPONENTS OF THE INTUITIVE EATING PROCESS

A. Detoxification.

Before one can develop the sense of what the body needs, the body must be purified. When we use salt, coffee, nicotine, and other stimulants, the body begins to crave these substance. Similar cravings and convenience habits develop when we eat sugar, highly processed foods, and fast foods. These cravings camouflage our natural inclinations.

Once we clean out the residues of these unnecessary foods and chemicals, we begin to sense what the body really needs. To establish this true sense, or this intuitive relationship to our nutritional needs, detoxification of some kind is necessary. Detoxification is the process of cleaning and purifying our bodies by the use of foods, juices, herbs, fasting, etc.

Detoxification is not a new idea. Religions around the world have long recommended fasting to the masses. It is mentioned in the New Testament, for example, that our bodies are "temples" of the Spirit and that we should therefore keep them clean. Fasting is one age-old way to accomplish this.

Many foods are full of unnatural additives and preservatives. These literal poisons can be stored in the body for years, and when they are finally released into the bloodstream (as happens when we begin a detoxification program). The blood can become quite thick and that can cause sluggishness or other disease symptoms. These reactions to cleansing are actually a positive sign, what we call the *healing crisis*. But if we are not prepared for them, we can easily become alarmed and attempt to regroup our strength by falling back into our old patterns — stimulating ourselves with our addictions again. That is where education comes in. In what school can you learn about how to properly detoxify the body and how to handle a healing crisis? This book will be that school.

Detoxification is a necessity, and there is a right way and a wrong of going about it. I will be guiding you through a detoxification program, but primarily I will be showing you how to design a program that suits your individual needs.

B. A Gradual Transition.

A slow, gradual approach to detoxification as well as to changing diet and lifestyle is the hallmark of the *Intuitive Eating* process. Too many people set themselves up for failure when they try to change their diet too quickly. This program, on the other hand, gives your body and mind a chance to adjust to the new tastes and the new body responses as well as a chance to adjust to the elimination of poisons from the system.

For example, every food and drink causes some type of stimulation or slowing down of the body's processes. Coffee is a stimulant while heavy foods can cause sluggishness. Sugar creates both stimulation and then, after causing a low blood sugar, leads to a slight depression. The body needs time to detoxify these food residues and rebalance itself. When one tries to travel the path of change too rapidly, especially as we get older, the body becomes disorganized, weakness develops, and the organs of the body become overstressed. A series of transitional diets will prevent this unnecessary stress.

Intuitive Eating will present you with three transitional dietary stages and supply you with recipes for implementing each one. You will be encouraged to remain at any stage as long as you want — learning to trust your body every step of the way. The stages will move you in the direction of more natural, energy-efficient foods, but it is never assumed that the final stage is the one stage that will suit everyone. Your personal goals for health and weight and strength, etc., will be your guiding principles. Some people may want to stop eating meat and dairy products, for instance, while remaining on chicken and fish. Others will choose a completely vegetarian approach. The diets are only offered to assist you in leaving behind what no longer serves your goals.

The body will heal itself at its own pace. It takes time to purify the blood, clean out the debris in the intestines, strengthen the immune system, and detoxify the liver and kidneys. If you rush these stages recuperation will be lengthy and you will only delay the accomplishment of your goal.

C. Eating for Low Stress and Energy Efficiency.

A low-stress, regenerative diet using enzymes, raw fruit and vegetable juices, and pre-digested foods will supply the body with the maximum energy for the minimal amount of digestive "work." These elements refine your body so that your nutritional intuition become second nature. These elements together are what make this approach unique.

Many diets that are commonly taught are not regenerative at all, i.e. they do not contribute to longevity. I will be giving you information here that will clearly explain the difference between regenerative foods and degenerative foods. This approach will orient you to begin to *choose* your foods based on how they contribute to optimum health rather than simply *react* to your conditioning by eating what tastes good, smells good, what is convenient, or what is right in front of you.

Don't be discouraged in thinking you are going to have to make big sacrifices to "give up" your favorite foods, either. After you have been detoxified to a certain point your body will simply crave different foods — i.e. more low-stress foods. You will find that this change in your relationship to food affects other aspects of your life as well. *Intuitive Eating* is a lifestyle, not simply a dietary program.

As you practice the *Intuitive Eating* system you will start to realize that the time of day in which you eat will have a direct effect on the energetic efficiency of your food. Some foods digest better according to when you eat them, and while there are some general guidelines I can share with you, this is also an individual phenomenon. For instance, I choose to eat my protein foods in the middle of the day because proteins seem to slow me down and deplete my energy if I eat them in the morning. You will figure out what works best for you.

One of the principal ways in which we overstress the system is by overeating, particularly when the body is already stressed with some condition of fatigue or illness. Any excess of food causes an oversecretion of digestive juices and enzymes. If the body can't handle the excess, this food does not get digested properly and ferments in the colon. Evacuation is then retarded and constipation is the result. Most physiologists now agree that two light meals a day (provided they consist of high-density, nutritious foods) are sufficient to provide all the nutrients necessary for the body to carry on all its functions. Americans and other citizens of industrialized countries are going to premature graves because they persist in eating more than their systems require. *Intuitive Eating* will help all of us in reorientating our eating habits to preserve our life and health.

D. Positive Mental Attitude and Self-Responsibility.

The role of the mind in influencing health is becoming more widely accepted every day. Current estimates are that upwards of 85% of all diseases have a strong psychosomatic component, meaning that they are intensified, if not completely caused, by the ways in which we think.

Every thought vibrates through the body as an electrical impulse. Whether these thoughts are positive or negative they will create corresponding conditions of health or disease. Yet how rarely is the mental state of the patient considered in diagnosing a common cold or allergy, for instance. My experience has convinced me that to the extent that the individual cannot deal with emotions and spiritual stresses, he/she becomes receptive, or susceptible, to viruses and bacteria.

In a study done at Harvard Medical School, Dr. Roger Meyer and Robert Haggarty observed sixteen families (a total of one hundred individuals) for a period of one year. They found that both streptococcal illnesses and respiratory diseases were four times more common following periods of emotional stress.[2]

Certain emotions stimulate or depress physiological function and hormonal secretions in the body. Hostility, anger, and hate increase the output of cortizone, which alters the immune system. At West Point, studies indicated that overstressed individuals had weaker immune systems because of the oversecretion of adrenalin hormones, cortizone production in particular.[3] In a third study, when medical students were taught how to meditate and relax it was found that their T-cells (cells that recognize foreign substances and toxins in the body) actually increased.[4] The opposite was shown when people were analyzed after they experienced a shock, like a death in the family.[5] Poor functioning of the essential T-cells is constantly found in cases of depression, stress, anxiety, and fatigue.

The role of belief in health is demonstrated conclusively when you consider the effectiveness of the placebo, or "sugar pill." In one double-blind study it was shown that valium was no more effective than a placebo in treating anxiety. When the doctor and patient knew that valium was being used the drug was 80% effective. When the doctor and the patient didn't know, the valium's effectiveness was reduced to 35-40%.[6]

Anything which gives an individual an increased sense of personal control increases self-healing — and that includes a feeling of love, an acknowlegement of respect by their health care pratitioner, and the recognition that they have a choice about the treatment, i.e. a sense of participation in the process. *Intuitive Eating* puts that sense of control back into our own hands.

You no longer have to be the victim. You can be the determining factor of whether you will be sick, weak, and emotionally unstable, or strong, healthy, and living every day to the fullest. But to gain that degree of self-control you must be open to truth, and to change. Old ways of negative thinking and "negative eating" will keep you stuck. They are precisely why we have more physical and mental diseases today than in any other time in human history.

Before we are going to experience global peace we must start with ourselves, and this means eating properly and learning methods of controlling our thoughts and our inner world. I believe that life is spiritual and that we are evolving on an inner plane of consciousness just as we are evolving externally. These emotional changes that we go through will manifest as physical changes, not only in the personal body, but also in the planetary *Body* as a whole. Great changes will be brought on by the ways in which we think. The Earth will benefit if each one of us takes charge of his/her life. *Intuitive Eating* is one significant way to support that.

E. Learning About Yourself.

As you follow the transitional steps suggested in this book you will develop a whole new relationship to the messages that your body is giving. You will honor yourself as you learn about yourself.

For example, when you are tired you will often find that heavy protein and starch meals will only make you more tired and rob you of valuable energy, whereas a fruit meal, or skipping a meal entirely, will energize you. Your body will give you the feedback that will be undeniable.

When you are thirsty your body will be signaling for liquid foods that help it to overcome dehydration. Your experience, coupled with your refined nutritional education, will tell you that drinking coffee, tea, or cola will not satisfy that need in the way that purified water will.

You will begin to feel which foods produce heat (like high-protein or starch foods) and which foods will cool you down, like melons and other types of fruit. You will come to know the difference between mouth-hunger (which is really a psychological craving) and genuine stomach-hunger, and you will want to make it a practice to eat only when genuine hunger is present.

During times of illness the body will be crying out for help in rebalancing itself, and you will learn what those cries are really for. You will instinctively know, for example, what is causing a condition of constipation, and how to rememdy that.

In Chapter 3 and Chapter 8 you will be introduced to a simple method of urine testing which will indicate the Ph balance in your system and alert you to the types of foods you will need to eat to correct any imbalance.

After detoxifying and then applying some of the methods of eating suggested in this book you will notice changes both in your looks and in your eating habits and cravings. Each day your senses will become keener until you will once again trust your own intuition about your body's needs. There will be no more guesswork. Your judgement will be your guide.

HOW TO USE THIS BOOK

Intuitive Eating is divided into four parts —

PART I. Motivation and Definition (Introduction and Chapter 1);

PART II. Education (Chapters 2-5);

PART III. Action Steps and Dietary Plans (Chapters 6-12);

PART IV. Appendices.

Part II, which you are about to begin, brings you some of the latest research and nutritional information. It explains how to combat the negatives of our environment, such as water, indoor and outdoor air pollution, and even the electrical imbalances that surround us and cause disease. This section further covers the proper use of nutrition against disease as well as primary education about common food fallacies and the essential role of enzymes in the human dietary process.

Part III will explain, in layperson's terms, exactly how to make dietary changes. We will call these changes "transitional steps" because when you change your diet to a more regenerative type of eating it will not be beneficial to do it all at one time. There are three major stages and each stage is an education within itself and should be implemented slowly. These stages, moreover, will put everything you've learned in this book into a system of eating and lifestyle changes.

By the time you reach Part III, hopefully you will have made the necessary commitment to improve your life, realizing that your health is your responsiblity. You will then be ready to move beyond degeneration, beyond maintenance, and into regenerating your body and mind. That's the promise of *Intuitive Eating*.

In Part IV you will find handy charts, and additional scientific data that will aid and substantiate the process you will be undertaking in making *Intuitive Eating* a way of life.

A SPECIAL NOTE TO PAGE SKIPPERS

If you are one of many people who like to skip over the educational sections of a book and jump right into the "how-to-do-it" part, please take the time to read the chapter on Enzymes in Part II. This is one of the essential and unique features of the *Intuitive Eating* system and I don't want you to miss it.

PART 2

EDUCATION

CHAPTER 2

Environmental Causes of Disease

BEFORE we investigate the dietary causes of disease, we will begin with the environmental causes of health problems.

Environmental factors such as air and water pollution, plus electromagnetic fields that surround us in our homes, are hidden hazards, less talked about by physicians and laypersons simply because this information is not yet as widespread as dietary information. This does not mean it is less important, but many doctors don't have ways to diagnose and treat imbalances caused by environmental toxicity and electromagnetic forces.

The body is wise; it heals itself. When this healing process is interfered with, the body becomes weaker, the immune system begins to fail, and sickness results. There is growing agreement that symptoms of what we call disease are primarily the result of toxicity, deficiencies, and imbalances in our lifestyle and our environmental surroundings. Nutrition, lifestyle, physical and mental uniqueness, and the environment in which we live—these will be the specialities of the physician of the future. He or she will have to be a compassionate healer, using heart, hands and mind to heal the sick. He or she will learn from patients, not just professors. For this to happen, both the layperson and the doctor must be educated, and some re-educated. It is still very difficult for any health professional to convince his/her patients that the pain they are experiencing is caused by the food they're eating or the environment they live in, especially when a drug gives them such quick relief.

Let's examine the hazards in our lives to get a clearer picture of what we're up against.

ELECTROMAGNETIC POLLUTION

> Any new theory first is attacked as absurd, then admitted to be true, but obvious and insignificant. Finally, it seems to be important; so important that its adversaries claim that they themselves discovered it.
>
> - *William James*

Most people are not aware that they live in an electrical universe, that their bodies are surrounded by electro-vibratory fields which form and develop all physical bodies. The human body contains an estimated 200 quintillion cells (that's a 2 with 32 zeroes added to it). Each cell is an electrical universe in itself, containing enough information to fill an encyclopedia. When we consider this invisible matrix of interrelating fields, it is obvious that the human body is awesomely designed by an all-knowing, ever-present, divine, creative power.

Each cell is made up of protons, electrons, and other small electrical particles moving at the speed of light, yet never interfering with each other. George Lakhousky[1], a French scientist, postulates that the cell is an essential organic unit which acts like an electromagnetic resonator, emitting, absorbing, and radiating several frequencies. The nucleus of the cell consists of tubular filaments (chromosomes and mitochondria) made of insulating materials and filled with a conducting fluid containing the same mineral salts found in sea water. These filaments are thus comparable to oscillating circuits, with the capacity to store energy and induce their own frequency and current. Lakhousky realized that each cell worked as a conductor, with energy flowing through it. This created a magnetic and electromagnetic field unique to each cell depending on its form and function. He further believed that the cells of all living organisms wage a continual war against microbes, which he described as a "war of radiations." If the radiations of the microbe *win,* the cell ceases to oscillate at a healthy level and eventually dies.

It is important that our cellular-electrical bodies vibrate at their given frequencies. Doctor Gerber's book, *Vibrational Medicine*[2], clearly shows that the human body is a process of interacting, multi-dimensional energy systems that are constantly interacting with each other in an harmonic fashion. If these systems become imbalanced, pathological symptoms can manifest on the physical, mental, emotional and spiritual planes. For the body to return to a high level of health the energy fields must be balanced and the source of interference eliminated.

Scientists can now monitor the energy of the body. An EKG (electrocardiogram) monitors the electrical activity of the heart. An EMG (electromyograph machine) shows the flow of electricity along the nerves in the muscles. A polygraph (lie detector machine) measures the electro-activity of the body, brain, skin, respiratory system and muscles in response to stress. Biofeedback devices monitor the brain waves to allow a person to consciously control the brain waves, heartbeat, temperature, blood supply, and digestive capabilities.

We cannot deny what the Chinese have been telling us for 5,000 years—that the body is electrical, with energy pathways called "meridians" that can be used to diagnose and treat ailments. In 1960 Professor Kim Bong Han[3] proved that meridians existed by injecting radioactive phosphorous into a rabbit at specific acupuncture points, and monitoring the uptake of the substance into surrounding tissues. He discovered that the isotope substance was actively taken up along a fine tubule system, approximately .5 to 1.5 microns in diameter, which followed the path of the classical acupuncture meridians. (See: Doctor Gerber's book *Vibrational Medicine,* pp. 122-123, for more about acupuncture meridians.)

All life pulsates in time with the earth, and artificial fields cause abnormal reactions in our bodies. Doctor Becker, one of the most respected scientists in the world, and author of *Body Electric*, states,

> We now live in a sea of electromagnetic radiation that we cannot sense, and that never before existed on this earth. ELF (electrical low frequencies) electromagnetic fields vibrate about 30-100 hertz. If weaker than the earth's fields, it interferes with our bodies' biological cycles. Chronic stress and impaired disease is the result. Recent studies of mice exposed for 30 days to 60 cycles electro-fields whose strength was similar to those found near high-voltage transmission lines, revealed changes in hormone patterns, body weight and blood chemistry, producing all the signs of chronic stress. But also, the study showed increase in degenerative disease, particularly those related to decreased competency of immune system, such as cancer.[4]

Basically, we are plugged into the universe. Natural electromagnetic fields surround our bodies and move through us constantly. The sun, moon the planets, in fact all living things and inorganic substances generate electromagnetic fields because everything is made up of electrical particles (electrons, protons, etc.). The earth and our physical bodies vibrate at about the same pulse, which is 7.43. But when the body comes into contact with artificially generated electrical fields, we become electrically imbalanced. Power lines leading to our homes, all electrical appliances, radio waves, telephones, automobiles, buses, planes, video display terminals, computers, electric blankets, radar, motorcycles, CB radios and more, produce electrical currents which interact with the membranes of every living cell.

Manfred Kohnlechner, a German medical doctor, described the effect of modern communication systems on the health of the inhabitants of a rural area in Bavaria. The people of this area were incredibly healthy, surpassed only by the health and longevity of the Hunzas, at least up to the time of the installation of power lines, microwave towers, TV and radio. Just six months after the introduction of these foreign electromagnetic fields, these healthy people began to die of cancer and heart attacks. They began to develop cavities in their teeth, which were totally unheard of in the past.

VDT's (video display terminals) first came under suspicion in the late 1970s and early 1980s when 12 unexplained miscarriages and birth defects were found in women who worked with computers.[5] In one group of computer operators working for Sears in Dallas, 8 out of 12 pregnancies ended in miscarriages, or in neo-natal deaths. In 1988 the Kaiser Permanente Medical Care Program did a study of 1583 California women who worked 20 hours or more a week with VDTs. These women stood an 80% greater chance of miscarrying than women who did similar work without VDTs.

In the July-August 1986 issue of *American Health,* Nancy Shute discussed a study that linked high-current power lines and transformers to cancer in children. She also cited a study by the Maryland Department of Health and Hygiene which found an unusually high percentage of electricians, electrical engineers, and utility repairmen among 951 men who died of brain tumors.

Your office and your home are filled with electrical wiring devices and machines which create EMF (electromagnetic fields). These unnatural energies, especially those produced by alternating currents of 60 cycles per second are suspected to cause depression, suicide, cancer, leukemia, psychosis, cataracts; and the list grows daily.

Here's What You Can Do:

They are ways to protect yourself from some electromagnetic pollution. There are life-field polarizers which you can carry in your pocket, and larger ones for your home. They absorb, concentrate, and radiate infinitely a broad spectrum of wavelengths. They are available from: Environmental Polarity Research, Temecula, CA.

Tessler watches and other devices are available from E.L.F. Cocoon, Route 1, Box 21, St. Francisville, Ill. 62460. (618) 948-2393.

Suggested books:

Cross-Current: The Pearls Of Electro-Pollution, by Dr. Robert Becker, M.D.[6]

Current Switch: How To Reduce or Eliminate Electromagnetic Pollution In Home and Office, by John and Trish Banta. (To order call (408) 372-8626, or write Baubiologie Hardware, 207B 16th Street, Pacific Grove, CA 93950.)

And don't forget *Vibrational Medicine* by Dr. Gerber. (Santa Fe, NM: Bear and Co., 1988).

THE AIR WE BREATHE

Each human being breathes between 15,000 and 20,000 litres of air per day. Meanwhile, millions of pounds of toxic chemicals are routinely emitted into the air each year. Air pollution, however, is the least regulated medium in terms of toxic releases. Estimates are that 1700 cancers per year in the United States are caused by air emissions. This figure does not take into consideration the health effects of hundreds of other chemicals that have been identified as causing cancer, birth defects, sterility, nervous disorders, kidney or liver damage, headaches, nausea, skin rashes, respiratory diseases, eye, nose and throat problems, and other conditions.

Industrial pollutants from power plants, incinerators, and automobiles have turned our skies, lakes, and rivers into toxic dumps. These air toxins have killed trees, crops, birds, fish, wildlife, and insects. They have altered the weather patterns, destroyed the earth's protective barrier from the sun's harmful rays, and threatened virtually all living organisms on this planet. In many cities across the United States people are warned to avoid exercising outdoors because of the dangerously high ozone levels. Pregnant women or people over 60 years of age are cautioned against going out at all. The day may not be too far off when children will be walking to school with ultra-violet-ray protectors and respirators.

Federal and state laws have focused mainly on water and land pollution. The federal Clean Air Act has not been strong enough over the last 19 years, as the EPA has set standards for few of the 70,000 toxic chemicals in use. In July of 1988 the Emergency Planning And Community Right To Know Act, also known as Title III of the Super Fund Amendment and Restoration Act, required major industries to release information on the kinds of toxic chemicals that are being released into our air, water, sewage systems and treatment plants, and landfill areas. According to the information provided by the industries in New York state alone, 87,000,000 pounds of toxins were reportedly released into the air. Forty percent, or 33,480,788 pounds of these emissions, were from cracks in valves, pipes, open chemical tanks, etc. They are, therefore, unregulated! Sixty percent of these chemicals were released from industrial stacks. When the report was released in New York, only 683 of the 14,500 industrial plants had submitted their toxic release information. A further example of the limitations of this law and the information it allows is that the information was based on the industry's own estimates, with no governmental verification.

Here's What You Can Do:

The Title III Act, the Right To Know law, is a valuable and powerful tool that citizens can use to protect the environment. It gives individuals a right to know and to demand tougher laws and safer practices. Industries are not required to provide toxic release information directly to the public, but the Environmental Conservation and the local Emergency Planning Committees are mandated to provide this information. To request this information for yourself, please contact USEPA, P.O. Box 70266, Washington, D.C. 20024-0266, Attention: Public Inquiry. Or you can call EPA Right To Know Hotline, at 1-800-535-0202.

Once you've acquired this information, educate your community. Use this information to build cases against companies to reduce their emissions. You can request that the company test around its site for toxins. If they refuse, call DEC (Department of Environmental Conservation) and ask them to test the groundwater, soil, and air emissions of the suspicious companies. It's a good idea to compare companies in your area to see which ones have reduced toxic emissions. Then make public statements over the radio, T.V., or newspapers asking why other companies haven't followed suit. Good luck!

INDOOR AIR

Indoor air pollution is a major cause of disease and an area of widespread ignorance. I include it here because I want you to get a complete idea about how to live a healthy life. Unfortunately, some people just throw up their hands when they read about our toxic air, water, and food. They feel defeated and do nothing about it. This attitude only makes things worse, however, not only for the individual, but for everybody's children. We must all start doing something. Simply by putting air purifiers in your house and using water systems, which I will talk about later, you can help prevent major health disorders.

Consider the fact that the average person spends about 90% of his/her time indoors. Further consider that 80% of all building materials consist of artificial products, like concrete, plastics, steel, aluminum, substances which are chemically treated with toxic paints, etc. Over 50,000 chemicals are currently used in modern technology. Some are already known to cause cancer and mutogenic diseases. There is actually a disease called SBS (Sick Building Syndromes) and BRI (Building-Related Diseases). Five hundred thousand work days are lost yearly because of these types of health damaging poisons in the air, in the walls of our homes, and in the buildings we work in. Allergies, asthma, dermatitis, headaches, and fatigue are a few of the problems we must consider.

Because of their size and the fact that their respiratory rates are 10 times faster than those of adults, children are particularly vulnerable to health problems from household and building toxics. Most of the air pollutants are heavier than air, so they hang lower to the surface of the floor, meaning that they're much closer

LIST OF 63 PESTICIDES FOUND IN GROUNDWATER ACCORDING TO THE EPA

LIST OF 20 ORIGINAL PESTICIDES

Alachlor
Aldricarb (sulfoxide & sulfton)
Atrazinde
Bromacil
Carbfuran
Cyanazine
DBCP
ACPA (and acid products)
Dicamba
1,2 – Dichloropropane
Dinoseb
EDB
Fonofos
Metolachlor
Metribuzin
Oxamyl
Propachlor
Symazine
Terbufos
1, 2, 3, –
Trichloropropane

NEW LIST OF 43 PESTICIDES

Aldrin
Ametryn
Alpha – BHC
Atratone
Gamma – BHC
Cabaryl
Chloropyrifos
Chlordane
Chlorothalonil
DDD
DDE – degradent of DDT
DDT
Dacthal
Diazinon
Dieldrin
Disyston
ETU – degradent of Maneb
(EBDCs)
Endosulfan
Endrin
Heptachlor
Hexazinone
Isofenfos
Lindane
Linuron
MCPA
Malathion
Metalaxyl
Methyl Parathuion
Para-nitrophenol
Paraquat
Parathion
Pentachlorophenol
Picloram
Propazine
Silvex
Sulprofos
TCP – degradent of
Trychlopyr
Toxaphene
Trifluralin
1, 3 Dichloropropene
2, 4 D
2, 4, 5 T
2, 6 Dichlobenzoic acid

to the nasal passages of a child. At the same time, children's bodies are not as well-equipped to process toxic chemicals, so the risk factors are increased.

Every year five to ten million household poisonings are reported. Most of the victims are children. These poisonings are the result of accidental ingestion, or from toxics splashed in their eyes, absorbed through the skin, or inhaled through the nose and mouth. These poisons are found in chlorine bleach, fabric softeners, spray starch, children's sleepwear, mothballs, insect sprays, pesticides, scented toilet paper, toothpaste, cosmetics, shampoos, microwave ovens, supermarket milk, produce, aluminum cookware, tobacco smoke, fireplaces, etc.

Let's look at wall-to-wall carpets, for example. Almost all carpets are made from synthetic fibers derived from petroleum. Petroleum is bad enough, but then the carpet is treated with stain-resistant or fire-resistant chemicals. They will then most likely be saturated with fungicides and pesticides, too. Once laid on the floor, the fibers begin to emit powerful fumes. NASA has banned all such chemicals from its space capsules. These chemicals cause allergies, headaches, and malformed cells.

Once a carpet gets old it begins to emit dust and fibers into the heating systems. This causes sinus and respiratory problems for many people. Shampooing or steam-cleaning can aggravate health conditions by adding more chemicals to the indoor air.

Here's What You Can Do:

There is not enough room in this manuscript to completely cover each and every subject, so I suggest you read a book called *The Non-Toxic Home*[7], by Deborah Lynn Dadd. It's a terrific book and gives plenty of suggestions on how to live in a safe indoor environment.

WATER

Water is necessary for human and animal life. In fact, 60-70% of the adult human body is composed of water; 90% of a baby's body is water. Pure live water is the major liquid that the body uses to dissolve and eliminate its own cellular waste. Water lubricates the body and keeps us limber. Without the proper amount of water we become fatigued and our metabolism becomes sluggish. The problem is that most people do not know what type of water to drink. Normal tap water is loaded with chemicals, pesticides, chlorides, gasses, inorganic minerals and other carcinogenic substances.

Chlorine is a case in point. Seven out of ten Americans drink chlorinated water, yet this chemical was identified as a potential health hazard over 15 years ago. Scientists have discovered that chlorine forms carcinogenic compounds called trihalomethanes when it mixes with decaying leaves and other organic compounds. The National Cancer Institute studied 3,000 people newly diagnosed with bladder cancer[8]. They found that drinking chlorinated water may double the risk of this illness, which strikes about 40,000 people a year.

The EPA (Environmental Protection Agency) has set standards for chlorine in our water, but not its toxic byproducts. Up until the date of this writing, only four toxic byproducts from the trihalomethanes class have been recognized. But there are many more that must be considered. Even though there have been safety limits set for some of these chemicals, few studies have been done on the results of absorbing these same chemicals through the skin by showering and bathing. Another consideration is that we also inhale these toxic gasses while showering.

Nitrates which commonly find their way into our water supply via sewage, feed lot waste, and agricultural runoff, are also considered carcinogenic. One-fourth of the private wells in Iowa, Kansas, Minnesota, Nebraska, and South Dakota had excessive levels of nitrates[9]. In fact, the EPA has found excessive amounts of nitrates in over one-half the well-water across the country. Inside the mouth, stomach, and bladder, nitrates are transformed into nitrosamines, which act as potent carcinogens in rats. In babies, these nitrates are converted into a substance that keeps red blood cells from absorbing oxygen.

Lead is another major problem in water. Lead seeps into our water systems from old plumbing, paint, and dishware. A recent study estimates that 54% of low-income black children and 12% of white middle-class children have enough lead in their bodies to gnaw at their intelligence, impair the memory, and cause slow reaction time and poor concentration[10]. These levels are enough to steal up to three or four points from a child's I.Q. Among other things, that sort of shift can produce 76,000 more retarded children and 44,000 fewer gifted kids.

Doctor Randolph Byers, a Harvard professor and pediatrician, treated inner-city children who had cut their teeth on nails and leaded paint on cribs and windowsills. These children developed pale skin, vomiting, and listlessness (because of lead poisoning). Some of these children were studied for years after this incident to see if mental problems can develop from lead poisoning. In the study done at Harvard, only 2 out of 20 children weren't having serious academic problems[11]. Several had not learned to read, even by the age of 8.

The chart that follows lists 63 pesticides found in groundwater by the EPA. You can look them up to see just how toxic they are. Many of these chemicals get into the water systems from our "modern lawn care," which is really just toxic pesticides in weed and feed products applied to the lawn. Spraying companies add to the problem. The word *pesticide* (cide) means *kill.* These chemicals are called *biocides.* They are poisonous to pets, insects, neighbors, and your family. (My little boy was sick for 10 days, with vomiting and fever, when my neighbors sprayed their lawn.) Some of the most common symptoms of pesticide poisoning are sore nose, tongue, and throat; burning skin and ears; rash; earaches; muscle pain; twiching; seizures; temporary paralysis; eye pain; blurred vision, and the list goes on.

Here's What You Can Do:

There are many ways to keep the water pure in your home. Three of the most popular methods are activated carbon filters, reverse osmosis units, and the distillation process. The problem is that these water purification systems leave the water dead. Water that has rolled over the hills and rocks in streams is "live" water. It has an electromagnetic charge, which it picks up from the air, sun, and movement in a spiral configuration. For information on *live water* purification systems, write to The International Institute For Baubiologie and Ecology, Inc., Box 387, Clearwater, FL, 34615, USA. This method adds oxygen back into the water, making it once again *live water*, which cleans our bodies, stimulates cellular metabolism, and purifies the lymphatic system. Some of the latest reverse osmosis systems claim that oxygen is added back into the water. Unfortunately, at this point in time these methods are the most advanced but also the most expensive.

I'll leave it to you to research the best water system for your home. Anything is better than tap water! At my house I have a carbon filter that handles all the incoming water, so even my shower and bathing water is clean. Then I add a reverse osmosis unit to the sink in the kitchen. That filters drinking and cooking water that has already been filtered through the carbon unit. It is a good idea to have two units to ensure good water.

To find out how toxic the water is in your area, you can call the American Council of Independent Laboratories for suggestions, (202) 887-5872. They can refer you to reliable labs to do testing on your water. You can also contact the EPA Hotline in your state or city.

SOIL DEFICIENCIES AND THE CAUSE OF DISEASE

More than 25 years ago the great French scientist Alexis Carrel said that chemical fertilizers, by increasing the abundance of crops without replacing all the exhausted elements, i.e. minerals, in the soil, had indirectly contributed to the change of the nutrient value of cereals. These changes not only affect cereals but all the grasses, fruits, and vegetables. The more chemical fertilizers are used, the more impoverished the soil becomes. These imbalances in our soil cause metabolic changes in human cells.

The relationship between soil, plant, and human health is a fascinating subject. The plant is an intermediary by which certain elements of rocks, decomposed vegetation, and minerals are assimilated and made available for vital human processes. The inorganic substances of the atmosphere—carbon dioxide, nitrogen and oxygen—are also selected by the plants, combined with earth substances, and built up into protein, sugar, starch, fat, and organic cells. The earthworm is one of the most important considerations in terms of human health and disease. The worm ingests materials such as seeds, decaying plants, larva, and eggs. It helps keep the soil nutritious by secreting substances back into the soil which the plants can use during their own metabolic activities. The decaying bodies of worms become an excellent source of nitrogen, which amounts to one ton per acre every seven months.

When chemical fertilizers are used, the worms literally leave the soil. Many of these chemicals kill the earthworms and alter the nature of other microbes until they become virulent instead of beneficial. The same thing happens in the human body. Inorganic substances, drugs, and chemicals upset the body's internal pH and metabolism, and what was once a healthy bacteria can turn into an infectious microbe. (See Chapter III for more about this.)

The soil can vary in nutrients from city to city, state to state, or from country to country. (Keep in mind that a lot of our food is shipped in from cities all over the United States.) A comparative study[12] was done in 1948 between two cities in upper Bavaria. The inhabitants of Riegsee had 32% incidence of goiter, as opposed to just 13% in the city of Aidling. In Aidling the butter had 65% more vitamin A than the butter in the city of Riegsee. To verify this study, grass that the cows grazed on in Aidling was tested and found to contain 60% more carotene than the grass at Riegsee. These cities are only one mile apart.

Another study was done by Professor Schuphan at a German research center[13]. To show how important properly nourished soil is to human health, Schuphan grew tomatoes and carrots on soil receiving either manure alone or manure plus a complete mineral food. The tomatoes and carrots grown on soil fertilized by manure and minerals had 58% more carotene than the foods grown on just manured soil. To take this study further, he fed infants the food grown on both soils and found that the children who ate the vegetables grown on manure and mineraled soil had four times the amount of vitamin A in their blood serum than the group eating just the deficient foods grown in manure alone. (Vitamin A has been considered an anti-cancer nutrient by the American Cancer Society.)

Dr. Max Gerson's work on cancer therapy shows how soil becomes deficient after using the same land for continuous cropping. Oats and buckwheat have been analyzed for their mineral content over a 10-year period. The potassium level of one crop measured out at 37.38% the first year. Ten years later a crop from the same field had only 11.69% potassium. In other words, that is a loss of two-thirds of the nutrients. When we become deficient in potassium, we open the door to many acute and chronic diseases. Anemias can be caused by similar copper and iron deficiencies; poor teeth by potassium and calcium deficiencies; skin and bone problems by deficiency of potassium and calcium. For 30 years Professor Czapek collected information about the mineral content of potatoes[14]. He found that whenever artificial fertilizer was used there was generally an increase in the potato crop, but at the same time a deficiency in water, potassium, calcium ions, and sodium chloride in the potatoes.

We must conclude from these observations that unless the soil is properly cared for, disease will always prevail in the human body. We must not only consider what we eat, but where the food came from, how it was processed, and whether it was irradiated or not.

CHEMICALS IN OUR FOODS

A large number of diseases are caused by the chemicals that are added to dairy products, meat, and eggs. There are more than 55,000 chemicals now in commercial use, some 3,000 added to our food, and more than 700 found in common drinking water.

Farm animals are no longer raised by traditional farming methods. Instead, they are mass produced by assembly line farming. The problem is that factory farm animals have 30 times more saturated fat than yesterday's graze-fed animals. Livestock today are also subject to large quantities of toxic chemicals, artificial hormones, growth stimulants, pesticides, and antibiotics.

Cattle, pigs, sheep, and other livestock are routinely dosed with a chemical called Toxaphene to kill the parasites they develop in crowded, unsanitary conditions. This substance is a member of the deadly family that includes DDT, Kepone, Dieldrin, Heptachlor, and PCB's. In the most microscopic dose it produces cancer, birth defects, and causes bones to dissolve in lab animals. Dr. Adrian Goss, the chief scientist for EPA's Hazards Evaluation Division, has this to say about Toxaphene: "It is abundantly clear that Toxaphene is an extremely potent carcinogen. I have never encountered an agent purposefully introduced into the environment which had a carcinogenic propensity as clearly marked and as pervasive."[15] But still each year over 1,000,000 cattle are dipped in or sprayed with Toxaphene.

Another point to consider is what antibiotics are really doing to the animals, as far as protection against bacteria. The continuous feeding of antibiotics to livestock breeds strains of bacteria, including salmonella, that are resistent to drugs. As a result, diseases (salmonellosis) which used to be treatable with antibiotics are becoming increasingly dangerous. Over 4,000,000 cases of salmonellosis poisoning occur annually in the United States. The National Research Council of the Academy of Sciences states, "Salmonellosis is one of the most communicable disease problems in the United States today."[16] Tragically, salmonella bacteria is only one of many bacteria increasingly resistent to antibiotics. Today 90% of staphylococci are resistent to penicillin. The promiscuous use of antibiotics is creating new diseases and symptomologies. In times to come there will be only one way to treat these diseases, and that is by prevention, i.e. by avoiding the foods that are impure. Recent studies indicate that 95% to 99% of all toxic chemicals in America's diet comes from meat, fish, dairy products, and eggs[17].

The use of antibiotics has increased the growth rate of animals, thereby leading to a reduction of cost and more money by weight paid for the slaughtered animal. But this has also led to a general depression in food quality. For example, eggs derived from caged battery chickens may be lower in Vitamin B12 and folic acid than free-ranging chickens. Whether the animal is high in protein or micronutrients does not seem to matter much anymore. You would think that the farmers that feed their animals would want the end product to be of high quality. Yet, cases have been reported where farmers have allowed their cows to eat chicken droppings from henhouses. One American farmer was quoted as saying that he doesn't feed his pigs for 90 days, thereby saving $9300 each year on feed. He just lets them eat the droppings.[18] To economize, some farmers feed their livestock a blend that consists of 75% sawdust mixed with ammonia. Some factory farms mix raw poultry and pig manure with corn and stalks for pig and cattle feed, and animal waste is processed and sold as food supplements. Currently, scientists are working on ways to recycle animal waste and human waste as food for animals.[19] That means recycling antibiotics and other additives in the already inadequate food supply of animals.

In a book called *Food Chemical Sensitivity*, Singer and Mason state that, "There are a number of human diseases, namely cancer, heart disease and gallstones that originate in the meat packing plants of this country. Animals that contract cancer are processed into pig and chicken feed and recycled back into the animal chain. These new techniques necessitate the use of antibiotics, steroids and . . . agents which adversely affect human behavior and health."[20] We now know that people who are food sensitive (allergies) are not actually allergic to a food, but to the chemicals that are contained in the food. The Journal of the American Medical Association, 1982[21], contained a story of a woman who experienced asthmatic attacks after eating restaurant food. The doctors found that she was allergic to bisulphite, which is an additive in foods. There have been seven deaths reportedly due to sulphite hypersensitivity.[22]

In the United States alone it is thought that 450,000 of the nation's asthmatic sufferers may be experiencing reactions to food additives. Food coloring, such as Blue #2 and FDC Yellow #5 often have adverse effects such as hypersensitivity, skin rashes, asthma, upper respiratory infections, runny nose, reduction in blood pressure, shaking, and nausea.

Given the quantity of poisons we put into our foods you may wonder how much is affecting our children. Forty years ago cancer in children was a rarity. Today, more children die of cancer than from any other disease. Children eat much more food relative to their body weight than adults do. Consequently, their food-chemicals-ratio is actually higher than that of adults. There is excellent research cited in John Robbins' book, *Diet For A New America*[23], showing that infinitesimal concentrations of pesticides cause birth defects in animals. Who can dispute that these poisons are affecting our children's immune systems, internal organs, and learning abilities?

Another frequently asked question is, "How good is fish for human consumption?" Authorities agree[24] that human contamination with PCB's comes mainly from eating fish. Fish absorb large concentrations of toxic chemicals from their environment since they breathe the water that they swim in. They are constantly accumulating toxins. The EPA (Environmental Protection Agency) estimates that fish can accumulate up to 9,000,000 times the level of PCB's from the water in which they live. Shellfish continually filter water, some up to 10 gallons an hour. In one month, an oyster can accumulate toxic chemicals at concentrations of 70,000 times the amount in the water that it lives in. A recent government report said that 100% of human sperm samples show concentrations of PCB's[25]. They also found a correlation between high levels of PCB's with low sperm count. In 1976 the EPA found concentrations of DDT and PCB's in 99% of mother's milk. Dairy and meat products account for 95% of the population's intake of DDT. Meat contains 14 times more pesticides than plant foods, and dairy products contain 5 1/2 times more pesticides than plant foods do.

The problem continues and gets worse when you start adding up the effects of everyday usage of not-so-important chemicals, and drugs such as alcohol. Alcohol can cause zinc and Vitamin B6 deficiencies by impairing their absorption. Antacids can lead to the breakdown of bones. Aspirin affects Vitamin C absorption, which leads to bleeding gums. It also affects iron absorption. Tetracycline, an antibiotic, binds with calcium and can cause darkening of the teeth in children, and also decreases iron absorption which leads to fatigue and anemia.

Here's What You Can Do:

For more information, please purchase *Diet For A New America* by John Robbins[26], and *Food Chemical Sensitivities* by Robert Burst, PhD[27]. Your allergies, digestive problems, asthma, skin problems, and fatigue symptoms, and those of your children may be caused by the chemicals in your foods. Many times I've seen sick people recover overnight when they eliminated eggs, meat, and dairy products from their diet. If you suspect food allergies, also suspect the chemicals in your food as being the culprit.

Go to your local health food stores and ask for the names of physicians who deal with food sensitivities and allergies. Read the other books referred to in this chapter. Refer back to the sections in this chapter which mention EPA laws and take action to implement them.

We must go back to nature to find the answers. We must live on pure food and pure water, and study natural living and eating. It is simple and easy, and in some cases, life-saving. In chapters to come I will discuss how to eliminate these foods from your diet, and I will guide you in general detoxification and transitional diets.

RADIATION

Irradiated food is one of the newest hazards of our times. The process of irradiation is done with nuclear waste material. This country has no satisfactory place to store these nuclear wastes, so they are now putting them into our foods. Foods exposed to these nuclear wastes will absorb them. These wastes have already been related to kidney, bladder, and other cancers in the body. As if that wasn't bad enough, irradiated food is deficient. The enzymes which are so important for our immune system are totally destroyed .

We are also exposed to other environmental radiations, like radioactive fallout, which is airborne radioactive particles that have fallen on foods, water, and soil, leakage from nuclear plants, cigarette smoke, X-rays, radon gas, and radiation from other medical devices such as mammographs and CAT scans. It might surprise you that cigarette smoke contains radium 226 and potassium 40. Some other radioactive elements are found in commercial fertilizers used in tobacco farming. These low levels of radiation over a long period of time can damage cell structures, and cause free radicals (see the section on free radicals in Chapter 4. These free radicals can produce severe radiation sickness and contribute to cancer. Physicist John Gofman from the Atomic Energy Commission concluded by his research that radioactive exposure is directly related to the increase of cancer[28].

Here's What You Can Do

Several things can help protect against radiation. The body will absorb minerals before it will absorb these radioactive elements. For example, with plenty of calcium or iodine in the body, the tissues will not tend to absorb additional strontium-90. The body is selective, and knows what it can use best. In addition, certain foods will *chelate* (draw out) radioactive materials from the intestines and other tissues. Sea vegetables, which contain sodium alginate, will do this. At the research laboratory at McGill University in Canada, sodium alginate reduced the amount of strontium-90 absorption by the bones by 53-80%. Wakame, kimbo, and kelp also contain sodium alginate and can be beneficial to the body. Sodium alginate combines with metal pollutants such as barium, lead, plutonium, and cadmium; green algae binds with Cesium 137. Two to three ounces a week of sea vegetables are a maintenance dose. Since sea vegetables contain iodine that can cause overstimulation of the thyroid, those with thyroid disease or heart conditions are advised to consult their physician before taking seaweed supplements.

Other foods that help protect from radioactive elements are Miso (paste from soy beans), garlic, Siberian ginseng, bee pollen, liquid chlorophyll, and echinacea. We can avoid eating foods high on the food chain, like animal products, since cow's milk is 15 times more concentrated with radioactive elements, and beef is 30 times more, than leafy green vegetables. Fish is 15 times more concentrated.

Find out about the current legislation regarding irradiated foods. Check in your local health food store to learn how you can help prevent this catastrophe. To have a healthy planet you must enter the battle against these ludicrous acts.

CHAPTER 3

Nutrition Against Disease

UNDERSTANDING the cause and prevention of disease will be our main concern in this chapter. It will be approached from an age-old, but radically different perspective than is generally held by contemporary allopathic medicine.

The material contained here is taken from a personal interview I conducted with Dr. D.J. Scott, D.M., D.C. of Strongville, Ohio. Dr. Scott is both a personal friend and a long-time teacher of mine who has been in practice for over 40 years. His approach is to get people well, no matter what it takes. Dr. Scott is an expert in the use of fasting and nutrition in fighting disease. I am deeply grateful for his contribution to this book.

THE CAUSE AND EFFECT OF DISEASE: *A NEW PERSPECTIVE*

Dr. Scott:

When considering disease you have to think about what's triggering this acute phenomenon that you're looking at. However, the acute phenomenon is probably an indication of the hypersensitivity that has been acquired as a result of a lot of defense mechanisms that have been insulted and offended. That's one of the places where modern "allopathic" medicine differs from a more nutritionally-based approach.

Professor Antoine Bechamp, for example, thought that bacteria and the viral forms were an *effect*, and not a cause of disease. We're really a viral soup. We're transporting viruses in many forms in our organism, but they're in harmony with the organism. So therefore they live with the organism in health. When the manifestations of life become altered toward the direction of disease, by insult (such as air pollution, water pollution, food pollution, pesticides, herbicides, anything like this) whether it be biochemical, mechanical, structural injury, or emotional, it disrupts the nervous system and therefore the functional capacity of the organism to adapt.

Anything that is not consistent with life becomes an influence which life must either *adapt* to or *defend* itself against. (Even the *adaptation* mechanisms are essentially *defensive* in nature.) So when allopathic medicine looks at organisms in the body that are related to disease, they find this organism under the microscope, or they isolate it by culture and then they say, "See that? That organism is causing your disease." In the realm of biology, that would be like saying, "Those flies in the garbage can make the garbage can dirty." It would be like saying that the maggots on the dead horse killed the horse. So it's putting the cart in front of the horse. It's confusing the whole world of biology.

In the world of biology, in the world of life, everything is orderly. Everything is consistently predictable and reliable. So when the organisms that are normally consistent with health and life are present, they're non-offensive. But as soon as life is altered to the extent that there is some element of disease present, and the body starts defending, repairing, healing, it produces symptoms—like an abnormal secretion on the membranes of the body. Those abnormal secretions then produce, or contribute to, the production of a change in the microorganism. They alter their form to be consistent with the conditions that are present—the disease conditions. So now those same organisms mutate somewhat, adapt somewhat, to these new abnormal conditions. Now they're called abnormal organisms, pathogens, disease-causing bacteria. The typical physician says, "We have to get a drug to destroy that." And that's the starting point—at the effect. Medicine approaches these conditions by trying to kill the flies rather than cleaning up the garbage. These conditions are not the disease's cause. They are the effect of the disease.

The body ultimately has to do the healing. It produces the medium—a culture for organisms to thrive in so they can raise families and propagate. When the body itself provides a culture in the form of abnormal disease secretions, then the organisms which propagate will be of a type which are so-called "pathogens," or the flies. They're the abnormal type of organisms. Medicine calls them the causes of disease; we in hygiene call them the effect of disease. I think our principle is consistent with all nature. The large macroorganisms like hyenas and vultures consume dead and dying material; the microorganisms consume dead and dying material. Through nature all diseased or dead forms go back to the soil, and microorganisms are the key to that process. Those microorganisms are also part of the living body, consuming diseased or dead forms. When death sets in there's an instantaneous flooding of the whole body with microorganisms. So it's the same whether it's the interior environment of the body, or the exterior environment of the planet. The same laws exist.

In my early years of practice I was still experimenting with remedies and thought I could remedy people into health. The mega-vitamin mentality is part of that remedy mentality. It's a belief that you can swallow something and it will solve your problems. Or inject something to get well. Or cut something out to get well. It's always a *remedy* approach rather than *elimination of causation* approach.

It is scientific to eliminate causes. It is scientific to provide for needs. It's consistent with life to provide life's needs in accordance with its needs, not in accordance with our notions, our beliefs, our superstitions. It comes back to whether you believe in mega-doses of vitamins or mega-doses of drugs, or mega-doses of anything. What you believe in is what you do. If what you do doesn't work then you'd better change your beliefs.

Today I'm not trying to dose people into health; I'm trying to nourish them into health, because it's consistent with life. Many of the people I saw early on in my practice actually got well much quicker when they stopped their vitamins, when they stopped their supplements, because they were becoming allergic to all these concentrated mixtures. They were producing intoxication and adding to their disease. Once I realized that, then all I did for thousands of people was just stop them from taking their vitamins, and put them on wholesome food. People instantly start to get better when they stop causing disease.

FOOD IS MEDICINE

Because we're constantly changing the environment all the time, with new chemicals, new poisons, new drugs, the defense mechanisms of the body are constantly changing. These new forms of insults and assaults on the living organism are causing the body to go through all sorts of gyrations and defensive mechanisms to try to protect and preserve itself.

I've been in practice 40 years, and in those early years it seemed very easy to get sick people well. I used to take the most horrendous diseases and just "fast" them and "feed" them appropriately with raw fruits and vegetables, and it was miraculous to watch how extremely ill people got well. Today it's more of a struggle to get those same results.

Food has a lot to do with it. The state of the immunity of the populous in general has been offended by so many things—immunization, drugging, insults on the environment, both internal and external. As a major contributing factor, I would say that the chemicalization of our food has altered the responses of the organism.

So many of our fruits and vegetables come from California. Since the Mediterranean Fruit Fly episode in California I have observed a radical change in food sensitivity to fruit, in particularl. In my programs we used to use fruit in such great abundance. We have to be more careful with the use of fruit today. It might also be due to the fact that the state of California has literally been saturated with malathion—one chemical used to destroy and conquer the fruit fly.

It's hard to find a pure food these days. It's also hard to find ripe food. Food that's tree, vine and plant-ripened is tremendously different from food that was ripened off the plant. That's one reason why today we're more careful in our selection. Some foods are characteristically picked green and unripe, and other foods are characteristically picked ripe. Those are fewer and fewer all the time.

Essentially all of life, whether we're talking about human life or microbiological life, or animal life, plant life—any form of life—has to find its sustenance in its food. The only way you can support any form of life is by maintaining its nutrition. We need to distinguish between nutrition and food. Food essentially provides the elements of nutrition. But nutrition supplies the needs of life. It's impossible to sustain life without good nutrition. For a period of time you can sustain human life in a state of malnutrition or faulty nutrition, or offended nutrition, but it's a lower quality of life, and it's usually a diseased state. So if we're going to overcome disease, we must overcome the nutritional failures, like the lack of excellence in the food quality, for one thing. Another big failure is in the lack of excellence in the digestive efficiency of the organism to translate food into nutrients. There's a big failure in the area of excretion of metabolic waste, which is a byproduct of the food-processing within the organism. So we need to deal with these areas—of food, digestion, and excretion in the maintenance of human life. Food is the first line of offense in turning disease around—turning the organism around from disease to health—because there is no health problem that doesn't have an associated nutritional derangement. All of life, in all its expressions, must be maintained by nutrition, and nutrition means translating food into nutrients available to the organism, to every living cell in the organism.

It all comes down to intelligent selectivity and intelligent rejectivity—mechanisms which the organism itself programs into its nutritional regulation. The organism itself decides what it will accept and what it will reject. It's my observation that in excellent health you'll see people who use a wide spectrum of foods without too much offense to the organism. But when their health breaks down, or progressively deteriorates, especially in the acute phase of illness, the body rejects food totally for a period of time. Like in high fevers, for example, the body doesn't want any food. Any food that you consume at that time will only add to the fever. But as the organism progresses through the various stages of degeneration—deterioration into degeneration—and finally terminal disease, there is a progressive failure of the organism to utilize nutrients efficiently, and the progressive increase in the production of toxic elements from food. As you move in the direction of nutritional failure you move in the direction of intoxication; you move in the direction of the body selectively rejecting food. If the body is selectively rejecting food that tells you right away that there's a condition going on, a hypersensitivity of some type. That is probably the earliest place to start changing and reversing this whole process. In order to restore nutritional efficiency an individual must change eating habits and lifestyle.

THE PROCESS OF DISEASE

If we were to chart life—with perfect health at the top of the chart and death at the bottom of the chart—rarely would an organism leap from perfect health all the way to death in an instant of time, except as a result of some violence or accident. But progressively, over the years, as we age and deteriorate and experience disease, we go down through the chart.

An initial loss of perfect health would be characterized by a degree of fatigue. The cells of the organism are no longer fully restored by rest and sleep and nutrition; so now they are somewhat less efficient. We call that *enervation*. Enervation meaning loss of nerve energy, loss of vital energy. That's the first sign of an imbalance. As we progress downward on this scale of life towards death, we go through various stages of enervation. The cells of the living organism progressively become more exhausted in their capability.

As vitality goes down (meaning the efficiency with which life carries on its processes) the exchange of nutrient utilization and excretion goes down. Then defensive activity tends to go up because the body's going to always, as long as it's alive, attempt, by defensive mechanisms, to restore balance within itself. So it may give you a sense of fatigue; it may give you a sense of pain; it may give you a sense of distress in one form or another. That distress is a message to your brain that comes from the cells. Now your consciousness is aware of symptoms. But initially, it all starts with decreased vitality. You may not even be aware of that early fatigue. You may not feel it because your sense of awareness isn't that acute until it deteriorates further. By the time you are aware of the physical fatigue you're probably three or four stages down the chart already.

The next stage would be toxicity. With this failure of living cells to carry on that process of nutrition, excretion, absorption, and utilization, plus disposing of the waste products of that metabolic process, the cells are less efficient in utilization and excretion, and become somewhat toxic. Now they are not only enervated, they are offended by their own waste products of nutrition, which are the byproducts of metabolism. The consequence of a living cell becoming toxic is its activity becomes intensified. So it speeds up its metabolic processes to attempt to compensate for this level of failure, and it's in a further state of excitability, a state of irritation. It's actually the defense mechanism of that cell responding to the toxic state.

So now we get into accumulation. Months or even years have gone by and we're starting to accumulate the waste in the system. Now we approach the degenerative states. Toxemia (poisons in the body) becomes magnified. In inverse proportion to the decline in the efficiency of the body, there is an increase in intoxication from metabolic waste. Normal waste that the cells are putting out and accumulating is added to the accumulation of whatever other poisons you were taking—drugs, caffeine, alcohol, pesticides. All that is accumulating and affecting the living cells with excitability and irritability and intoxication. If you treat the symptoms with more poisons called medicine or drugs, you are adding more defensive need to this organism.

The moment the body in high vitality is insulted and offended and toxic, it implements its defensive responses, i.e. acute, intensive responses. This is not an intense attack by some outside thing called a bacteria, but rather an intense defense response, which could be a high fever, a lot of vomiting, pain, an eruption on the skin, or diarrhea, i.e. some defense mechanism which says, "Get this poison out of here and let's get back to normal and get on with life."

When you are in high vitality the body mobilizes a violence of intensity to deal with this toxic and offensive state immediately. But as the vitality goes down, that ability to mobilize the "army," to mobilize the defense, to solve this problem and to win the "war," can't happen very efficiently. You still mobilize some defensive effort, so therefore you move with decreasing vitality, but then you move into chronic disease, which is the inability to mobilize enough defensive action to solve the problem—the toxic and enervation process.

WHO'S IN CHARGE?

I'm sure there are real "inherited" conditions which are at play here, but I think true genetic conditions are pretty rare. Unfortunately, many doctors love to tell people what they want to hear, like, "It's not your fault that you've got a problem, it's your grandma's fault," or "It's not your fault. It's the kid's fault." "It's anybody's fault but your own." But that's not true. You've got to change yourself if you're going to change your organism. The only way you can practically change your organism, or what it's doing to itself in health or disease, is to change what *you're* doing to it. Mainly, what you're doing every day of your life—eating food. It's the most practical thing in this world. A lot of these disease conditions could be avoided. You don't necessarily have to die of the same disease your parents died of. You can avoid the causes of disease and live out a normal lifetime before the biological clock of this mortal organism finally just runs down.

If you look at pathology, you see why we die early. In fact, famous doctors have said, "It is not surprising that people die. The question is, why do they live?" The lives of many are so pathological, so degenerative. The only way we can change that is to change the environment in which we live. Mainly, our own internal environment. We can all survive quite well in an external environment which is only half-way reasonable, if our internal environment is sustained. That's where our nutrition comes in. That's how to sustain life. There's no use in destroying the clock prematurely. *If we're going to live out our genetic lifetime, our genetic capabilities, we must live within our tolerances.*

FASTING AND OTHER LIFE-SUPPORTING APPROACHES

In all of nature, fasting is as common as feeding. Most forms of life, except for humans, practice fasting frequently. Humans fast between meals, whether they realize it or not. But they should use it to a greater extent than they do. I think of fasting only as one more way of helping to support life, to maintain life. Fasting should not be used indiscriminately. Feeding should be used when it's appropriate, just like you should wear clothing when it's appropriate, and you use activity when it's appropriate. Everything that has a normal relationship to life has a normal and appropriate use.

The person who follows a natural hygenic lifestyle will maintain a high level of sensitivity in the immune system, have acute defensive mechanisms, and produce intense symptoms everytime the organism is offended. That person should immediately abstain from a meal or two, or fast for a day or two, or a week or two, when these acute symptoms arise.

Remember, fasting is only one more way to support life. Air is a way to support life. You need to breathe to support life. You need rest and sleep to support life. You need activity and exercise to support life. You need food to support life. So there's a way to support life with all these associated needs of life. They must be used appropriately to support life, and misuse of fasting, just like misuse of food, is going to be harmful, not beneficial.

Some people who do a lot of fasting say, "Fast till your tongue is clean," but I think that is an extremely unreliable indication. Some elderly people and some chronically ill people who are way down the ladder of vitality may not live long enough to get a clean tongue. They may be dead! If you're waiting for a clean tongue, you're going to have a corpse on your hands!

You always want to support life and its needs, whether its need is fasting, or whether its need is feeding. If its need is feeding you want to feed it in the form that it tolerates and accepts the food. It's common sense. It's consistent with life. The more life deteriorates, the more you need to provide its needs in easily available forms. Otherwise you're going to force things upon it that it isn't capable of using.

Forty years ago when I started fasting people I'd get calls from people who'd been to Yale and Harvard, and they'd say, "What's that crazy doctor in Strongsville doing, anyway." It's amazing how doctors can be educated into fear and superstition just like the layperson can be. I started using fasting because it worked. I read about it and studied about it. I studied the whole hygenic literature. I was particularly inspired by *Toxemia Explained*, by Tilden[1] and have since discovered that a lot of his ideas are right, but a lot of them are wrong. There's a lot of things that, with time and with learning, we're altering our concept on, but nevertheless the principles were clinically sound.

I came back from the military in World War II with a lot of liver damage. Drugs that we'd been given in the South Pacific to protect us from malaria gave us hepatitis, and all types of other serious conditions. It was a very toxic drug. It contained such a toxic dye that it could turn a white undershirt brilliant yellow with just one pill of it in a volume of water. We all turned yellow from this toxic dye that was supposed to be protecting us from malaria, but was really just poisoning our bodies. It's a residual poison. It just accumulates in your lymphatic system so abundantly that eventually you turn yellow from it. Some of us seemed to be more susceptible, less capable of metabolizing it and excreting it than others. It took me years of repeated fasting to get rid of that stuff. In fact, it's only in the past few years that I don't taste that drug anymore when I fast. In the early years when I would fast, that drug would come out so offensively. (It's just the most foul-tasting stuff that you can imagine. You taste it in your mouth and your saliva. The mucous that you cough up and blow out is all saturated with this yellow stuff.) So, little by little, each fast diminished the excretion of that, and little by little the system cleared itself.

I had developed severe allergies, colitis, ulcers, arthritis. As I was studying this natural lifestyle thing, looking for answers, looking for supplements, I was already convinced that the poisoning we call medicine was the wrong way to go. So I didn't go back to that as a solution. Rather, I searched for ways to solve my problems, and remarkably, as I learned about my problems I was able to help more people.

Today I feel wonderful compared to the way I used to feel. I'm still susceptible to arthritis, so I don't go off the track. I don't go off these programs very far. When you live this lifestyle, your immune system is very sensitized, very acute. I know to fast when my body produces acute symptoms, because at that point I know it's going to be offended, and it's fighting back, it's mobilized.

A SENSITIZED IMMUNE RESPONSE: *THE PRICE OF HEALTH*

Once you intensify the sensitivity of your immune system, as you want to if you want health, you're going to have an intensely sensitive immune response to everything that's offensive to life.

That's the only way you're going to learn intellectually and intuitively how to avoid things that are offensive (*and the only way to experience Intuitive Eating).* After they've been on a good diet for a long time, a lot of people say, "Jeez, I had one glass of wine, or one beer, or one cup of coffee, or I took a puff off this cigarette, and my body just went crazy. I got very hyper, I got a reaction . . . in other words, before when I was using coffee or beer, or smoking all the time, or drinking, it didn't bother me." Once you've cleaned out your immune system, however, the body really attacks the poisons. You really feel the strength of the energetics of the immunity in the body, and that's marvelous. It's not negative. It is very important.

You have the choice of eliminating the causes of disease with building a good defense system, or you have the choice of suppressing all your symptoms with poisons called medicine. In suppressing symptoms, however, you suppress your immune responses, and when you suppress your immune responses, you can no longer mobilize a defense effort sufficient to resolve your "poisoning."

The other choice is to maintain your health by an intensely sensitive immune system, and the best way to do that is by using primarily raw food in your diet. As you sustain the life principle of immunity, you will have an acute response to toxic and offensive conditions. Everytime you offend or insult or damage your organism in any way, it's going to instantly spring into defensive action which is uncomfortable. It's going to produce symptoms. People who use medicine, for example, as soon as they feel uncomfortable from a cold or flu they take aspirin, which suppresses the body's defensive action. People who do a fast, on the other hand, allow that defensive response to accomplish its purpose, which is to restore normalcy in the body.

It's so simple. It's so logical, once you see through what you're doing to yourself. The logic is to fast a day or two, a meal or two—whatever it takes to allow the body to restore harmony again. The happiest thing this organism wants to do during your whole lifetime, is be symptom-free, and it can be symptom-free unless you damage it, offend it, insult it, or do something that evokes a defensive reaction.

Symptoms are always a defense action. Symptoms are not an attack—the body doesn't attack you, your heart doesn't attack you. Your body protects you, it defends you, it repairs you, it heals you. It always mobilizes its defense action to protect and heal and repair, not to destroy. Whether the symptoms are pain, or swelling, or fever, there is really only one disease, and that one disease is a defense action, and that one defense action is inflammation. Every time a tissue is intoxicated and irritated it will evoke a defensive action called inflammation. That inflammation will be characterized by fever, redness, swelling, and pain. Pain lets the brain know there's something wrong. Fever and swelling and redness are all part of the immune response to repair the damage. So it all goes together.

Now, if you do something to stop the inflammation, you take an anti-inflammatory, you'll be stopping the defensive mechanism and suppressing your immune system. Then the inflammation goes into an ulcer instead, because now you're destroying the cells you were trying to heal. So now you have a void. You have cells which are not defending themselves. You also have a different stage of disease—a chronic stage.

Eventually the body tries to repair that damage, the ulceration, by scarring. It replaces the dead tissue with scars—nonfunctional tissues. Now you have fibrosis, or hardening of the arteries, arthritis, sclerosis of the liver, or sclerosis of the brain, or something. You've got a destruction of living cells which are being replaced by scar tissue. Some of those cells may mutate, and begin to form abnormal cells under these same suppressed conditions. Then it's tumors, and some of those tumors may become malignant, which will be cancer. All as the result of interfering with the whole process of repair and healing!

If you fast and support life and stop offending, you allow the body to accomplish its purpose and repair the damage with its natural defense mechanisms, which is what all disease is, in spite of all the complications.

DIGESTIVE EFFICIENCY: *THE KEY TO HEALTH*

It's not uncommon for doctors themselves to be causing disease by adding things to a diet, or doing other things that the body rejects. If your body rejects what you're consuming—be it food, drugs, supplements, herbs, anything—it's only going to add to your disease, or change the form of your disease. It's not going to correct the problem. Any food that you cannot metabolize is toxic to the human body. A nutritionist today should at least be aware and be able to define when a person digests one food better than another food, because ultimately, to sustain nutrition, one must digest the food eaten. If you can't digest beans, you had better not eat beans. If you can't digest raw juice, you had better not eat raw juice. It's important to find the food that we can digest. Overall, however, I'd say juicing should be a tool because fluids are a necessity of life, and juices contain our sugars, minerals and electrolytes. Liquid is an important part of life. It's the single most important thing, and in the juice form it's most easily digested.

It's like a blood transfusion for some people. When their energy gets so low and their vitality gets so low that they can't support their life much longer on common foods, if they can absorb the nutrients from juice the results are almost miraculous. Gradually that person is restored to nutritional vitality and nutritional health, the excellence of health. It may not always be necessary, but at the point when a person might acutely need a form of food that's easily available to them, juices can be just the thing. Fluid, glucose, and electrolyte minerals are the most important single need as your health deteriorates, and those are all in juices.

The best water would be in juice form because it's living water. You can easily overcome dehydration with juices. It's the best way, in fact, because it supplies the minerals. Pure water, as such, doesn't overcome dehydration very successfully. Whereas with water which contains electrolytes (as juices do), you will retain that water and you'll get into water balance because of the metabolism of the electrolytes. Enzymes also are necessary. Every living cell probably has at least a thousand different enzymes in it, if it is healthy. It is important to support those living enzymes that even the body itself produces, and it's important that you supply nutrients in a form that the body can utilize and in a form which is consistent with the life form that you're talking about. Providing nutrients in *utilizable form* is absolutely essential to the restoring of life and health in life.

People get well on raw food if they can digest and assimilate that raw food. They get better much more efficiently, much more quickly, much more vitally on raw food than they do on cooked food. On the other hand, there are certain disease states where cooked food is necessary as a transition. So I don't exclude cooked food; I only exclude it because it's less efficient in sustaining life than raw food is. But when you're near death, cooked food might be an essential for a time until healing can be supported. All good things have to be used intelligently, that's all. Anything that has proved helpful in human experience shouldn't be totally excluded. It should be included intelligently. It's all a matter of balance.

We need to find out what is the common denominator in all the approaches to nutrition. Why is it that a system sometimes works in one setting and not in another? There is a problem with systemitizing everything. I call it "ritualizing." You can't live life by rituals. You've got to live it by intelligent decisions that are made choice by choice as you go through it. It's important to be wise enough to choose when to use the lacto-vegetarian diet, or when to use an all-vegetarian diet, when to use an all-raw diet, when to use an all-cooked diet. There are some common denominators that we have yet to discover, but the clearest one so far is that humans, by design, by nature, by instinct, are raw-food eaters—raw fruits and vegetables. When we try to monkey with the design of nature, especially in the diseased state, we're going to create a lot of problems for ourselves.

HEIGHTENING SELF-AWARENESS

Everybody in the world of science knows that the body has innate intelligence in its choice and utilization of food, i.e. its absorption of nutrients from the intestinal tract, and its distribution to the whole system. Every living cell has this intelligence, especially in the gut. What the scientific community hasn't come to agree on and to understand is that the very principle of intelligent selectivity implies that there is a converse, i.e. intelligent rejectivity. This is a very important principle to understand.

When the body rejects food, it sort of "trashes" it. It decomposes it in the gut with bacterial action, by fermentation, putrefaction, decomposition. This causes toxic products like alcohol and cedic acid, and others, to be absorbed into the system. This "gut rejectivity," which I call this process, is more prevalent as people get progressively more ill. As people deteriorate in health there is more *rejection* of food than there is *acceptance* of food, more *rejectivity* than *selectivity*, and therefore more toxification as a consequence of mal-metabolism of food.

This mal-absorption, or this absorption of toxic, or mal-metabolized, or incompletely digested molecules from food, becomes a toxin in the body which the organism must dispose of. These materials, which have entered the bloodstream through the gut wall are now adding to the toxic irritability of the cells of the body, so the body evokes a defense mechanism. It attempts to dump this waste out through the urinary tract because that's the quickest route out, and so you'll find a lot of this debris in the urine.

To get a feeling and an understanding for this mechanism of excretion, we measure the byproducts of toxic mal-metabolism in the urine. We try to quantify it, using a precipitating agent called ferric nitrate. We put freshly passed urine in a test tube, add the drops of ferric nitrate, and notice that where there's a toxic offense, based on mal-metabolism of food, there frequently is a great deal of debris in the urine, which is visible immediately. The goal of this is to demonstrate something so that the mind comprehends what is inappropriate. For instance, if I swallow a certain food and an hour or two later I see all this debris in the urine, my mentality, my intelligence has to say this is not the best for me. I should choose a food that my body accepts more appropriately. Then there won't be so many waste products from metabolism spilling in the urine to protect me. Why should I be evoking all these defensive responses that constantly have to protect me? So I want to be conscious of which foods my body chooses to call *acceptable*, and I want to avoid those foods which my body chooses to call *unacceptable*.

We are all a little different, because we all have different stages of vitality. We have different stages of disease, different stages of health, different stages of emotional health, all of which are important to good digestion. We have different stages of fatigue, which also make a difference in how well we handle food. The goal is to digest the food so that your body will utilize it. If the body is selectively saying, "I don't want this food," it's better to see it early, when it's only in evidence in the urine, rather than wait till it's an ammonia, or it's evidenced as a massive secretion from the lungs. We need to understand our personal tolerance and our individual limitations. Urine testing is one way of helping us to understand. I'm not saying it's the whole answer—not at all. But it's part of the answer.

• • • •

Humbart Santillo, N.D.:

Thinking that America is a well-nourished country is a joke. Despite the high levels of education and research, 80% of the nation's population may be afflicted with malnourishment, according to Dr. Cheraskin and Dr. Ringsdorf[2]. A study done at Jersey City Medical Center showed that 83% of the patients admitted to the hospital had at least one or more vitamin deficiencies, and 68% had two or more deficiencies. Missing one nutrient is like missing one link in a chain, like an orchestra performing without its main instrument.

Metabolic functions are controlled by nutrients. A whole chain-reaction of metabolic events can be disturbed, and over a long period of time severe illness may result. The longer the period of time that a deficiency exists, the more serious the problem can be. Sometimes many symptoms will manifest, making it seem like several maladies are being experienced. But when the proper nutrient is taken, it almost seems miraculous how fast the body heals itself. This also goes for mental conditions that may be caused by being malnourished.

Nutrients, ideally, are supplied by our foods. But many lack the education to know what to eat, and how much, to supply these essential links. In the next chapter you will have an opportunity to study the building blocks of nutrition so that you can build a better foundation for your life and health.

CHAPTER 4

Your Nutritional Primer

INTRODUCTION

THE ABC's of Nutrition are not easy, and to try to explain them simply is a worthy challenge. In this chapter I have attempted to give you just enough data about nutrition to help you to feel more confident in designing your own diet, and to hopefully allow you to talk about your process of *Intuitive Eating* with some credibility. If I've done my job well you will also be motivated to want to learn more.

The topics covered in this chapter are Fats, Carbohydrates, Protein, Fiber, Minerals, and Vitamins. The subject of Enzymes, one of the primary elements for consideration in *Intuitive Eating*, will be discussed at length in the next chapter.

As you read ahead here try not to get discouraged if you come across a concept that is difficult to understand. Just keep going. Often you will find that things get clearer as you read on. Anyway, it is not necessary to know all the details of chemistry etc., to begin to appreciate what these nutrients are, what they do for the body, and how to supply them optimally.

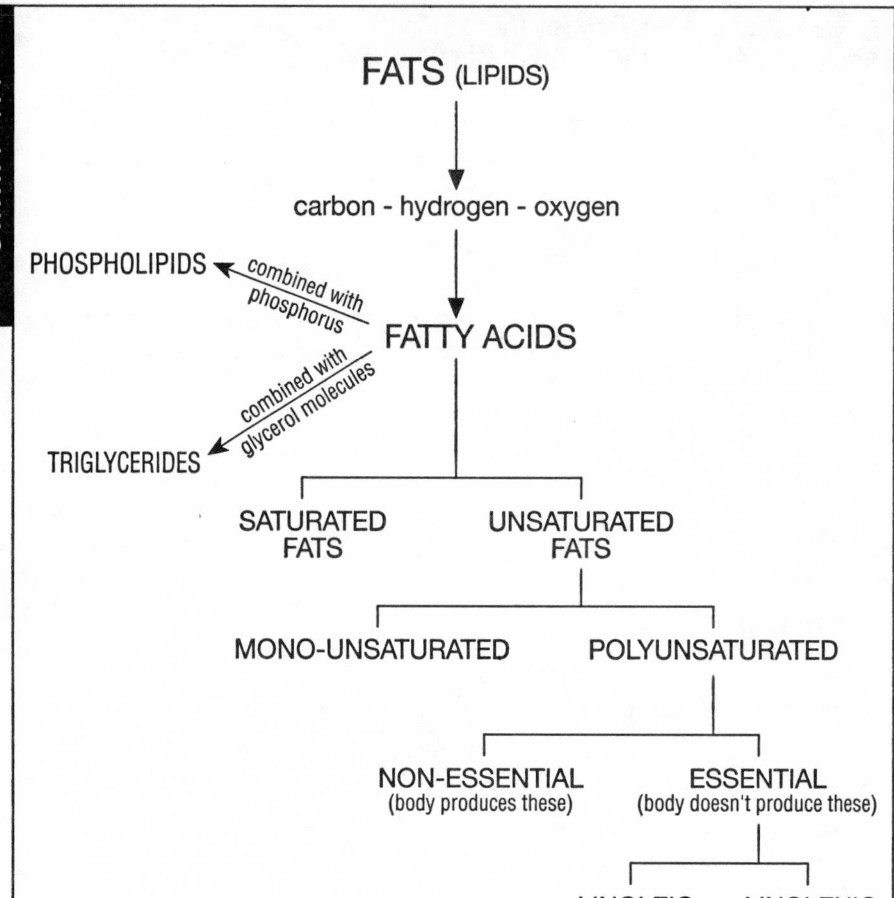

UNDERSTANDING FATS

Diseases of fatty degeneration will kill approximately 75% of the people in affluent societies. To get to the root of the problem we must study the different types of fats to discover which ones are necessary to include in our diet and which ones to avoid.

Fats may be defined by their basic structure. (See Chart 4.1) All fats are made up of carbon, hydrogen, and oxygen. (These are the same elements that comprise carbohydrates, but in fats the relative hydrogen content is much higher.) There are many types of fats, all made up of the same elements but in different amounts and in different structural (molecular) designs.

Fatty acids are the primary componants of fats; in fact, we can consider them the building blocks of fats. Fatty acids are all made up of carbon, hydrogen, and oxygen, but the differing amounts of each give us many different fatty acids.

Some fatty acids are necessary and good for us, others accumulate in the body and can be detrimental. Some fatty acids are joined and combined with glycerol molecules (a combination of a sugar-alcohol substance) and form fats called triglycerides. Once again, some triglycerides are good for us, while some are definitely not.

There are two major groups of fatty acids we must be concerned about — the saturated and unsaturated fatty acids. The difference between these two types is the ratio of hydrogen atoms to carbon atoms. The next section will explain these types further, but for now keep in mind that saturated fats are solid fats, with higher melting points; unsaturated fats are usually of liquid consistency.

Unsaturated fatty acids are further subdivided into monounsaturated and polyunsaturated fats (which you have probably heard a lot about). Two important polyunsaturated fats are linoleic and linolenic fatty acids. These are called *essential* fatty acids because the body doesn't produce them on its own, and hence we must supply these in our diets. Fatty acids that the body can produce on its own are called *non-essential* fatty acids. Let's take a closer look at the story behind fats in our diet.

SATURATED FATS

Saturated fats, the simplest kind of fatty acid, are usually found in animal foods, such as beef, pork, and dairy products. These fatty acids are made up of an arrangement of carbon atoms hooked in a chain, with each carbon atom attached to a hydrogen atom. Since each carbon atom has a hydrogen-atom-partner clinging to it, it can't take on another partner, so it is said to be *saturated*.

Saturated fats have a high melting point and tend to stick together to form a solid mass, like in margarine, vegetable shortening, and cocoa butter. Sticking together, they tend to aggregate in the bloodstream, forming droplets of fat and hard plaque which gets deposited on cell walls and in organs and arteries causing cardiovascular disease and diseases of fatty degeneration.

Fatty degenerative conditions are characterized by the appearance of fatty materials in cells where fats are normally not found. Arterioschlerosis (deposits of fatty material in the arteries and heart) is an example. When arteries lose their elasticity and narrow because of the accumulation of these unnatural fats, high blood pressure develops. This puts excess stress on the kidneys and heart, and leads to both kidney and heart disease.

Besides the saturated fats we get from animal food, refined sugars and starches are converted to fats in the body. This definitely intensifies the fat problem due to the large quantity of refined sugars and starches in the typical diet.

UNSATURATED FATTY ACIDS

Unsaturated fatty acids differ from saturated fatty acids in only one respect. They are also made of carbon and hydrogen chains hooked together, but in this case not all the carbon molecules are attached to hydrogen molecules. A few carbon molecules stand alone. Since they do not have hydrogen-molecule-partners, these fats are called *unsaturated.*

Unsaturated fats break up easier and do not aggregate in the bloodstream. They have lower melting points and disperse much more readily than saturated fats. Unsaturated fatty acids can also move easily within the membrane of the cell. (For those who want a more scientific explanation of this, unsaturated fatty acids have double bonds and form a kink at the double bond position. They all carry a negative charge, which means that they repel each other and will therefore not stick together.)

Mono-unsaturated fats are those that have only one double-bond. Some "monos" are detrimental and others are quite beneficial. For example, palmitoleic acid, found in the coconut and palm kernel oil, can lead to health problems because it interferes with the essential fatty acids. Oleic acid, on the other hand, is the most important mono-unsaturated fat, and it is good for us if eaten in small amounts. Found in olives, almonds and other seeds, and in plant skins, this fluid oil helps keep the arteries clean and elastic. It is also produced in the skin and pores of humans. In excess, however, oleic acid also can inhibit the function of our essential fatty acids.

POLYUNSATURATED FATS

Two of the most essential fatty acids — linolenic (LNA) and linoleic acid (LA) — are poly-unsaturated. There are many different poly-unsaturated fats, and like all the other classifications of fats we have talked about thus far, some are good while others are harmful. The poly-unsaturated fats present in refined and hydrogenated oils, for instance, are some of the worst! The heating and refining process actually alters them in such a way that they become destructive to human tissues.

For our purposes poly-unsaturated fats will be considered as either "healthy" or "unhealthy." The healthy ones can also be called *natural* poly-unsaturated fatty acids — LA or LNA are examples of this type. Technically they are referred to as *cis-fatty* acids because the arrangements of their molecules are in a *cis* configuration. (This means that both hydrogen molecules are on the same side of the carbon molecule involved in its bonds. This helps hold the fatty acids together.)

Unhealthy poly-unsaturated fatty acids are also called *trans-poly-unsaturated* fatty acids (TFA). (Two identical atoms or groups are attached to opposite sides of a molecule.) TFA are produced by high temperatures. When the fat is heated to 160 degrees Centigrade, or higher, the hydrogen molecules switch to the opposite side. This switch alters the original structure of the molecule so the fat is no longer a natural fatty acid. The *trans*-configuration is more stable than the *cis*-configuration, but it no longer fits properly into cellular membranes and enzymes. It tends to change the ability of the cell to absorb certain nutrients while it allows destructive substances into the cells. The protective barrier to the cells is systematically destroyed. Trans fatty acids interfere with enzyme systems that metabolize natural fatty acids, and can cause fatty acid deficiences.

Trans fatty acids are very difficult for the body to break down. They work more like saturated fatty acids, i.e. they stick together, causing plaque deposits in the liver and arteries. They also cause blood platelets to stick together, thus increasing the risk of strokes and heart attacks.

Ninety-five percent of trans fatty acids come from hydrogenated oils, and the rest from beef, butter, margarine, and shortenings. Partially hydrogenated oils also contain trans fatty acids. (The process of hydrogenation, and other facts about fats and cholesterol, will be covered later in this chapter.) These trans fatty acids can increase cholesterol levels by 15% and triglycerides (also explained later) by 45%. Taking flax seed daily helps reduce the accumulation of saturated fat and reduces trans fatty acids.

All in all, you can understand how some poly-unsaturated fatty acids can be detrimental to health. It's confusing at times because we also know that that poly-unsaturated fatty acids lower blood cholesterol, which many people are looking for. What actually happens is that poly-unsaturated fats drive large amounts of cholesterol from the blood to the liver and then into the gallbladder, through the colon. This contributes to the formation of gallstones, and is related to bowel cancer.

Poly-unsaturated fats can also thin the blood and create excessive bleeding. Eating an excessive amount of poly-unsaturated-fatty-acids (PUFA) can be dangerous. They is why I suggest a diet high in complex carbohydrates, low in fats (approximately 10-15%), and low in protein. (The Pritikin Diet suggests about 10% total fat intake and 10% protein intake, and 80% complex carbohydrates.)

ESSENTIAL FATTY ACIDS — LINOLENIC ACID AND LINOLEIC ACID

These two essential fatty acids are both poly-unsaturated. They are essential since the body cannot produce them, therefore they must be supplied by the diet. Other fatty acids which can be made from these two (like arachiodonic acid which can be found in meat), are made from linoleic acid.

Deficiencies of these essential acids result in liver damage, hair loss, kidney problems, drying up of glands, infections, miscarriages, retardation, arthritis, tingling in the arms and legs, weakness, impaired vision — in other words, almost anything.

Safflower oil is 80% linoleic acid (LA); linseed oil, made from flax seed, is 60% linolenic (LNA) and 20% LA. These oils attract oxygen and sunlight in the body and spread out over a large surface area. Consequently, they do not aggregate in the blood. They carry toxins to the kidneys, intestinal tract, and lungs, where they are naturally eliminated. These oils also give us mental vitality. They carry oxygen to all the cells in the body, so food can be burned as energy. They transfer oxygen to all the cells, including the brain.

LA is involved in hemoglobin production and helps hold protein in the membranes of the cells, and thus control the passing of nutrients and fluid in and out of the cells. Both LA and LNA generate bio-electric currents which travel along from cell to cell. LA and LNA help people recover from muscle fatigue after exercise by reducing lactic acid to water and CO_2.

Essential fatty acids are precursors (your body takes the precursors and builds the hormone) to a family of hormone structures called prostaglandins. Prostaglandins control cellular functions, lower blood pressure, and inhibit blood fats from sticking together. The brain, retina, inner ear, adrenal gland, and testicle tissue all need fatty acids which are produced from LNA and LA. At levels of 12-15% of the total calories, they increase the metabolic rate and thus increase the burning of calories so necessary for weight loss. They are necessary in the body so it can absorb and store sunlight. The diet should contain approximately

3-6 grams of essential fatty acids daily to avoid deficiencies, and 9-30 grams for people who are under stress, obese, or experiencing some of the previously mentioned symptoms. Oils of seeds and nuts are good sources of fatty acids. The best source, flax seed oil, can be easily made by grinding the seeds in a coffee grinder. Ground flax seed can then be added to your juices, or sprinkled directly on your salads.

Safflower oil is another good source of LA but does not contain LNA. The best oils for human consumption are flax seed, pumpkin, soy, and walnut oil. Each of these contains both LNA and LA. These seed oils are dispersed in our tissues and help to break down and dissolve saturated fatty acids and cholesterol.

To be effective, however, oils have to be fresh — i.e. not exposed to light, oxygen, or heat. These three agents destroy the essential fatty acids. Clear glass or plastic bottles will not preserve the nutritional quality of your oil.

TRIGLYCERIDES

Over 95% of all the fats we eat are in the form of triglycerides — i.e. fatty acids combined with glycerol molecules. They are, therefore, the main class of food fats. Most of the stored fat in human and animal tissues is stored as triglycerides. They also serve as the body's reserve of the essential fatty acids, LA and LNA, and carry them around in the body. Some triglycerides carry saturated fats like the ones found in beef and pork, which are detrimental to the body. Flax seed oil, on the other hand, carries LA and LNA.

When we consume triglycerides the body breaks them down into glycerol and fatty acids, takes what it needs for its various functions, and then reconstructs the remaining elements back into triglycerides, and stores them. Triglycerides form a layer of insulation around the body and internal organs to protect them from shock. (The body also takes excess sugar and turns it into triglycerides and stores it in the body, which is why we gain weight from excess sugar intake.)

When the brain needs glucose for its functions, the body breaks down the triglycerides and uses the glucose. Triglycerides store essential fatty acids which are used for prostaglandin production. They are also used by the brain cells, adrenal glands, retina of the eye, and the testes. Since triglycerides tend to clump together they can cause a build up of arterial plaque, high blood pressure, heart and kidney problems.

DIGESTION OF FATS

Most fats are digested in the small intestine, which can digest about ten grams of fat every hour. Here the fats are mixed with bile, which is made in the liver out of cholesterol. The bile mixture is then concentrated and stored in the gallbladder. The bile emulsifies the fats, breaking them down to small fatty droplets. The pancreas then secretes its fat-digesting enzymes on top of any fat in the small intenstine (duodenum). These enzymes split off the fatty acids from the triglycerides, the cholesterol, and the phospholipids (*lipid* means fat or oil, *phospho* means the lipid contains phosphorus).

The digested fatty droplets, called chylomicrons, are absorbed through the small intestine wall into the lymphatic system. These chylomicrons transfer their fats to HDL (high density lipo-proteins) which circulate in the blood. Then they are taken to the liver. The liver makes smaller "fatty packages" of these fats, called VLDL (very low density lipo-proteins), or LDL (low density lipo-proteins). These VLDL and LDL transfer fatty acids to the cells. Once the cells have all the fat they can handle, the excess LDL, with their cholesterol and triglycerides, circulate in the blood. Eating excessive amounts of fat, therefore, will increase the amount of excess LDL in the blood, and these can accumulate in the blood vessels causing cardiovascular disease.

Lecithin is a phospholipid which makes up 22% of the high density lipo-proteins. The amazing characteristic of lecithin is that it keeps cholesterol from depositing in the arteries, and prevents and dissolves gallstones and kidney stones. Lecithin is necessary in the liver for proper detoxification. It also supplies choline to the body, which is necessary for liver and brain function. Most seeds and nuts contain lecithin.

CHOLESTEROL

Let's talk about cholesterol. Cholesterol is absolutely essential to our health. It is a natural substance found in the human body — in the liver, skin, brain cells, adrenal glands, blood, and bile. It is necessary for hormonal production. In fact, cholesterol is considered to be both a fat and a hormone (sterol). Chemically it is closely related to sex hormones and adrenal gland hormones. It is synthesized by the liver, intestines, and other tissues, and converted to steroid hormones, bile acids, and pro-vitamin D-3. It is the building block for cell membranes.

The body produces 500-1000 milligrams of cholesterol daily, which is about all anybody really needs. Nonetheless, most people add an additional 500-1000 milligrams of cholesterol to their diet every day, chiefly from animal flesh and animal products (plant foods do not contain cholesterol), and that is where many problems arise. We don't need that much cholesterol.

Some of the excess cholesterol will normally be eliminated through the liver, gallbladder, and intestines. What cannot be eliminated remains in the body and is deposited in the tissues and arteries. Fat and calcium accumulated in this cholesterol begin to harden, a process is called atherosclerosis (hardening of the arteries). This build-up can accumulate to such a point that it can plug an artery. If this occurs in an artery that nourishes the heart, the heart can be deprived of oxygen, nourishment, and blood. Such a heart will eventually cramp (heart attack), and begin to die.

The excessive consumption of cholesterol is not necessarily the whole problem, however. Some cultures consume large amounts of animal fats and do not have cholesterol problems. But they also exercise daily, eat most of their foods raw, and live outdoors.

Cholesterol can be a big problem if the liver breaks down for any reason. Then it will not be able to handle large amounts of cholesterol. If constipation is a problem, this can block the elimination of cholesterol and other toxic substances. A high protein diet can also cause cholesterol troubles.

There is an average body content of 150 grams of cholesterol, 7 grams of which are found in the bloodstream. This cholesterol in the blood, along with triglycerides, phospholipids, and proteins, are found in carrier vehicles of which there are several with different jobs. These carrier vehicles are also called plasma lipoproteins — the most important of which are called low density lipoproteins (LDL). These carry cholesterol from the food and liver to the cells. Another plasma lipoprotein — high density lipoproteins (HDL)— takes cholesterol from the cells back to the liver where the excess is changed to bile acids and cholesterol. Then it's carried into the intestines to be eliminated from the body.

Any fat, good or bad, in excess, can cause problems in the body, because it forces the liver to produce excessive amounts of bile acids. Excessive bile (because of the excess amount of fats that are brought to the liver where the liver produces this bile) is converted into carcinogens by bowel bacteria. This excess acid is often associated with the cause of bowel cancer.

One way of measuring blood cholesterol is to measure the amount of HDL and LDL in the blood. Both these lipo-proteins are necessary, but you want more HDL in the blood than LDL. HDL takes unused cholesterol back to the liver to be processed and excreted. High HDL indicates that the blood is getting rid of the excess cholesterol and preventing it from accumulating. A high LDL, on the other hand, indicates that the body is becoming overloaded with fats. So, what's important is the ratio between these two, not just a total cholesterol reading.

Choosing your foods carefully, as well as getting the right amount of physical exercise, are important factors in controlling blood cholesterol. Saturated fats and cholesterol from a meat-based diet increase LDL and cholesterol levels. This causes the blood platelets to stick together and stress the liver's production of bile acids, thus increasing our risk of cardiovascular disease.

All cholesterol comes from animal tissues; meat, dairy, and eggs are the worst offenders. They not only have high fat content, but they lack fiber which helps control blood fats (see the section on Fiber later in this chapter). It would be smart to eat less saturated fats and sugars and more unsaturated fatty acids that help control cholesterol problems and cariovascular disease. Cholesterol is lowered by increasing LNA and LA. Exercise also lowers cholesterol by burning fats. Dairy products contain a high percentage of saturated fatty acids which can cause allergies, constipation, cholesterol problems, and a host of other difficulties. A strictly vegetarian diet seems to be the best approach to controlling blood fat difficulties.

HYDROGENATION OR COLD-PRESSING

During the hydrogenation process natural oils are heated to a temperature of 120-210 degrees Centigrade (248-410 degrees Fahrenheit) and combined with hydrogen gas. This process saturates all the fatty acids with hydrogen molecules. Now they cannot be digested or dissolved in the body naturally. If you remember, unsaturated fatty acids are not saturated with hydrogen, so they can be easily broken down in the body. In other words, they are natural and still in their *cis* configuration.

Hydrogenated fats do not spoil, so even though they contain *trans* fatty acids, which cause toxic reactions in the body, they have a longer shelf life, which is greatly appealing to manufacturers and grocers. Some margarines contain an average of 31% *trans* fatty acids. Vegetable shortenings may have 37.3% *trans* fatty acids, with an average of 20% *trans* fatty acids in vegetable oils.

For years I've used "cold-pressed" vegetable oils thinking that was the healthy thing to do. "Cold-pressing" means that no external heat has been added during the processing of the oil, but it doesn't mean that heat might not have been used *before* the processing. Nuts and seeds are often preheated to high temperatures to deodorize them before the cold processing. Not only that, during the grinding of the seeds, heat is produced by friction while the material is being crushed and rotated. Heat is necessary for the oil to run out of the press. In Switzerland it is illegal to call an oil "cold-pressed" because of this process, since the oil that runs out of the press is usually between 85-95 degrees Centigrade. Inside the press the temperature is even higher. The higher the temperature, the faster the oil can be broken down by heat, oxygen, and sunlight. The fatty acids then turn into *trans* fatty acids, and are now unnatural oils.

Look for unrefined oils that have been mechanically pressed but have not been exposed to sunlight. Oil should be sold in cans or dark glass containers and kept in a cool place.

FREE RADICALS

The theory of free radicals gives us a logical explanation for how they can be a contributing factor to cardiovascular disease, cancer, and aging. A free radical is a molecule with an unpaired electron. This unpaired electron is free to jump around at will, looking for a partner to join up with. During this process, it can destroy other elements in the body. There are naturally-occurring free radicals in the body, but the body has natural ways of controlling these. Unnatural free radicals (electrons), on the other hand, can cause faulty metabolism.

Oils that are exposed to heat or sunlight will often have electrons knocked loose. This freed electron can then go knocking other electrons apart, and this process can be repeated 30,000 times by just one electron before it stops. This means that the fatty acid in the oil will be altered, i.e. denatured. Frying food causes free radicals to be released, and turns an unsaturated fatty acid into a trans fatty acid. Oxygen destroys oils by a similar process. Light increases the activity of oxygen and causes the release of electrons, creating more free radicals. Light actually destroys oils 1,000 times faster than oxygen does.

In the body, vitamin E, carotene, vitamin C, B6, bioflavonoids, zinc, silenium, and sulphur-containing amino acids protect the body from free radicals. They are called antioxidants. These nutrients, plus enzymes, confine and direct free radicals so they complete their natural chemical reactions. So the key here is to include these nutrients in your diet, and avoid fried and heated oils. Keep in mind that free radicals cause the body to age rapidly, because they attack and destroy living tissues, particularly proteins in the blood, cellular membranes, and fatty acids.

CARBOHYDRATES: *SUGAR AND STARCHES*

All sugars (which include glucose, fructose, galactose, maltose, in beer, and lactose, which is in milk), all syrups, and honey, are rapidly absorbed and quickly turned to fats. Starches are just sugar molecules bonded together. In the body when starches are digested by enzymes, these bonds are broken down to simpler sugars.

The worst kind of starch is from refined sources, which include pasta, white rice, enriched flour, cornstarch, tapioca, and most breakfast cereals. These refined carbohydrates are digested and absorbed quickly, and can overload the blood with glucose, but this is only part of the problem. Since refined foods lack important vitamins and minerals, the body cannot properly burn them, and so they are usually turned to fat. Because they lack these nutrients, they must steal them from the body's store of vitamins and minerals. The body cannot properly metabolize these refined foods, and this can cause long-term deficiencies.

Carbohydrates that are not refined are left in their whole state, like whole grains, potatoes, corn, rice, and vegetables. These are called complex carbohydrates because they contain vitamins, minerals, and fiber. Because they require time to be broken down to simple sugars, these sugars are released slowly into the blood over a long period of time. This prevents overloading the blood with glucose as refined foods do.

When complex carbohydrates are cooked or ground they are easier to digest. Consequently, they will cause a faster rise in blood sugar than the raw forms will. So, diabetics and hypoglycemics should have a balance between raw, uncooked carbohydrates like fruits, vegetables, whole grains, and some cooked grains. Candies, cakes, ice cream, sugar, etc. should be avoided by everybody.

The body has two ways in which to deal with excess blood glucose. It spills it into the urine, causing diabetes, or it can store the sugar as fat. High blood-glucose triggers the pancreas to secrete insulin, which stimulates the conversion of sugars to fatty acids, or triglycerides. These fats are stored in tissues and organs and can cause strokes, heart attacks, and an increase in blood pressure. They can be stored and used as energy sources later on too, but are not essential. Excess sugar and starches can also be converted into cholesterol, a major health problem for many people.

The body can turn sugars and starches to fat, but cannot turn some fats back to sugars. This is why exercise is so important in order to burn the excess fat. When the simple sugars needed for energy are not available in the diet, the body must use protein for this purpose. This is why people often crave excessive protein when their diet is high in refined carbohydrates.

DISEASES CAUSED BY REFINED CARBOHYDRATES

Refined sugar, as we have suggested, is rapidly absorbed into the body. Insulin is secreted by the pancreas, removing this excess sugar from the blood. This must happen rapidly when glucose rises unnaturally fast. The blood-glucose may then fall too rapidly, causing low blood sugar (hypoglycemia). When this happens, the adrenal glands secrete their hormones which stimulate both the release of sugars from the tissues, and the synthesis of glucose from proteins.

After years of this "yo-yo" chemistry, the adrenal glands or the pancreas weaken and degenerate. If the pancreas weakens it secretes less insulin, and glucose overflows in the blood (diabetes). If the adrenal glands weaken and become exhausted we cannot respond to stress normally, and we become susceptible to

CHART 4.2

THE GLYCEMIC INDEX FOR SELECTED FOODS*

• 100%

Glucose

• 80% - 90%

Cornflakes
Carrots**
Parsnips**
Potatoes (instant mashed)
Maltose
Honey

• 70% - 79%

Bread (wholemeal)
Millet
Rice (white)
Weetabix
Broad beans (fresh)**
Potato (new)**
Swede**

• 60% - 69%

Bread (white)
Rice (brown)
Muesli
Shredded Wheat
"Ryvita"
Water Biscuits
Beetroot**
Bananas
Raisins
Mars bar

• 50% - 59%

Buckwheat
Spaghetti (white)
Sweet corn
All-Bran
Digestive biscuits
Oatmeal biscuits
"Rich Tea" biscuits
Peas (frozen)
Yam
Sucrose
Potato chips

• 40% - 49%

Spaghetti (wholemeal)
Porridge oats
Potato (sweet)
Beans (canned navy)
Peas (dried)
Oranges
Orange juice

• 30% - 39%

Butter beans
Haricot beans
Blackeye peas
Chick peas
Apples (Golden Delicious)
Ice cream
Milk (skim)
Milk (whole)
Yoghurt
Tomato soup

• 20% - 29%

Kidney beans
Lentils
Fructose

• 10% - 19%

Soya beans
Soya beans (canned)
Peanuts

*The glycemic index is the area under the two-hour blood glucose response curve for each food expressed as a percentage of the area under the curve after taking the same amount of carbohydrate as glucose. 50 gm. carbohydrate portions were used in most cases except where specified. Results are the means of 5 to 10 normal, nondiabetic individuals.

**25 gm. carbohydrate portions tested.

***Reprinted with permission from Jenkins, DJA, *Diabetes Care* 5:634, 1982.

disease. This cycle causes emotional imbalances and unnatural food cravings for more sugar, sweets, and coffee.

For those of you who have blood sugar problems this glycemic chart will help you. (See Chart 4.2.) The foods listed on this chart are listed in the order that they raise blood glucose levels. Everything has been rated relative to the absorption of glucose. For example, glucose would raise the blood sugar level 100% two hours after meals. Cornflakes would raise blood glucose 80-90% two hours after meals. Bread and millet raise blood glucose levels 70-90% two hours after meals. Now look at the foods that only raise blood sugar 20-29%, like kidney beans and lentils.

If you are hypoglycemic or diabetic you wouldn't want to use foods that raise blood glucose (sugar) too high. You would concentrate on foods that raise blood glucose 60% or less, depending on the severity of your condition.

When I was hypoglycemic, carrot juice would weaken me. So I avoided it until I strengthened my adrenal glands and pancreas. Now I drink at least 20 ounces of carrot juice daily with no ill effects.

Because these excess sugars can be turned into fats, these fats are deposited in our organs and blood vessels causing fatty degenerative diseases. These saturated fats cause anoxia (lack of oxygen) at the cellular level, which leads to all types of diseases. Chronic diseases like cancer are always associated with low oxygen levels in the body. The answer here is to use high-fiber, natural, complex carbohydrates so the sugar is slowly released into the bloodstream. This food is doubly advantageous because it helps with proper elimination because of its high fiber content. Refined carbohydrates remain in the colon for a long period of time because they lack the necessary fiber. Consequently, they ferment, causing gases, diverticulitis, hemorrhoids, and other intestinal problems.

FIBER

Fiber is a non-digestible, complex carbohydrate, sometimes called "bulk," "roughage," and "residue." When whole grains are refined, much of the fiber is removed and therefore many nutrients are lost during the refinement process. This is especially true for the B vitamins which are extremely important for mental health. During World War II, when Denmark stopped refining its flour, the death rate dropped, with a marked decline in heart disease, cancer, diabetes, and kidney problems[1]. These diseases are all linked with a lack of fiber (from bran and cellulose of plants) in the diet.

There is no fiber in meat, fish, poultry, shellfish, eggs or cheese. And yet, these foods make up a large percentage of the American diet. Lack of fiber leads to constipation—white bread eaters, for instance, receive 87.5% less fiber than the whole-wheat bread eaters.

Dr. Roger Williams, former director of the Clayton Foundation Biochemical Institute, once conducted an experiment in which rats were fed standard white bread. Within 90 days, two-thirds of the rats were dead, and the others had stunted growth.

A lack of fiber can cause chronic constipation, diverticulitis, appendicitis, stomach and duodenal ulcers. After fiber-deficient food is digested, little bulk residue is left in the intestines to form the stool for bacteria to live on. The result is hard, marbly stools, and harmful straining. Straining at the stool increases the pressure of the blood in the veins, both in the legs and the rectum. This leads to hemorrhoids and varicose veins. Straining can also lead to hiatal hernias, by pushing the stomach up into the chest cavity, causing a large opening in the diaphragm. After years of trying to pass small, hard stools, pouches are blown out in the bowel. These pouches are called diverticuli. They become infected, and may bleed. The condition is then called diverticulitis. Thirty-five percent of the people over 60 in affluent countries have this condition.

Irritable colon syndrome (spastic colon) is another common condition. The symptoms of this condition are lower abdominal pains, diarrhea, mucous discharge, and small stools (thin and narrow). When a high fiber diet is used, these symptoms generally improve.

Dietary fiber dilutes, inactivates, and binds cholesterol, bile acids, carcinogens, and other toxic substances in the bowel. This action inhibits the absorbing of these toxins into the bloodstream, and reduces their contact time with the bowel wall. This explains why people on high-fiber diets have less colon cancer, heart disease, cholesterol problems, and gallstones.

When a person is on a low-fiber, high-calorie diet, the sugars are rapidly absorbed into the blood, and can cause hypoglycemia and diabetes. High fiber diets retard the absorption of these sugary and starchy substances, which makes this factor very important in the prevention of such diseases.

Other diseases found in affluent societies which relate to a low-fiber diet include Crohn's Disease (inflammation of the bowel), colitis, and blood clots in veins and lungs. A high-fiber diet is suggested for all these conditions. It is also excellent for people who want to lose weight since fiber fills the stomach, and takes away excessive hunger.

Fruits and vegetables are high fiber foods. Psyllium seed powder, available at health food stores, is extremely high in fiber and is commonly recommended as an excellent laxative. (Always follow directions on the container, or consult your physician or health professional when using laxatives.) See Appendix E in this book for a breakdown of the fiber content of foods.

PROTEIN—AND THE CONTROVERSY ABOUT IT

Proteins are made of amino acids—in other words, amino acids are the building blocks of protein. Amino acids are what the body uses to reconstruct its own protein, and to maintain bodily tissues and hormones. As proteins are broken down during digestion, these amino acids are absorbed into the bloodstream through the vili of the small intestine.

There are eight essential amino acids. Essential amino acids are aminos that the body cannot produce and make within itself, so they must be contained in the foods that are eaten; without them protein deficiencies will result. So, foods that contain the eight essential amino acids are considered complete protein and are necessary.

Most fruits and vegetables contain all the essential amino acids that are necessary for growth.

One of the chief arguments in the field of nutrition is how much protein do we really need, and what is the best source of protein? Many of you may still be under the impression that meat protein is the best. Experiments have proven that one can secure all the protein that is necessary from vegetable and fruit sources, and that the use of meat is both unnecessary and harmful. Meat also brings impure substances along with excessive protein into the body. Excess protein puts a stress on the digestive tract, kidneys, and liver, and lowers the body's nerve energies.

Eating too much protein, especially animal protein (eggs, meat, cheese, etc.), places the body into a "luxurient metabolism" when the catabolic (degenerative processes) of the body are stimulated. "Luxurient metabolism" means the body is stimulated into a rapid burning off of the excess protein. This process gives us a sense of false strength. Uric acid, which is a byproduct of meat, metabolizes and acts as a stimulant (false strength), and is very irritating to the nervous system. In order to protect itself from the excess uric acid, the body steals calcium, as a buffer, from the teeth and bones, and combines it with the uric acid to form calcium urate crystals, a less irritating substance, but one that can also lead to kidney stones and rheumatic disorders. There are two things happening here: the body is overstimulated, giving us a false sense of strength, and calcium is being depleted. Both these factors are considered to be a major part of the aging process. This aging effect is seen in heavy meat-eating tribes, such as the Eskimos and the Masai of Africa, where the average lifespan is approximately 25 to 45 years of age.

In his book *A Cancer Therapy*[2], Dr. Max Gerson, M.D. reports that he discontinued the use of animal protein in the diets of his cancer patients because animal protein had damaging effects. He noticed that the detoxification process was retarded and the healing process was delayed when meat was used. His experience with diabetic patients further revealed that additional protein burdened the kidneys and liver, and caused an increase dosage of insulin. Spasms of the diaphragm, and overstimulation of the G.I. tract and nervous system were also observed.

The estimated amounts of protein needed by the human adult have been shown to be as little as 2.5% of our daily calorie intake. This amount is equivalent to less than 20 grams a day—two-thirds of an ounce. The World Health Organization has estimated a slightly higher daily minimum of protein, approximately 5% of the daily caloric intake. I believe that even this is a little high, although it is only half of what had been estimated years ago by Liebig and Voit, which was 118 to 160 grams of protein daily[3].

A working person generally consumes about 3000 calories a day. Five percent of this would be 150 calories of protein. Since each gram of protein is equivalent to 4 calories, this represents 37 grams of protein daily. This amount of protein would be easy to get using most fruits and vegetables, seeds, and nuts. (Three thousand calories of rice alone would provide 60 grams of protein. Three thousand calories of white potatoes is equivalent to 80 grams of protein.)

During the first World War, Denmark was surrounded by German submarines and could not receive shipped foods. The inhabitants de-emphasized animal proteins and lived basically on apples, potatoes, and other vegetables. The death rate during this time was reduced by 40%.

The old fallacy of eating large amounts of protein is dead. Ragner Berg of Sweden, and Jaffe of the University of California, have shown that perfect health can be maintained on just 25-35 grams of protein daily[4]. There are natives living in the South Seas who are enormously healthy, living on only 15-20 grams per day. I myself have existed on 20 grams or less of protein daily since

1977. With this low-protein diet I have overcome allergies and arthritic symptoms, and lost 75 pounds of unnecessary weight. I exercise at least 90 minutes daily, lecture in 200 cities a year, study music, and still only sleep 4 1/2 hours a night. I never have a runny nose or experience fatigue, unless I overwork.

Dr. Ralph Bircher[5] claims that a low-protein diet has demonstrated that the body needs 10-20% less oxygen and a 30% lower calorie-intake. This conserves the resources of the body. High protein diets, on the other hand, tend to accelerate the turnover of protein in the body, put the cells into high activity, and promote stress and premature aging. Cancer is characterized by this rapid protein synthesis.

Keep in mind that 70% of the body's protein is supplied by recycling of discarded proteins from the cells and tissues of the body and the remaining 30% is supplied by the diet. Arthur Guyton's *Textbook of Medical Physiology*[6] mentions that 30-45 grams of protein are entirely adequate for adults. Any food in excess immediately places the body on a danger alert.

The habit of overeating puts the body into a "burnout syndrome" and diseases unfortunately follow. The worst foods that tend to cause problems are beef, pork, fish, poultry, eggs, and all cheeses. Too many nuts, seeds, and legumes can also cause problems. Furthermore, animal sources may contain drugs, chemicals, a high fat content, and unknown substances that have been injected into the animals while they are still alive. These "mystery toxins" eventually find their way into the bloodstream of the human race. Meat-eating is a risky affair.

In the September 3, 1982 issue of the "New England Journal of Medicine," researchers Dr. Barry M. Branner and Timothy W. Meyer state that "undigested protein must be eliminated by the kidneys. This unnecessary work stresses out the kidneys so much that gradually lesions are developed and tissues begin to harden."[7] In the colon this excess protein-waste putrifies into toxic substances called indols, skatols, and hydrogen sulfide, etc. Some of these substances are reabsorbed into the bloodstream and are eventually found in the urine. These substances irritate the bladder and kidneys, and cause an unnecessary loss of vital energy. And we wonder why we experience unexplained fatigue!

While we are discussing disease, one of the first symptoms is that blood vessels, large and small, become blocked with metabolic waste products. The system undergoes a hardening process known as arteriosclerosis. Uric acid and cholesterol are among the wastes that harden the body. Another substance that hardens the arteries and capillaries is called amyloid. Amyloid is a waxy, fatty-type substance which intrudes upon the cell spaces, joints, ligaments, and soft tissues. This substance is mainly made of protein by-products. Two amino acids which are richly contained in these amyloid deposits are *tryptophane* and *tyrosine.* (These deposits are 5-10 times higher in meat protein than vegetable protein.) At Harvard University, studies indicated that the amino acid *methionine* contributed to hardening the soft surfaces of the arteries. Methionine is three times higher in cow's milk than in breast milk[8].

For many years it was thought that nature made a mistake in not putting enough protein in mother's milk. Amino acid studies were done on rats, attempting to find out the correct amount of protein needed by humans. In proportion to their size/weight, rats need 3 1/2 times the amount of protein needed by humans, because rats grow to adult size much faster than humans. Therefore, they need more protein relative to their size/weight. The protein of rat's breast milk is 10 times more concentrated than human breast milk. Human breast milk has 1-2 grams of protein per 100 milliliters, and the baby doubles its weight in 180 days. Rat's milk is 8-11 grams of protein per 100 milliliters, and a rat doubles its weight in 4-5 days. This interesting research was done by Dr. MacDougal and reported in his book, *The MacDougal Plan*[9].

The body is wise. It takes care of its own, and the more naturally we feed it, the better it will be.

The body needs amino acids, whether they are from vegetable sources, fruit sources, or meat sources. But when you consider the high fat content of meat, and the fact that it is high in protein, hormones, chemicals, antibiotics, and so on, it's hardly a question of which protein is superior. Consult Appendix F in the back of this book to learn the protein content of a wide variety of foods. Specifically, notice which foods contain all the essential amino acids.

OSTEOPOROSIS

Osteoporosis, meaning "porous bones," is a condition that affects vast members of aged people in our culture. It is characterized by demineralization of the bones to a point where falling can break a leg, hip, shoulder, or arm. Sneezing can even break a rib, and the body is usually bent over and becomes stiff, and even rigid. Many probably consider it natural to the aging process, but this is a fallacy planted in the minds of the American public. I used to believe that osteoperosis was caused by insufficient calcium in the diet. It is now proven, beyond a shadow of a doubt, that osteoporosis is caused by a high protein diet.

I began to consider why this condition is unheard of among the Vilcabanbas of Peru. At the age of 100 years, members of this tribe are still bending over hoeing their gardens daily with great flexibility. The Hunzas and the Yucatan Mayas also have no signs of osteoperosis. This is because they are all on a low-protein, vegetarian-based diet. Around the world, studies have shown that osteoporosis correlates directly with protein intake. The greater the intake of protein, the more calcium is lost in the urine. In fact, in countries that use dairy products in large amounts, like the U.S., Finland, and Sweden, osteoporosis is very common. The Bantu tribe of Africa utilize a low-protein diet, mainly vegetarian. They consume 47 grams of protein daily, with only 350 milligrams of calcium, and are free of osteoperosis.

The National Dairy Council of the U.S. suggests that we need 1200 milligrams of calcium daily, or we will become calcium deficient. The difference is that where high protein diets are consumed, protein leaves a high uric acid residue in the body which must be neutralized by calcium. So of course it seems as if more calcium is needed. The body steals calcium from the bones and teeth to carry on this activity to neutralize the uric acid. The African Bantus, who live on a low-protein diet, have little osteoporosis, but their genetic relatives who live in the United States, eating a standard American diet, have levels of osteoporosis equivalent to the rest of the American population.

If osteoperosis were caused by a deficiency in calcium, how would one explain why the Eskimos, who consume 2000 milligrams of calcium a day, suffer from a high rate of osteoporosis? The answer is simple. They also consume 240-400 grams of protein daily from fish, whale, and walrus.

Some interesting research was reported in the March 1983 issue of the "Journal of Clinical Nutrition." Researchers at Michigan State and other universities studied people aged 65 and older in the United States. They found that the group of male vegetarians had average measurable bone loss of 3%, while male meat-eaters had average measurable bone loss of 18%. Female vegetarians had an average measurable bone loss of 7%, and female meat-eaters had an average measurable bone loss of 35%[10]. So you can see the results of a high protein, meat-based diet. With as little as 75 grams of protein daily (less than 3/4 of what the average American meat-eater consumes) more calcium would be lost in a year than absorbed. This is another reason why I suggest that you keep your protein intake to around 20 grams daily.

MINERAL SALTS: *THE REGULATORS OF LIFE*

Besides the three classes of foods—carbohydrates, proteins, and fats—there are other substances that are body regulators and are used as building materials for bones, teeth, other solid parts of the body, and cellular tissues. These are called minerals. There are two types of minerals: organic minerals, meaning organized minerals, which come from food sources, plants, and animals, and can be used by the body. Then there are inorganic minerals, which come from tap water, medicine, etc. and overly-cooked foods. The body cannot use these and they are stored in the tissues. These eventually harden the body, can cause arthritis and arteriosclerosis, and may lead to kidney and gallstones.

The general functions of minerals, or mineral salts, in the body are:

1. They act as electrolytes, which carry electromagnetic currents through the body.
2. They act as specific building blocks.
3. They carry nutrients to the cells and help keep the osmotic pressure around the cells normal so fluids and nutrients can pass in and out of the cells properly.
4. They are the materials that help keep the blood and body fluids at a specific pH (acid-alkaline balance), especially the acid-alkaline balance of the bloodstream and other tissue fluids.

ACID-ALKALINE BALANCE

One of the least understood concepts of nutrition is a true understanding of what acid and alkaline balance really is. It is hardly ever talked about in 90% of the books written about nutrition. Yet, if the body cells are not bathed in fluid with a balanced acid-alkaline (pH), we die at the cellular level each day. Dr. Alex Correl kept a chicken heart alive for 28 years by controlling the acid-alkaline balance of the fluid that bathed it.

> For the cells of the body to continue living, there is one major requirement: the composition of the body fluids that bathe the outside of the cells must be controlled very exactly from moment to moment and day to day, with no single important constituent ever bearing more than a few percent. Indeed, cells can live even after being removed from the body if they are placed in a fluid bath that contains the same constituents and has the same physical conditions as those of the body fluid.[11]

Body fluids comprise 70% of your body weight. Fluid inside the cells accounts for 55% of the weight; fluid surrounding the cells is 10% of the body weight, and 5% of the weight is your bloodstream. Maintaining the pH (acid-alkaline balance) of these fluids is very important, as Dr. Alex Correll has pointed out. The normal pH of saliva should be between 6.8 and 7.4, gastric digestion (stomach) should be between 1.0 and 2.0, gallbladder secretions, or bile, between 7.0 and 8.5, the small intestine between 7.4 and 8.5. The pH of the large intestine is between 7.4 and 8.5, and the urine should remain between 6.2 and 7.4. If any of these pH's are abnormal, digestive enzymes are rendered inactive, food does not get digested properly, and allergic reactions can result. Not only that, but food-bound microorganisms such as yeast, bacteria, parasites, molds, viruses, etc., are liberated in the body, which puts a stress on the immune system.

Foods are categorized into two groups: acid foods and alkaline foods. By "acid-forming" or "alkaline-forming," nutritionists mean the condition that foods cause in the body after the food is digested. This is determined by the elements that the foods contain. If foods have a large percentage of acid elements, such as sulphur, phosphorous, choline, and iodine, they are acid-forming. If the food contains large amounts of sodium, potassium, calcium, magnesium, and iron, the food is said to be alkaline-forming. All foods have some of both of these types of substances, but one or the other will predominate.

Acid-forming foods are not the same as foods that have small amounts of acid in them, like lemons, limes, grapefruits, and other citrus. Although these foods have organic acids in them, these mild acids are cleansing to the system, are oxydized into $C0_2$ and water, and do not create an acid effect on the body fluids. They also contain high concentrations of alkaline minerals which, after digestion, increase the body's alkaline mineral reserves. The problem with citrus fruits is that, if they are not properly grown, or grown in deficient soil and are not ripened properly, they may contain large amounts of acids. These fruits, then, can produce an acid effect on the body simply because they lack the alkaline minerals usually present in the soil. In other cases, because a person's diet has been so acid-forming over the years, any foods containing even small amounts of acid may not be oxydized properly because the bloodstream is already too acidic. In that situation I suggest using a vegetable-based diet, with the addition of vegetable juices like carrot, celery, parsley, and beet, to quickly bring large amounts of alkaline minerals into the system.

Basically, after food is digested it leaves a mineral ash. The minerals left in this ash determine whether the food is acid or alkaline. Chemists have done this by burning the food, then taking the ash and dissolving it in water, which has a neutral pH. Then, the pH of the solution is measured. The result is either acid or alkaline, which tells whether the food will have an acid or alkaline effect on the body.

The pH of the bloodstream is slightly alkaline (7.4). This alkalinity must be kept constant. Even a minor variation is dangerous. Even if the body falls to a pH of 6.95, this can result in a coma, or even death. If it becomes too alkaline, for example a pH of 7.7, convulsions can occur. With a low-acid blood, the heart relaxes and ceases to beat; with too much alkalinity, it can contract and cease to beat.

An acid bloodstream is usually caused by a diet too high in protein. As we've suggested before, protein foods are very high in sulphur and phosphorous. As protein is metabolized and digested in the body, these elements remain as sulphuric or phosphuric acids. These acids are neutralized by the alkaline minerals, such as calcium, sodium, magnesium and potassium. Too much protein can cause a deficiency in these minerals, because they are constantly being used to neutralize these excess acids of a high-protein diet, instead of carrying on their normal chemical activities in the blood. If these acids are not normally neutralized, the kidneys must eliminate them, and too much acid on a regular basis can cause kidney damage.

Another thing that happens is that the body, to reserve its alkaline minerals, deposits these excess acid substances in the tissues and joints. The cells begin to degenerate, and diseases like osteoperosis, arthritis, and cancer can develop. Keep in mind that the cells naturally produce acids on their own as part of their function. During exercise the body also produces lactic acid, but these acids are taken care of normally without producing any problem, unless one is on a high-protein diet. Then, even the natural acids produced by the body can start to accumulate. This is one more reason why we should remain on a low-protein diet.

The nucleus of a cell is naturally acidic. The cytoplasm, which is the fluid that surrounds the cell, is alkaline. These two opposite poles create an electrical potential at the cellular level. When the blood and extra cellular fluid becomes acidic, the cytoplasm also can become acidic, and the energy of the cell is reduced. We feel fatigue because we are dying daily at the cellular level. Our physical existence depends on the health of our cells. So you can see how important it is to keep the proper acid-alkaline balance in the body at all times.

On a high acid diet, we can become mineral deficient, even if we are taking mineral supplements. This is because our minerals are being used to neutralize the excess acids in the blood instead of carrying on their normal functions. We are mainly concerned with deficiencies in calcium, potassium, magnesium and sodium. These are the major acid-buffers in the body. A shortage of calcium can lead to weak bones and teeth, osteoperosis, bleeding, soreness in the muscles, irritability and loss of teeth. A decrease in sodium can cause weakness, salt hunger, loss of weight, and digestive disturbances. Potassium deficiencies can lead to weak muscles, heart irregularities, bloating, and infections. Magnesium deficiencies can lead to weak bones and teeth, brain and nerve problems, weak lungs, and poor elimination. Consult the chart 8.3 in Chapter 8 to learn what foods are acid and what foods are alkaline. In general, your diet should consist of 80% alkaline foods (which is basically 80% fruits and vegetables), and 20% acid-producing (I suggest most grains, seeds, and nuts instead of meat, dairy, and egg products). There will be other information on acid and alkaline in Chapter 8.

PHOSPHOROUS TO CALCIUM RATIO

Protein is not the only problem with a high meat diet. Animal products, with the exception of dairy, are high in phosphorous, but they all have low calcium-phosphorous ratios. Animal products are low in alkaline minerals—magnesium and manganese—

and low in vitamin C, but they are high in sulphur, phosphorous, and fat. When phosphorous is high in the diet (a high phosphorous to calcium ratio), bone deterioration is inevitable. When calcium is high (calcium to phosphorous ratio), this promotes strong bones and teeth. When the phosphorous is high in the blood, the body must balance it with calcium, so calcium once again is removed from the bones and moved into the bloodstream to take care of the problem.

Taking calcium supplements and increasing dairy product usage only adds to the problem. The excess calcium doesn't get absorbed properly into the bloodstream, and dairy only adds more phosphorous to the system. The typical American diet contains 20-100 times too much phosphorous, choline, and sulphur, and this tends to acidify the body. So the body must buff these acid minerals with potassium and calcium. This can cause an increase of potassium in the bloodstream.

Another problem is that when calcium is removed from the bones, the kidneys put a halt on calcium excretion. The excess that should have been excreted by the kidneys is now in the bloodstream, and is eventually deposited in the soft tissues and joints, causing arthritic conditions.

The traditional American diet is very acidifying to the system with its high intake of eggs, milk, meat, and cheese. Fruits and vegetables, on the other hand, produce an alkaline effect in the body, because of the alkaline minerals that they contain. When fruits and vegetables were added to the diets of men consuming 140 grams of protein a day, calcium loss was reduced by at least 25%[12]. (I am not suggesting that anyone eat that much protein, but this research does make a statement.) Fruits and vegetables should be 80% of the diet, while acid-producing foods (like meat, milk, or cheese—if you choose to use them—and seeds, nuts, and legumes) should comprise 20% of the diet.

Taking extra calcium doesn't solve the problem. In 1984, the "British Medical Journal" published research indicating that additional calcium is irrelevent to bone loss[13]. The study used three groups of post-menopausal women. One group received less than 550 milligrams of calcium a day; another group got 550-1100 milligrams of calcium a day; and the third group took over 1100 milligrams of calcium a day. After two years, the research showed that virtually all the women in these groups had the same amount of bone loss. Women who took 2000 milligrams of calcium daily had the same amount of bone demineralization as women taking no calcium supplements. As usual, the problem is in the diet.

There is a definite link between osteoperosis and kidney disease because on a high protein diet the protein must be eliminated by the kidneys. This excess protein puts a stress on the kidneys and causes deterioration and even kidney stones. Foods, like fruits and vegetables, that have a high calcium-phosphorous ratio are much more compatible with the body. Furthermore, the calcium is more accessible and easier to absorb. Green leafy vegetables, such as kale, parsley, mustard greens, endive, etc., are all good sources of calcium.

A WORD ABOUT CHROMIUM

During the refinement of wheat products and sugar cane, chromium, zinc, iron, magnesium, B vitamins and vitamin E are stripped away and lost. Chromium, for example, is a glucose tolerance factor needed to burn and utilize sugar in the body. Refined flour only contains 13% of the chromium found in the whole wheat. This leaves the food high in calories, but lacking enough chromium to utilize the sugar. Consequently, one may suffer hypoglycemia, or be mimicking pre-diabetic symptoms and fatigue because the body is not capable of metabolizing the sugar for energy. One of the main symptoms of hypoglycemia is depression and drastic mood changes, making chromium an important nutrient for mental stability. See Appendix C-3.

VITAMINS

The word "vitamin" derives from the Latin *vita* meaning life, and *amines*, a word that relates to a nitrogen-containing compound. Vitamins are substances, naturally existing in all foods, which are essential to the digestion, metabolism, and maximum health potential of the foods in which they are naturally found. That is one reason why it is essential to get our vitamins from our foods, rather than try to supplement them. It is one of the strange paradoxes of modern life that we refine and cook our foods to the point where the vitamins are depleted or destroyed, and then run to the pills to attempt to add them back to our diet.

In the past hundred years since vitamins were "invented"—i.e. isolated and named—much research has been conducted to determine what each one supplies to the bodily system. Vitamin E, for example, is necessary for the health of the pituitary, adrenal glands, and kidneys. It is used extensively in the treatment of burns. Vitamin K, also known as Menadione, was only discovered in the later 1950s. It is essential in the coagulation of the blood and is therefore called the anti-hemmoraghic vitamin.

It is beyond the scope of this book to provide a thorough treatment of the subject of vitamins. But the food charts in Appendix D at the back of the book will give you thorough lists of the vitamin content of your foods. So, I suggest you familiarize yourself with them.

For years now, I have been interested in both the mental as well as the physical effects of vitamins, and the various conditions that result when these vitamins are missing in our foods. Mood changes, allergies, and depression affect most of the population. I believe, and many agree with me, that these conditions have to do with what we eat, or don't eat. I would like to cite a few examples, stressing how important it is that we eat the type of diet that will give us all the vitamins we need in the form and quantity we need them.

Niacin, or vitamin B-3, part of the B-vitamin complex, assists in the breakdown of fats, proteins, and carbohydrates in the body. A deficiency of niacin produces symptoms such as palegra, weakness, diarrhea, dermatitis, and nervous mental disorders. In its role as a co-enzyme, niacin helps in the oxydation of sugars, which is essential for brain metabolism. In 1966 Dr. Pfeiffer used niacin to help raise histamine levels in the bloodstream. This relieved symptoms such as paranoia, hallucinations, and other mental problems[14]. Niacin is also helpful in treating alcoholics who have schizophrenic symptomologies.

It is a well-known fact that vitamin C is essential for strong bones, cartilage, and connective tissues. During times of stress, vitamin C is depleted from the tissues, particularly from the adrenal glands. Research has indicated that as the adrenal-cortical activity (stress) increases, the concentration of vitamin C and cholesterol decreases in the adrenal glands. When the adrenal glands are deficient in vitamin C, this upsets the adrenal gland production of hormones (steroids). Adrenal insufficiencies can trigger emotional imbalances. Experiments using an EEG have proven that the use of vitamin C improves biochemical factors in the brain and acts as an anti-anxiety factor in schizophrenia[15].

Inositol, another B vitamin, is contained in the spinal cord, brain, and cerebral spinal fluid. Some studies have indicated that it may have anti-anxiety effects similar to librium. Patients who have used Inositol have sometimes stopped the use of valium. Inositol has been used with schizophrenic patients and hypoglycemics who have high levels of serum copper and low levels of zinc. It has also been used as a sedative, and to reduce anxiety problems.

Vitamin B-12 has a structure similar to hemoglobin (with iron at its center) and to that of chlorophyll, the green pigment in plants. There are several forms of B-12, called cobalamins, but the most active is hydroxycopalamin. B-12 is stored in the liver, kidney, stomach, muscles, and brain. When B-12 is missing in the diet or in the body, the bone marrow is unable to produce mature red blood cells. Red blood cells carry oxygen to all the cells in the body, including the brain. When red blood cells do not mature properly, they become enlarged, and are then called megaloblasts (megaloblastic anemia). The most common symptoms of

B-12 deficiencies are mental difficulties, shortness of breath, lack of appetite, neurological disturbances—such as peripheral neuritis, spinal cord changes, and tingling in the extremities—auditory hallucinations, intolerance to noise and light, paranoia, mental depression, and psychoses.

AND ENZYMES?

The consideration of Enzymes, the next essential nutrient, is so vital to the understanding of the process of *Intuitive Eating* that I have devoted the entire next chapter to it.

CHAPTER 5

Enzymes and Health

THROUGHOUT my years of experience as a health practitioner, author, and researcher I have developed a certain understanding that there is no singular formula, food, or health product that is a "cure-all." Even though I intellectually felt this to be true, I firmly believed that there was something that every person could use during therapy, or as a health supplement, that could act as foundation and adjunct to both medical and non-medical therapies. Now I feel my wish has come true! I found that food enzymes were what I have been searching for. If you are interested in longevity, vitality, superior health, overcoming sickness, or if you are having trouble losing weight, and feel that after taking vitamins and minerals for years you haven't really benefitted as much as you would like to, this chapter should be of special interest to you.

Years ago, Viktoras Kulvinskas, author of *Survival into the 21st Century*, sent me a book written by Dr. Edward Howell, called *Food Enzymes for Health and Longevity.*[1] This book explained to me why some therapies work and why some don't—because of enzymes. The entire chapter that follows is a condensation of Dr. Howell's book, used with permission.

Enzymes are needed for every chemical action and reaction in the body. Our organs, tissues, and cells are all run by metabolic enzymes. Minerals, vitamins, and hormones need enzymes to be present in order to do their work properly. Enzymes are the labor force of the body. In 1966, a Scottish medical journal stated, "Each of us, as with all living organisms, could be regarded as an orderly, integrated succession of enzyme reactions."[1]

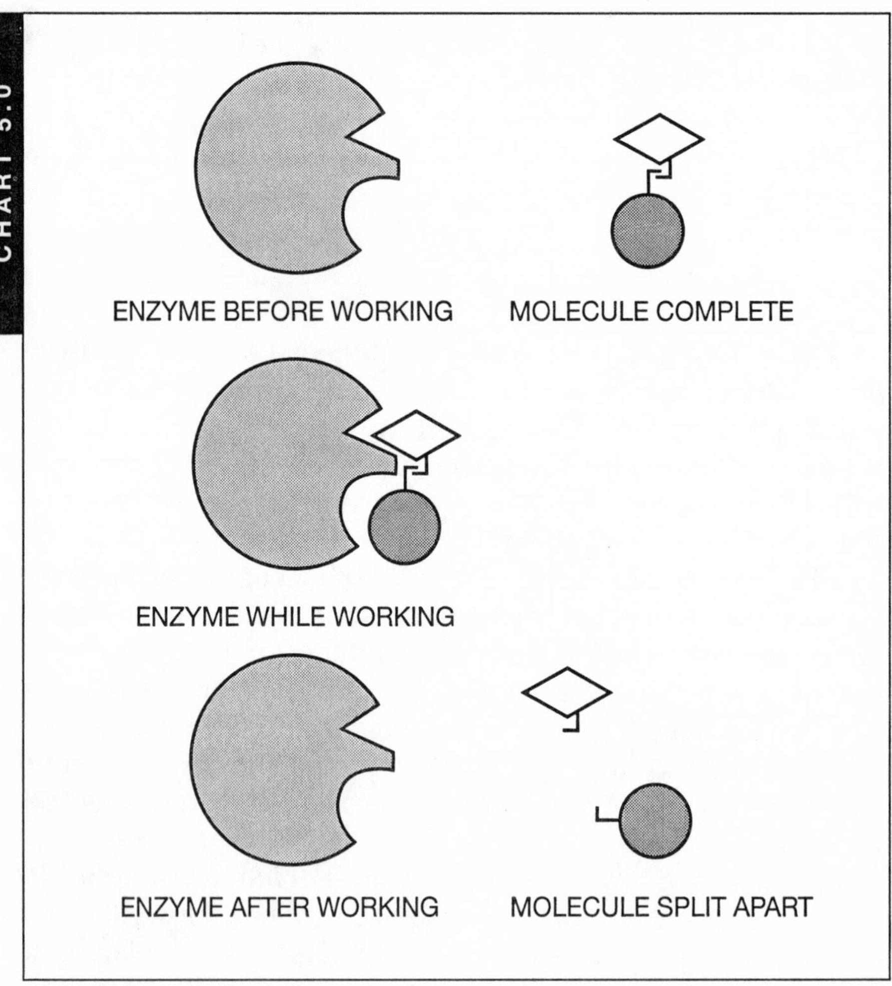

From The Chemicals of Life, by Isaac Asimov
Illustration by John Bradford
Published by New American Library, New York and Searsborough, Ontario 1954

WHAT AN ENZYME IS

It has always been thought that enzymes are protein molecules. This is incorrect. Let me clarify this by giving you an example: a light bulb can only light up when you put an electric current through it. It is animated by electricity. The current is the life force of the bulb. Without electricity we would have no light, just a light bulb, a physical object without light. So, we can say that the light bulb actually has a dual nature: a physical structure, and a non-physical electrical force that expresses and manifests through the bulb. The same situation exists when trying to describe what an enzyme is within our body structure.

Let me try to define enzymes and a few properties about them. An *enzyme* is said to be a protein molecule, and each enzyme acts in certain ways in the body doing specific jobs such as digesting food, building protein in the bones and skin, and aiding detoxification, to name a few. Once we cook food at high temperatures though, the enzyme is destroyed. It no longer carries on its designated function. Although the physical protein molecule is still present, it has lost its life force. Much like a battery that has lost its power, the physical structure remains but the electrical energy which once animated it is no longer present. A protein molecule is actually only the carrier of enzyme activity. In experiments described in *Chemical Reviews* (1933), the activity of one protein molecule was transferred over to another protein substance, leaving the original molecule devoid of its original activity[2]. This only proves further that an enzyme is the invisible activity or energy factor and not just the protein molecule itself. So, for clarity, let us agree that a protein molecule is a carrier of the enzyme activity, much like the light bulb is the carrier for an electrical current.

WHAT DO ENZYMES DO IN THE BODY?

Enzymes are involved in every process of the body. Life could not exist without them. Enzymes digest all of our food and make it small enough to pass through the minute pores of the intestines into the blood. Enzymes in the blood take prepared, digested food and build it into muscles, nerves, blood and glands. They assist in storing sugar in the liver and muscles, and turn fat into fatty tissue. Enzymes aid in the formation of urea which is to be eliminated as urine and also in the elimination of carbon dioxide in the lungs. There is an enzyme that builds phosphorus into bone and nerve tissue, and another to help attach iron to red blood cells. Male sperm carries enzymes that dissolve the tiny crevice in the female egg membrane, so it may gain entrance into it. An enzyme called streptokinase is used in medicine to dissolve blood clots. Enzymes in our immunity system attack waste materials and poisons in the blood and tissues. These few examples exemplify the importance of enzymes to our everyday body functions.[3]

The number of enzymes in the body is overwhelming, and yet each one has a specific function. A protein digestive enzyme will not digest a fat, a fat digestive enzyme will not digest a starch. This is frequently called *enzyme specificity*. Let us say: they are very intelligent when it comes to their activity and functions. Enzymes act upon substance and change it into another substance, either chemical, or a type of byproduct, but remain unchanged themselves. Any substance that an enzyme acts upon is called a substrate. The substrate is then changed from its original identity by the enzyme to another substance with a different identity. Each enzyme is believed to fit into a specific geometrical design as shown in Chart 5.0. Enzymes do a tremendous amount of work.

HOW DO ENZYMES GET THEIR NAMES?

Due to the volume of enzymes, there had to be a system of nomenclature which was devised by the National Enzyme

Commission. We now know that the names of all enzymes end in "-ase," and in most cases, the name of the enzyme will also reveal its function; thus, *protease* is an enzyme that catalyzes (acts upon) proteins, *lipase* is an enzyme which catalyzes fats, *cellulase* is an enzyme which acts upon cellulose, and *amylase* acts upon starches[4].

There are four categories of food enzymes. They are:

1. Lipase - which serves to break down fat
2. Protease (proteolytic enzymes) - works to break down protein
3. Cellulase - assists in breaking down cellulose
4. Amylase - which breaks down starch

Included in each category are a number of enzymes. For example, trypsin and pepsin act upon proteins, so they are proteolytic enzymes which fall under the category of protease. (The word *proteolytic* is just the singular form of the word *protease*.) Trypsin and pepsin do not end in "-ase" because they were named before the new nomenclature came into being. However, even these enzymes have been called *trypsinogenase* and *pepsinogenase*. Do not let the verbiage confuse you or cause you to lose interest in enzymes. The names are not important unless you are going to make enzymes a study. What is important is that you understand how to get enzymes into your body, their sources, and that without them life cannot exist. As we become enzyme deficient, the faster we age. The more we store up our enzyme reserve, the healthier we will be. We will learn how to increase our enzyme reserve later in this chapter.

WHERE DO WE GET OUR ENZYMES?

We usually think of enzymes as involved only in digesting our food so we can absorb it. Very seldom do we find informative material that demonstrates that enzymes are involved in every metabolic process. Our immunity system, bloodstream, liver, kidneys, spleen, pancreas, as well as our ability to see, think, and breathe depend upon enzymes. The lack of them in any of these areas can prove to be detrimental in degrees of depletion. Realizing that the lack of enzymes can be a predisposing cause of disease substantiates their importance. There is much literature which tries to establish that toxicity and genetics are the predisposing cause of disease. These are true statements, but the important thing to keep in mind is that all cellular activity is initiated by enzymes. Enzymes break down toxic substances so that the body can eliminate them without damaging the eliminative organs.

It is important that we preserve the body's enzyme level at all expense. There are two ways to preserve and replenish our enzyme level: by eating raw food and by taking enzyme supplements.

It is important to understand what happens when we cook our food. The difference between live (raw) and dead food is enzymatic activity. If you had two seeds and boiled one, which one would grow when placed in soil? There is no question that the unboiled seed would sprout because it has its enzymes intact. All foods provided by nature have an abundance of enzymes when in their raw state.

One characteristic of enzymes is their inability to withstand hot temperatures such as those used in cooking. Consequently, the enzymes are completely destroyed in all foods that are canned, pasteurized, baked, roasted, stewed, or fried. At 129 degrees Farenheit all enzymes are destroyed. Baking bread kills enzymes. Most butters have no enzymes because they are pasteurized. Canned juices may have vitamins and minerals, but the heating process has killed the enzymes. The roasted breakfast cereals that we feed our children are devoid of enzymes. When live food substances come in contact with heated water, the enzymes are destroyed quite rapidly. Dr. Howell states, "Enzymes are more or less completely destroyed when heated in water in the temperature range between 48 degrees to 65 degrees Centigrade. Long heating at 48 degrees Centigrade or short heating at 65 degrees Centigrade, kills enzymes. Heating at 60 to 80 degrees Centigrade for one-half hour completely kills any enzymes."[5]

Food processing, refining, cooking, and more recently the advent of microwaving are detrimental processes that are causing dramatic changes in the food that we eat. They have rendered our foods enzyme-deficient, causing imbalances in our organs, acting as a predisposing cause of disease.

Enzymes are always a part of animal and plant life. They are a component part of living matter. Animals in the wild consume large amounts of enzymes as a result of their raw food diets. This aids in the digestive process, taking the stress off organs such as the pancreas, liver, and spleen which would otherwise have to produce large amounts of enzymes. This causes unwarranted stress on these organs and body tissues, decreasing the longevity of the body.

There are three major classes of enzymes: metabolic enzymes (enzymes which work in blood, tissues, and organs), food enzymes from raw food, and digestive enzymes. Our organs are run by metabolic enzymes. These enzymes take food substances and build them into healthy tissue and have numerous other duties. One authority found ninety-eight enzymes working in the arteries alone. Since 1968, 1,300 enzymes have been identified. A shortage of these enzymes may cause serious health problems.

Nature has placed enzymes in food to aid in the digestive process instead of forcing the body's enzymes to do all of the work. It is to be remembered that we inherited an enzyme reserve at birth and this quantity can be decreased as we age by eating an enzyme-deficient diet. By eating most of our food cooked, our digestive systems have to produce all of the enzymes, thus causing an enlargement of the digestive organs. To supply such enzymes, the body draws on its reserve from all organs and tissues, causing a metabolic deficit. If each of us would take in more exogenous enzymes (those enzymes taken from outside sources), our enzyme reserve would not be depleted at such a rapid pace. This would keep our metabolic enzymes more evenly distributed throughout the organism. This is one of the most health-promoting measures that one could implement into his or her daily lifestyle.

The pancreas, which is of primary importance to our digestive system, secretes lipase (fat digestive enzymes), amylase (starch digestive enzymes), and protease (protein digestive enzymes). The question is: Does this organ produce all of these enzymes from within itself? At the University of Toronto, the pancreas was removed from sixteen dogs. These dogs were kept alive for months by the use of insulin and were shown to have normal levels of amylase in their blood streams[6]. The School of Medicine at Yale University, doing a similar study, found that six dogs had a rise in blood amylase amounting to twenty times the normal amount after the ligation (tying off) of the pancreatic duct[7]. In a 1936 "Journal of Enzymology," Fiessinger and Associates could not find a significant change in the lipase content of the blood of dogs fifteen days after the removal of the pancreas. The enzymes that maintain blood levels after the pancreas is removed come from other tissues and organs[8 9]. It is foolish to believe that an organ weighing just a few ounces (the average pancreas weighs only 85 grams) can supply the enormous amount of enzymes needed in the body day after day, year after year. It can be substantiated that the pancreas receives constituents (enzymes) from the blood and tissues. Dr. Willstatter has demonstrated the presence of amylase in white blood cells (leucocytes) and has also shown that the white blood cells have proteolytic enzymes similar to the secretions of the pancreas[10]. White blood cells have a greater variety of enzymes than the pancreas. Leukocytes travel through the body, destroying foreign substances in the bloodstream, working as part of the immune system, protecting us against disease. We lose enzymes daily through our sweat, urine, feces, and through all digestive fluids including salivary and intestinal secretions. Logic dictates that a pancreas weighing only a few ounces could not possibly be responsible for the production of all of the enzymes found throughout the body of a 150-pound man. Enzymes are found in every tissue of the body. Even when the pancreas is removed, the body still maintains a certain enzyme level.

Another point of paramount importance is that a percentage of enzymes which are taken orally, or the ones already present in raw food, can be absorbed in the intestines and utilized in the body's metabolic processes, helping to prevent enzyme depletion. Before we look at the absorption of enzymes, let's look at other substances that are absorbed through the intestines.

At the University of Illinois, compressed yeast fed to dogs produced positive yeast cultures in the liver, lymph glands, lungs, spleen, and kidneys, proving that whole yeast cells were absorbed[11]. Dr. Oelgoetz documented in the *American Journal of Digestion* that if patients with low levels of blood amylase are given an extract of whole pancreas which contains amylase, the normal blood level can be restored within one hour and remain normal for days after administration[12].

It is a well-known fact that unassimilated proteins, yeast cells, carbohydrates, and fats can be reabsorbed into the bloodstream, causing allergies, skin diseases, and other illnesses[13]. Dr. Oelgoetz proved that when pancreatic enzymes are adminsitered to patients having allergies accompanied by low blood levels of enzymes, this level returns to normal and the allergy subsides. Functional digestive disturbances, hyperacidity, and skin problems were relieved the same way. Clinicians have effectively relieved a variety of skin diseases caused by incompletely digested food materials. The blood provides the ideal environment for enzymes to cause a partial breakdown of undigested materials.

The oral administration of proteolytic enzymes for inflammation and sports injuries have been used for years by Max Wolf, M.D. and Karl Ransberger, Ph.D. In one experiment reported in their book, *Enzymes Therapy,* certain enzymes were tagged with a radioactive dye to see if these enzymes could be followed through the digestive tract into the bloodstream. It was shown through electrophoretic investigations that the radioactive dye tagged to the enzymes could be found in the liver, spleen, kidneys, heart, lungs, duodenum, and urine[14].

If you would like more information showing how enzymes, taken orally, are absorbed and used throughout the body, taking the stress off other enzyme-producing organs, see the references for this chapter in the back of this book. For now, let's take a look at how the enzymes function in raw food and how they may aid in the digestive process, preparing bodily functions.

HOW FOOD ENZYMES AID DIGESTION

A human being is not maintained by food intake alone, but rather by what is digested. Every food must be broken down by enzymes to simpler building blocks. Enzymes may be divided into two groups: exogenous (found in raw food), and endogenous (produced within our bodies). The more one gets of the exogenous enzymes, the less will have to be borrowed from other metabolic processes and supplied by the pancreas. The enzymes contained in raw food actually aid in the digestion of that same food when it is chewed. One can live for many years on a cooked food diet but eventually this will cause cellular enzyme exhaustion which lays the foundation for a weak immune system and ultimately disease. Dr. Howell states, "Researchers show that cooked food with the fiber broken down passes through the digestive system more slowly than raw foods. Partially it ferments, rots, putrifies, throwing back into the body toxins, gas, and causing heartburn and degenerative diseases."

It is important to realize that the enzymes in raw food actually digest 5 to 40 percent of the food itself without the help of the enzymes secreted by the body. This is called energy conservation since the body does not have to supply 100% of the enzymes to digest the food. At the Institute of Animal Physiology, Agriculture College, Berlin, comparative experiments were done to show that the enzymes contained in raw food aid digestion. Fowl do not have amylase (starch digestive enzyme) in their salivary secretions. In one study, chickens were fed ground barley which has a good amount of pure starch in it. After five hours, the stomach contents of the fowl were analyzed showing that eight percent of the starch was digested[15]. It was also demonstrated by Dr. Boas that, as reported by Dr. Howell, "the enzymes in bananas were activated in the intestines to aid in the digestive process."[16] This also shows that not all enzymes are destroyed in the stomach, but merely inactivated there and then reactivated again in the intestines. This important point was also proven by Russian researcher, Dr. Matveev. He demonstrated that oxidase and catalase, which are enzymes supplied from carrot juice, were inactivated in the stomach because of the acidity, and then reactivated again in the alkalinity of the small intestines[17]. In summary, the enzymes in raw food digest a small percentage of the food. It appears then that all enzymes are not destroyed in the stomach as once believed, but are actually reactivated again to aid the pancreas in digestion in the small intestine.

We all suffer the consequences of a cooked food diet. As Dr. Howell demonstrates, the pancreas of an animal subsisting exclusively on raw plant food is much smaller relative to its body weight than a human's[18]. The pancreas of a human weighing 140 pounds, weighs 85-90 grams; the pancreas of a sheep weighing 85 pounds, weighs only 18.8 grams; the pancreas of a 1005 pound cow, weighs only 308 grams; and the pancreas of a horse weighing 1200 pounds, weighs only 330 grams. Calculated as a percentage of body weight, the following figures are presented.

	Body Weight Grams	Pancreas Weight % of Body Weight
SHEEP	38,505	0.0490
CATTLE	455,265	0.0680
HORSE	543,600	0.0603
HUMAN	63,420	0.1400

Notice how little humans weigh when compared to cattle and horses, and again in comparison, how much larger the human pancreas is. This is because the pancreas must enlarge because it is being overworked by consuming a cooked food diet devoid of enzymes. The fascinating point here is that in humans, the saliva contains amylase to aid the pancreas in starch digestion.

Herbivora (animals listed in the chart) have relatively no amylase in their saliva, and the pancreas still remains normal size without enlarging. The answer seems to be that the raw food of herbivora supplies active enzymes which participate in digestion, taking stress off the digestive organs, the pancreas, and in fact, the whole body's metabolism.

A similar experiment was reported in the *Phillipine Journal of Science* (Vol. 52) as performed by the School of Hygiene of Public Health in 1933. The school performed 768 postmortum examinations of Phillipinos. The observations showed that the pancreas of a Phillipino was twenty-five to fifty percent heavier than that of a European or American, because cooked rice was the Phillipino's staple food and was eaten as much as three times a day. This caused the pancreas to be overworked, secreting large amounts of enzymes, particularly amylase, and causing an enlargement of the organ. An enlarged organ is often a pathological condition, showing the beginning signs of degeneration.

It is a fact that a cooked food diet shows a larger outpouring of enzymes from our digestive organs. At first thought, it might be presumed that a hypertrophied (enlarged) organ is a desirable accommodation, but it has always been shown that enlargement of an organ is accompanied by the excessive function of that organ, followed by exhaustion and degeneration. Since the enzymes in raw food actually help digest the food they are contained in, and can be absorbed into the blood and used in other metabolic processes, we can assume that taking enzymes, or eating a large percentage of raw food, will help take the stress off not only the pancreas, but the entire body.

ENZYMES AND LONGEVITY

The comparative study of the enzyme content of the blood, urine, and digestive fluids of the human population can present some very important data. The average diet is predominately heat-treated and possesses only a fraction of its original enzyme content. It has been shown that young adults have a high value of enzyme reserve in their tissues. In older persons, the potential enzyme tissue reserve is much lower and essentially depleted. When a young person eats cooked food, there is a greater outpouring of enzymes from the organs and body fluids than in adults. This is because years of eating a cooked food diet has depleted the older adult, whereas the young adult's tissue reserve is still at maximum.

A further experiment in relation to saliva and its amylase content was performed at the Michael Reese Hospital in Chicago. Used in the experiment were young adults from the ages of 21 to 31 and another group ranging from age 69 to 100. It was shown that the younger group had 30 times more amylase in their saliva than the elderly group. This is why younger persons can tolerate a diet of white bread, starches, and predominately cooked food. But as our enzyme reserve is depleted over the years, these same foods can cause illnesses such as constipation, blood diseases, bleeding ulcers, bloating, and arthritis. In older individuals, the enzyme content of the body has been depleted and these foods are not properly digested. They ferment in the digestive tract producing toxins that are then absorbed into the blood and deposited in the joints and other soft-tissue areas.

A chronic disease is a disease that has lingered in the body for many weeks or months and sometimes years. It has been a constant drag on the body, depleting it of its enzymes, vitamins, minerals, and trace minerals. During chronic diseases, there is usually a low body reserve of enzymes. In 111 Japanese patients who had tuberculosis, 82% of them had lower enzyme contents than normal individuals. As the disease worsened, the enzyme level decreased[19]. Dr. Volodin, in the Archives Vendanugskrankh, found after studying the enzyme level of urine, blood, and intestines, that it was usually decreased in diabetics. Studies of feces showed incomplete digestion of meat and fats in many cases. In five of six diabetic patients, the lipase and trypsin (proteolytic enzyme) of the pancreatic juice was found to be decreased[20]. Dr. Ottenstein in a similar study pattern showed low blood amylase levels in skin afflictions such as psoriasis, dermatitis, and pruritis[21]. Another interesting experiment showed that 40 patients suffering from liver diseases such as cirrhosis, hepatitis, and cholecystitis (inflammation of the gallbladder), showed low levels of amylase. It was found that when there was a rise in the blood amylase level, there was an improvement in the general condition of each patient, as well as an improvement in the liver condition[22].

It is indisputable fact that during chronic disease we find a lower enzyme content in blood, urine, feces, and tissues. In acute diseases, and sometimes at the beginning of chronic diseases, the enzyme content is often found to be high. This shows that the body has a reserve, and the tissues are not yet depleted. Consequently, there is a larger outpouring of enzymes in the battle against disease. As the disease progresses, the body's enzyme content is lowered.

This correlation, between a diminished enzyme content during chronic disease and old age, is something that is often misunderstood. A low enzyme content in old age is often looked upon as "normal." A low content during chronic diseases is considered a pathological state. The truth of the matter is that age is not so much a matter of how many years one has been alive, but rather is a matter of the integrity of the tissues of the body. These tissues depend upon the amount of enzymes present to carry on the metabolism of every cell of the body. It is common to find a 60-year-old man or woman with a body of someone in his or her 40's.

There is a definite correlation between the amount of enzymes an individual possesses and the amount of energy he or she has. Increasing age shows a slow decrease in enzyme reserve. When the enzyme level becomes so low that metabolism suffers, death will finally result. Any time the metabolism is falsely stimulated by coffee, a high protein diet, or other stimulants, the metabolism increases, enzymes are used up, a false energy output is experienced, and the individual feels a sense of well-being. The end result will be lower energy, a more rapid burnout of enzymes, and premature old age. At Brown University a group of 158 animals were over-fed and they lived an average of 29.6 days. Another group was maintained on a starvation diet, given only small amounts of food and fluid and they lived an average of 39.19 days—an increase of about 40%[23]. This study should at the very least make each of us look at our own intake and determine if we are indeed over-ingesting.

A high protein diet is very stimulating to the body and can cause serious damage. When the diet consists of more protein than is needed, the excess is broken down by enzymes in the liver and kidneys. The major by-product of protein breakdown is urea which is a diuretic. The kidneys are caused to excrete more fluid. Along with water, minerals are lost in the urine. One of the most important losses is calcium. Experiments have shown that when subjects consumed 75 grams of protein daily, even with an intake as high as 1400 milligrams of calcium, more calcium was lost in the urine than was actually absorbed[24]. This deficiency must be made up by the body's calcium reserve which is taken from the bones. Deficient bones are a stepping stone to osteoporosis (a condition when the bones break easily). The aforementioned experiments all show that when excessive amounts of protein, or food in general, are eaten, there is a corresponding decrease in enzyme, vitamin, and mineral levels.

At the University of Toronto, a team of scientists showed that life runs its course in direct proportion to the catabolic rate. (The catabolic rate is the rapidity of the wear and tear on the body, or the rate of tissue breakdown. This is in direct proportion to the aging process.) This tissue breakdown is performed by enzymes. The faster the breakdown, the more enzymes are used up. Our enzyme reserve can be used up rapidly or it can be preserved. Taking enzyme supplements and eating raw foods are ways to add enzymes to our enzyme reserve and add to our energy level.

Dr. Howell further states that, "Enzymes are a true yardstick of vitality. Enzymes offer an important means of calculating the vital energy of an organism. That which we call energy, vital force, nerve energy, and strength, may be synonymous with enzyme activity." Our logic tells us that the building up and the breaking down of tissues is performed by enzymes. In other words, our metabolism is maintained by enzyme activity. When our enzyme level is lowered, our metabolism is lowered, and so is our energy level. Do not misunderstand this statement. We are not saying that the source of life is enzymes, but that there is a correlation between enzyme levels and the youth of the tissues of an organism and it's energy levels.

ENZYMES AND OUR IMMUNE SYSTEM

There is a connection between the strength of our immune system and our enzyme level. The greater the amount of enzyme reserves, the stronger our immune system, the healthier and stronger we will be. It has been clearly stated that enzyme activity increases during digestion and also during any other increase in metabolism, such as acute diseases. But what is the exact correlation between our immune system and enzymes?

Our white blood cells (leukocytes) are responsible for destroying foreign disease-producing substances in the blood and lymph fluid in the body. During acute diseases and infections, the white blood cell count increases to help fight off these pathologies. Dr. Willstatter, in an early enzyme research study, demonstrated that there were eight different amylase enzymes found in leukocytes[25]. Investigations also have shown that leukocytes contain proteolytic and lipolytic enzymes which are also common to those secreted by the pancreas. These enzymes act very much like the enzymes which are in our digestive tract (breaking down proteins, fats, and carbohydrates that have been absorbed by the blood, causing diseased conditions.)[26 27] Enzymes act as scavengers in the body. They latch onto foreign substances and reduce them to a form that the body can dispose of. They also prevent the arteries from clogging up and joints from becoming gummed up. It was always thought that the pancreas produced all of these enzymes, but as was mentioned earlier, this idea is erroneous. As small as the pancreas is, it couldn't possibly produce all of the enzymes found in the muscles, glands, and tissues, plus produce those used up daily in digestion, and those lost in the sweat, urine, and feces. Enzymes are produced by all the tissues and cells of the body. In fact, it has been shown that the enzymes found in the white blood cells act very much like the enzymes found in the pancreas, especially the proteolytic enzymes. Dr. Willstatter found it remarkable how closely the enzyme systems of white blood cells and the pancreatic gland agree with one another. Since the same enzymes are found in the white blood cells as are found in the pancreas, and since white blood cells transport these enzymes throughout the body, it seems that the pancreas and other enzyme-secreting glands receive a great portion of these enzymes via the leukocytes. After eating a cooked food meal, when digestive enzymes are desperately needed, the white blood cell count increases, seemingly to aid in the digestive process. Since every metabolic process is, at all times, interdependent and interrelated, this increase in the white blood cell count after the ingestion of a cooked meal, indicates a definite compensatory measure.

The body must supply a large amount of digestive enzymes because the enzymes that were once present in the food were destroyed by the heating process. Dr. Kautchakoff, in his book demonstrating the relation of cooking and its effects on our systems, showed that there was an increase in white blood cells after eating a cooked food meal[28]. This increase in leukocytes is needed to transport enzymes to the digestive tract. He also showed that after a raw food meal, there was no substantial increase in leukocytes, showing that the body has to work much harder to produce and transport enzymes for digestion after a cooked food meal. It is important to remember that enzymes in raw food aid in the digestive process and this takes the stress off having to borrow them from the body's enzyme reserve, particularly from the white blood cell count (our immune system).

A most important point demonstrated by Kautchakoff's experiment is that leukocytosis (increased white blood cell count) is a term which describes a medical pathology. Anytime the white blood cell count is increased to any great extent, it is considered that an acute illness or infection is present somewhere in the body. During acute diseases, enzyme levels rise. During chronic diseases, the body enzyme level is decreased. The pancreas and digestive tract are in a weakened state, as shown during diabetes, cancer, or chronic intestinal problems, to name a few. During chronic disease, the immune system also shows signs of great expenditure. The correlation is clear. Enzymes are found to be related to all diseases via the immune system, whether the disease is acute or chronic. Our enzyme levels must be maintained at any expense to help maintain vitality, endurance, and to prevent disease. If the pancreas output of enzymes is hindered, the whole body is affected. If a disease is present, enzymes are being used up to fight the condition and the pancreas is affected. You can see how eating mostly cooked food all our lives, or trying to overcome a chronic disease while still eating this type of diet can be detrimental.

RAW FOOD DIET AND PREDIGESTION

It is a tremendous advantage to know how to use raw foods and supplemental enzymes in the diet. Well-known naturalists such as Arnold Ehret, Dr. Ann Wigmore, George J. Drews, and Viktoras Kulvinskas are people who have shown the healing effects of raw foods. It is a fact that the enzymes in foods aid in digestion. This enzyme activity takes place in what Dr. Howell has called the enzyme-stomach, or the upper part of the stomach. (Anatomically speaking it is called the *cardial* and *fundic* parts of the stomach.) Here is where foods are predigested by enzymes. I will refer to this upper portion of the stomach as the enzyme-stomach. (See Diagram 5.1)

The enzyme-stomach is not unique to the human race. Cattle and sheep have no enzymes in their saliva, but have four stomachs. Only one secretes enzymes; the other stomachs let the enzymes within the food do the partial-digesting or pre-digesting. Dolphins and whales have three stomachs. One is devoid of enzymes where the food enzymes do the pre-digesting. As many as thirty-two seals were found in the enzyme-stomach of one whale at one time. Since there is no enzyme secretion in this stomach, how does all of the flesh get broken down into small

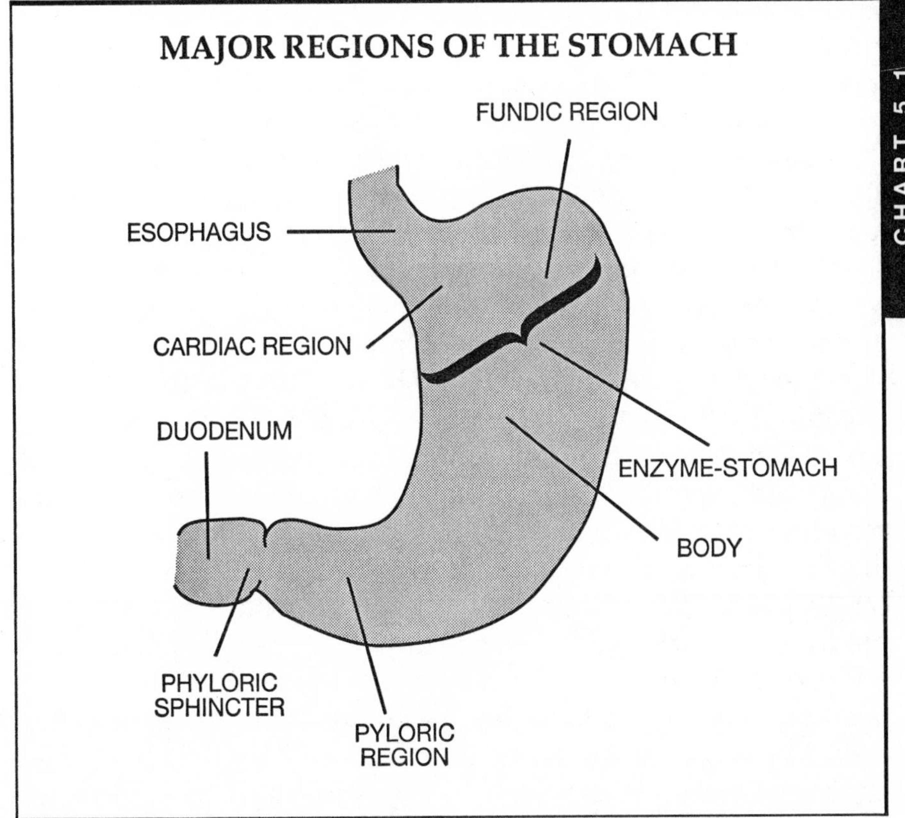

enough amounts to pass the small opening which connects the enzyme-stomach to the other stomachs? The enzymes contained in the flesh of the eaten animal itself seem to be the only answer.

We have already shown that enzymes help digest the food they are contained in if not destroyed by heat during cooking. These enzymes not only work in the stomach, but continue their activity in the small intestine. Popular opinion seems to be that the acid in the stomach destroys the enzymes in food. Research has shown this to be untrue. At Northwestern University it was shown that supplemental enzymes pass through the stomach uninjured. In one study the enzyme amylase (from germinated barley) digested starch in the stomach and then passed into the small intestine where it continued digestion.

It was also thought that only protein was digested in the stomach. Research by Dr. Beazell in the *Journal of Laboratory and Clinical Medicine*, showed that several times more starch was digested in the stomach than protein within the first hour. Olaf Berglim, Professor of Physiology at the Illinois College of Medicine, has also shown this to be true. He gave his subjects mashed potatoes and bread as a meal. Both foods contain large amounts of starch. After remaining in the stomach for 45 minutes, the contents were retrieved. Seventy-six percent of the starch in the mashed potatoes was digested and fifty-nine percent of the bread starch was digested. Research has shown that for the first forty-five minutes to one hour, a good percentage of food can be predigested in the stomach by food enzymes or supplemental enzymes before reaching the small intestine. At this time, the pancreas secretes its protein, fat, and starch-digestive enzymes into the duodenum (the first part of the small intestine). The pancreas can be put under tremendous stress if the food is not properly predigested at this point. It has to draw enzymes from the whole body to secrete the designated amount. The more digestion that takes place before the food reaches the small intestine, the better for the integrity, strength, and immunity of the whole body. The pancreas is one of the first organs to dysfunction during diabetes and other chronic illnesses.

The importance of this food-enzyme stomach, where predigestion takes place, cannot be overestimated. It is the upper part of the stomach where no acid secretion or peristalsis takes place for one-half to one hour after food is eaten. This is when supplemental enzymes and the natural enzymes contained in food do their predigestion.

Gray's Anatomy cites the authority Walter B. Cannon who demonstrated that the human stomach "consists of two parts physiologically distinct." *Gray's Anatomy* states:

> The cardiac portion of the stomach is a food reservoir in which salivary digestion continues; the pyloric portion is the seat of active gastric digestion. There are no peristaltic waves in the cardiac portion.

Predigestion by exogenous (outside) enzymes is widespread in nature. Our enzyme potential has other and more useful and taxing work to do than merely making endogenous digestive enzymes to digest food.[29]

The body is greatly relieved when predigestion takes place. The draw on metabolic enzymes is kept at a minimum. There is a law called the "Adaptive Secretion of Digestive Enzymes." This means that the more digestion that is accomplished by food enzymes or supplemental enzymes in the stomach, the fewer enzymes need to be secreted by the pancreas and intestines, conserving the body's enzymes for metabolic processes such as repairing tissues, organs, and other functions.

If the food is over-cooked and the enzymes destroyed, the only enzymes that get mixed with the food are the ones contained in the saliva. Some starch digestion may take place in the stomach from the saliva amylase. The protein is acted upon by the stomach pepsin, but mostly in the lower part of the stomach. In both instances, no help from outside enzymes is being demonstrated. The fat remains practically untouched, only waiting until it moves into the small intestine for the pancreatic secretions of lipase. The food remains in the food-enzyme stomach for its alloted time and practically no predigestion takes place, except for the starch. Cooked foods, especially those high in protein, can begin putrefying. The byproducts of putrefication are toxins that are absorbed into the bloodstream and deposited at body sites far removed from the intestinal tract. At this point, one can see how valuable enzymes are in helping to keep the blood clear of poisons. It has been estimated that 80% of diseases are caused by improperly digested foods and their by-products being absorbed into the body[30].

A diet containing mostly cooked food has proven to be detrimental in more ways than one.

> Cooking does not improve the nutritional value of food. It destroys or makes unavailable 85% of the original nutrients. Cooked food is totally lacking in enzymes; most of the protein has been destroyed or converted to new forms which are either not digestible by body enzymes or digested with difficulty; many of the vitamins have lost their vitality. To purchase organic food and then to waste precious hours in destroying most of the nutrients is poor economy and unsound ecology. Francis Pottenger, M.D., carried out a 10-year experiment using 900 cats which were placed on controlled diets. The cats on raw food produced healthy kittens from generation to generation. Those on cooked food developed our modern ailments: heart, kidney and thyroid disease, pneumonia, paralysis, loss of teeth, difficulty in labor, diminished or perverted sexual interest, diarrhea, irritability. Liver impairment on cooked protein was progressive, the bile in the stool becoming so toxic that even weeds refused to grow in soil fertilized by the cats' excrement. The first generation of kittens was sick and abnormal; the second generation was often born dead or diseased; by the third generation, the mother was sterile.[31]

Zoologists know that captured animals fed a human diet develop human diseases such as gastritis, duodenitis, colitis, liver diseases, anemia, thyroid diseases, arthritis, and circulatory problems. I am not stating that everybody should exist on a raw food diet. Some individuals don't have the inclination nor the interest to even try, but improving one's diet by taking supplemental enzymes or eating a good quantity of predigested foods, can be beneficial. Naturally, predigested foods include sprouts and fruits. This means that the proteins, starches, and fats are already predigested and high in enzymes before they are consumed. Sprouting seeds is simple and beneficial to your health. Refer to Chapter 11 for more information about sprouting.

BODY, MIND, AND ENZYMES

It seems that our happiness depends largely upon the thoughts we think. Is is impossible to think positively at all times when we are toxic, stiff, and are experiencing low blood sugar levels. Our brain exists on large amounts of sugar and oxygen. When this supply is low, we experience a lack of concentration, insomnia, lethargy, irritability, and confusion.

A lack of enzyme, oxygen, and sugar supplies to the cells of our body can cause hypoglycemia. Hypoglycemia is a disorder resulting from low blood sugar, which is the fuel for our cells. Authorities have estimated that anywhere from *10 million to 100 million Americans* are suffering from hypoglycemia. Since hypoglycemia is a malfunction of our fuel supply, every organ is then affected. Here's how: as the sugar level drops, the metabolism of every organ drops, resulting in fatigue and psychosomatic problems. The brain is nourished exclusively by glucose and oxygen. A drop in one's blood sugar can cause mental fatigue and depression. The endocrine glands, especially the pituitary, adrenals, thyroid, and pancreas, control the sugar level. The pancreas secretes insulin which causes a decrease in blood sugar. Insulin facilitates the movement of glucose (blood sugar) to leave the blood and enter the cells. Insulin also stimulates the liver and muscle cells to convert glucose into glycogen, which is a carbohydrate and the chief storage compound of sugar in the body. The adrenal glands secrete a hormone called epinephrine that, when stimulated, causes the stored sugar (glycogen) to break down into glucose which then enters the blood to raise the blood sugar. The thyroid gland secretes hormones that control the rate at which the body uses oxygen. Also its hormones increase the rate of energy released from carbohydrates. All of these glands are controlled by the pituitary gland, which, in turn, is controlled by an area of the brain called the hypothalamus. The hypothalamus receives information from all parts of the body via the nervous system. This includes (whether one is hungry or not) a person's emotional state, body temperature, and blood nutrient concentration, among other things.

It has been shown that the pituitary and other organs can enlarge, become exhausted, and then be susceptible to disease when a deficiency of enzymes is present. When there is a lack of blood amylase, blood sugar levels can be higher than normal. With the addition of the enzyme amylase, blood sugar levels have been lowered. In experiments done by Grubler and Myers, they showed that by giving amylase preparations to normal individuals who had eaten 80 grams of glucose, the blood sugar level was maintained[32]. Reports have shown that oral or intravenous injection of amylase causes a lowering of blood sugar levels in diabetics. Bassler showed that 86% of the diabetics who he examined had a deficiency of amylase in their intestinal secretions. After administering amylase to a majority of these patients, 50% of the diabetics who were users of insulin could control their blood sugar levels without the use of insulin[33]. Amylase seems to help the storage and utilization of sugar in the blood.

Cooked food, where most of the amylase and other enzymes are destroyed, has a tremendous effect on the blood sugar levels. At George Washington University Hospital, 50 grams of raw starch were fed to hospital patients. The blood sugar showed an average increase of 1 mg. per 100 cc. in one-half hour, a decrease of 1.2 mg. in one hour, and a decrease of 3 mg. in two hours. When 50 grams of cooked starch was given, the average increase in blood sugar was 56 mg. in one-half hour, then dropped to 51 mg. in one hour, then down to 11 mg. in two hours after eating the meal. In the diagram below notice the difference between the blood sugar levels when cooked starch and when raw starch, with the enzymes present, is eaten. The blood sugar in cooked starch rose to 56 mg. in one-half hour as opposed to the uncooked starch increase of only 1 mg. After two hours, the cooked food starch eaters' blood sugar level fell to 11 mg., a 45 mg. drop in blood sugar. This resulted in fatigue, anxiety, and the other aforementioned symptoms. The raw starch eaters only experienced a drop of 1 mg. to 3 mg. in two hours. A much more steady metabolic rate and emotional stability were experienced by the raw food eaters.

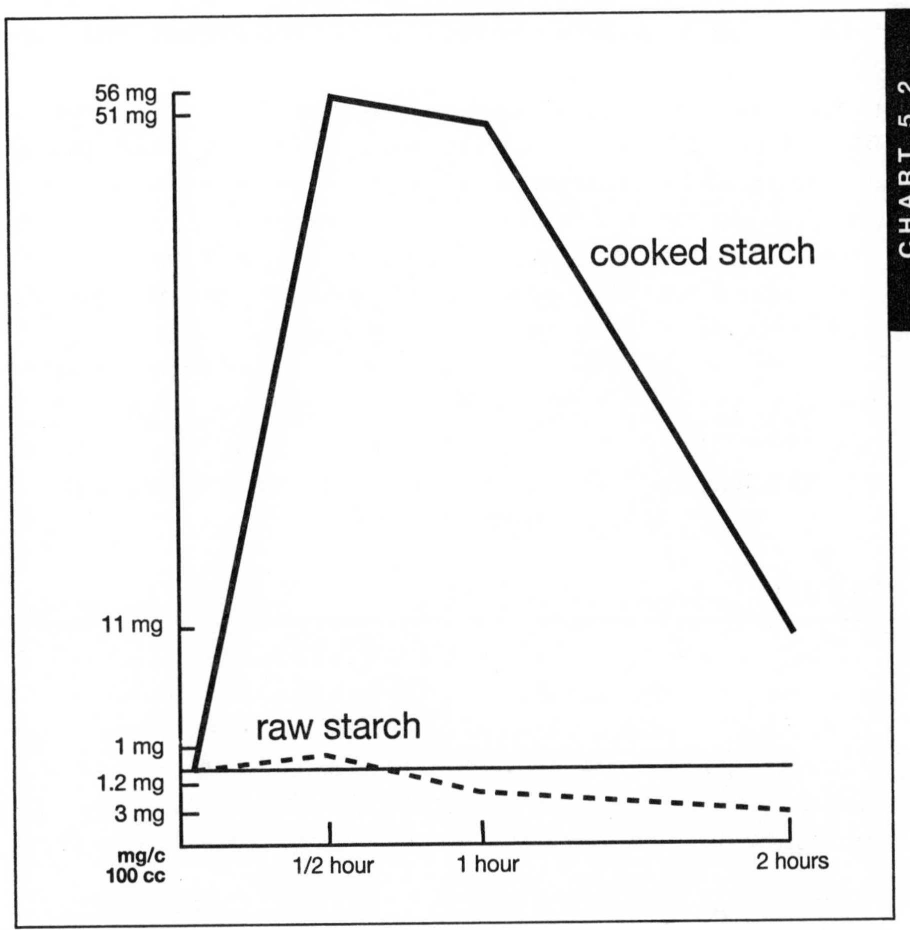

The endocrine glands need trace minerals and vitamins to function properly. A similar example of this is that of the thyroid gland needing iodine, and the adrenal glands needing vitamin C. Overcooked food is deficient not only in enzymes, but in nutrients also. These deficiencies cause many problems. The glands of the body are controlled by stimuli from the brain to secrete their hormones. When the blood sugar level drops below normal, the pancreas and adrenal glands are called upon to secrete their hormones. When there is a lack of nutrients in the blood which support the endocrine glands, the hypothalamus stimulates the appetite and causes a craving for food. The more that cooked food is eaten the more there will be hormone stimulation, resulting in overeating. Excessive eating can cause one to be overweight and obese. Obesity can be the cause of heart problems, high blood pressure, and many other diseases. Quickly rising and falling blood sugar levels in the body cause emotional swings and mental imbalances. Finally, the endocrine glands, deficient in their secretions from trying to keep the body metabolism normal, become exhausted. This state of exhaustion can be the foundation of both mental and physical diseases.

Enzymes have as much to do with our mental and physical health as any other element of nutrition. This is a subject that has not been given enough attention in today's literature. I hope this book will enlighten you as to the importance of food enzymes in your system as well as bring it to the public eye.

DETOXIFICATION AND ENZYMES

There are several methods that have been used to detoxify the body: fasting, purging, vegetarian-type diets, macrobiotic diets, the grape cure, and others. All of these have been successful to some people. At the same time none of these regimes will work all the time. The question is, what can be done to improve all of these methods of cleansing the body to make them more effective?

Anytime cooked food is eaten it must be digested by enzymes. The waste left over from the digestion of these foods and the toxins contained within the foods themselves, are broken down by scavenger enzymes in the body's immune system. The body draws enzymes from all of its tissue resources to do the job, decreasing its enzyme level. Concentrated foods such as heavy starches (breads and flour products), animal proteins, and fried foods, are more difficult to break down and consequently more enzymes are utilized. This is why, in most situations, a vegetarian diet is used for cleansing purposes. A good percentage of these diets are raw, which adds some enzymes to the body and to the food-enzyme stomach. Cooked vegetables and grains use some of the body's enzymes but are still easier to digest than more concentrated foods. The energy that is used to digest food and extract the nutrients, and eliminate the waste products while on a cleansing diet (especially if raw juices and predigested foods are used), is far less than the energy used to digest the everyday, traditional enzymeless diet. I have seen tremendous recoveries on predigested food diets that consist of raw sprouts, freshly-squeezed juices, fasting, soaked and sprouted grains, and soaked seeds and nuts that are blended before being eaten.

Two major changes take place in predigested foods: 1) the enzyme content sometimes increases 10-fold and 2) in the predigestion process the food is broken down into simpler components. Proteins are broken down into amino acids, starches into simpler sugars, and fats into fatty acids. This relieves the body of breaking down the more concentrated food elements and it also benefits from the increase in enzymes. This is conserving energy and enzymes for other metabolic functions. In other words, more energy and enzymes can be used in the healing process.

In the detoxification process, what we are trying to accomplish is the purification of the bloodstream and the balancing of the endocrine glands so that they will work in harmony instead of being overstimulated and exhausted. This purifies the organs and tissues, and takes the stress off the entire body. The foods that do not get digested properly can cause toxic reactions. For example, Dr. W. W. Oelgoetz had shown that undigested protein, fat, and starch molecules get absorbed into the bloodstream, and when the blood enzyme level is below normal, these obstructions can cause allergies. By giving the enzymes amylase, protease, and lipase orally to his patients, the blood enzyme level was normalized and alleviated the allergies[34]. (I can personally verify this, having had a history of numerous allergies as a result of living on a traditional Italian diet. I switched to a vegetarian diet and before long, my allergies were gone.)

We have discussed that enzymes are a part of our immune system. We have also shown that when there is a lack of lipase in the blood, cholesterol can accumulate. When there is a shortage of amylase, there can be sugar level problems and drastic emotional swings. So there is no need, at that point, to prove that enzymes are used for breakdown of toxins and foreign accumulation in our bodies. It would seem logical then that any diet that would increase the enzyme level would aid the purification process, especially when we now know that enzymes can be reabsorbed and reused in the body.

Much has been written about the so-called "healing crisis," and I will treat it again in Chapter 7. (For another thorough treatment of this subject please see my book *Natural Healing With Herbs*, Prescott, AZ, Hohm Press, 1984.) The "healing crisis" occurs when the system is overloaded with toxins and the body works to eliminate them through the skin, bowels, sinuses, kidneys, and lungs, producing such symptoms as rashes, lung and sinus congestion, constipation and diarrhea, and urinary tract problems. All of these can be symptoms of body cleansing. During these crises, enzymes are busy breaking down the accumulations of waste so that the body can rid itself of them. By adding enzymes during the crises, it would seem that it could only be an improvement and ultimately aid in the cleansing process. This has proven to be true in nature.

There are times when detoxification actually weakens the patient, even though a good cleansing diet has been prescribed. The tissues, releasing poisons that have been stored for years, may contain drugs that were ingested years before. If patients have a weak constitution, a chronic disease, and a submissive will, as soon as the first healing crisis is experienced, they tend to go back to their old diet thinking that the cleansing diet isn't worth it because it makes them feel worse, even if only temporarily. These people really are in need of enzyme support. Taking supplemental enzymes and using predigested foods will take much of the stress off their systems. They also need a good learning process in relation to proper eating habits, fasting, and the proper use of colonics and enemas. All of these things are adjuncts to healing. Bowel cleansing is one of the first things considered by natural healing practitioners. The bowel is the sewage system of the body and it too must be cleansed out. It has been estimated that 80% of all diseases start in the large bowel. What generally happens is that food that is not digested putrifies in the colon, producing byproducts that are reabsorbed through the intestinal tract and deposited in the joints and tissues of the body. It has been shown by Dr. Selle that by adding enzymes to the diet, the fecal bulk is reduced, transit time is speeded up, and the nitrogen compounds found in high protein foods that putrify into toxic gases can be reduced from 30 to 60%[35].

When poisons are eliminated from the tissues they then enter the bloodstream. These poisons cause the endocrine glands to secrete hormones which in turn stimulate the eliminative organs and result in a feeling of stimulation. When the glands become overworked and exhausted, there will be a feeling of exhaustion and recovery time will be necessary.

The point here is that enzymes can be used not only to maintain health, but also during detoxification programs. Enzymes can be used in both medical and non-medical approaches to healing. They can be the support system to all systems and to health-promotion processes.

CHAPTER 6

Eating for Life

From Degeneration to Regeneration

AFTER reading the last chapter on enzymes, which discusses the benefits of eating raw food, you will realize that some diets are regenerative while others add to the degeneration of the body. As we begin to design a diet that will support a life-long practice of *Intuitive Eating*, it is important to know the difference.

Most diets don't even suggest the use of enzymes. Some diets use little raw food. If a diet lacks raw food and enzymes, and is mainly a cooked-food diet with the use of vitamins, minerals, and other supplements, it is either a degenerative or a maintenance diet. It is degenerative if it includes meat, milk, cheese, other dairy products, and eggs. It's a maintenance diet if it is predominantly a vegetarian diet high in the use of cooked foods. A regenerative diet, on the other hand, is 100% vegetarian, high in raw foods, freshly made fruit and vegetable juices, and enzymes. This would be an excellent diet.

A high percentage of nutrients are destroyed by cooking. A personal friend of mine, Victoras Kulvinskas, author of *Survival into the 21st Century*, has quoted research which confirms that 50% of vitamin B, 96% of thiamin, 97% of folic acid, and 70-80%

of vitamin C is lost in the cooking process[1]. Scientists at Max Frank Institute for Nutritional Research in Germany have found that when protein-foods were cooked only 50% of the protein was left available for use by the human body[2]. Dr. William Neusome, at Canada's Department of Health and Welfare, Food Research Division, showed that cooking transformed certain fungicides into cancer-causing compounds[3].

Additional nutrient value is available when foods are organically grown. At Rutgers University, organically grown food was found to be considerably richer in minerals, particularly trace minerals, than non-organic food. Organic tomatoes have 5 times more calcium, 12 times more magnesium, 3 times more potassium, and 60 times more manganese than non-organic. Organic spinach has 2 times more calcium, 5 times more magnesium, 3 times more potassium, 70 times more sodium, and 80 times more iron.

A regenerative diet is usually between 60-90% raw food. Some people even exist on a 100% raw food diet, with plenty of enzymes, juices, and anti-oxident nutrients. Anti-oxident nutrients are free radical scavangers. (We discussed free radicals in Chapter 4, explaining how they damage the cells throughout the body and contribute to the aging process.) Anti-oxidents, such as vitamins A, E, C, the mineral selenium, and the co-enzyme Q-10, actually slow down the deterioration of fats in the body, including those in the brain, which is composed predominently of fatty acids.

Vitamin E deficiencies are common in America because of our refining of grains and the use of hydrogenated oils. Since it is a fat-soluble vitamin absorbed in the small intestine, many older adults lack vitamin E due to mal-absorption problems. Sixty percent of Alzheimer's victims have abnormally low levels of vitamin E in their blood[4].

With aging, the ability to bring oxygen to the cells through the lungs is often diminished. Free radicals, which are active molecules formed by biological or chemical reactions in our cells, can destroy the cell membrane of healthy cells and interfere with the cell's oxygen supply. An antioxidant is a nutrient that can neutralize free radical destruction. Co-Q-10 is an antioxidant that can help prevent this degeneration process.

Vitamin E, C, selenium, and enzyme Q-10, however, have been shown to slow the degeneration process down and thus retard the aging process. Moreover, anything that retards the aging process aids and strengthens the immune system. Doesn't this support the idea that aging and disease are really nutrient-deficient problems?

Selenium has produced up to a 30-fold increase in the immune system activity, and has slowed cancer growth in lab animals[5]. It has also increased antibody response against invading foreign proteins, which is usually part of the problem in allergic individuals.

THE IMPORTANCE OF CO-ENZYME Q-10

Co-enzyme Q-10, a relatively new substance, is sometimes referred to as a fat-soluble vitamin, or a co-enzyme. Every cell in the body needs co-enzyme Q-10 to produce energy. It boosts the disease-fighting capabilities of our immune system. Co-enzyme Q-10 can be found in foods such as spinach, broccoli, potatoes, rice, wheat, corn, almonds and chestnuts. Sometimes, however, due to extreme need, it is necessary to take co-enzyme Q-10 in supplemental form.

During the past decade there have been a number of studies that have shown Q-10's vital role in the prevention and treatment of many major diseases. To better understand how this co-enzyme works, realize that it is necessary for a cell to be alive in order to produce energy. Each of the hundred-trillion cells that make up a body must ingest and digest elements, and remove waste products. To perform these functions each cell makes its own energy by using oxygen to burn organic substances as foods. In each cell there is a tiny particle called the mitochondria. This is where the power and energy is produced. The energy then stimulates the metabolic processes of your cells. Co-Q-10 has been called the ignition of the cell, and has an important function in manufacturing ATP (adensoine triphosphate), a unit of energy used by the cell to perform its work. Without co-Q-10 in the cell, there is no spark—no ignition—no energy. Consequently, there is no life. When a deficiency in this essential nutrient exists, the cellular engine misfires and you experience fatigue. A severe deficiency of co-Q-10 will cause the engine of the cell to fail.

Dr. Carl Folkers, the father of co-Q-10 research, has theorized that when levels of co-Q-10 drop below 75% (a 25% deficiency), a number of diseases will surface. He also discovered that when levels of co-Q-10 drop below 25% of normal, death can occur at the cellular level. He believes that co-Q-10 is essential for human life. More exciting benefits of co-Q-10 were reported in an article published in the *Linus Pauling Institute of Science and Medicine Newsletter*. It stated that co-Q-10 strengthens the capillaries in the body, is a tonic for the heart, helps to normalize blood pressure, elevates energy, and contributes to extending the life of the cell.

Q-10 is a co-enzyme; it enhances the enzyme activity within the cell. It is usually synthesized in the liver from various foods that you eat. However, scientists have concluded that as we get older, our liver loses the ability to assimilate and synthesize co-Q-10. Consequently, deficiencies exist. Research has found that deficiencies in co-Q-10 leave you more susceptible to a list of health disorders. Co-Q-10 helps build the body's immunity; it promotes weight loss; it helps prevent and treat periodontal gum diseases; and it is necessary to increase stamina and endurance. That is why so many athletes are now using co-Q-10 as a supplement during their training.

An article by Dr. Toru Yananura, a leading Japanese research scientist, listed 60 clinical studies assessing more than 1200 patients on the effects of co-Q-10 against heart and blood-vessel disease[6]. In 42 studies that were concerned with the heart muscle, and heart muscle diseases, 77% (that's 470) of the patients treated with co-Q-10 showed clinical improvement. The dosages of co-Q-10 prescribed were never higher than 60 mg a day. More recent studies have indicated that doses of 100 mg a day may be more appropriate in heart disease. In other studies, patients with congestive heart disease were shown to improve dramatically when using co-Q-10. In fact, patients who were extremely weak, some in wheelchairs, were actually able to resume many of their normal activities.

Other research in Japan[7] indicated that 75% of cardio patients had significant deficiencies of co-Q-10. Between 70-80% of all heart patients given co-Q-10 have shown remarkable improvement. Dr. Folkers has said that a deficiency of co-Q-10 may be a major cause of heart disease. He showed that many severe heart arrhythmias (irregular heartbeat) could be directly related to a lack of co-Q-10.[8] In a 1981 study, 5 of 6 patients who had arrhythmia either reduced or totally eliminated it by using co-Q-10.[9] Angina, severe heart pain, can also be benefited by co-Q-10. Another Japanese study reported in the *American Journal of Cardiology* (56, 1985, pp. 247-251) showed that angina attacks were cut in half when patients were given 150 mg of co-Q-10 a day for a period of just four weeks.

Periodontal gum disease is a leading cause of tooth loss. Seventy-five percent of the population over 65 years of age lose some teeth due to periodontal disease. It is caused mainly by a plaque bacteria build-up in the mouth, and results in inflammation and degeneration of the gums. In 1971 Dr. Folkers pointed out that periodontal gum disease was caused by a deficiency of co-Q-10. In 1970, two U.S. Air Force dentists, Dr. Raymond F. and Edward G. Wilkinson, pioneered a study on co-Q-10 in treating gum disease[10]. They discovered that adding oral doses of co-Q-10 to the diets of patients who had periodontal disease produced measurable improvement in the condition of their gums. Other studies have confirmed that healthy gum tissues usually show a normal co-Q-10 level, whereas diseased gums show a deficiency of the nutrient.

BIOFLAVONOIDS

Bioflavonoids are an essential part of a regenerative diet. Bioflavonoids are the pigments in fruits and vegetables: the yellow in citrus fruit; red and blue in berries; red in some skins and peels; orange in skins and peels of lemons; peels and skins of grapes, grapefruits, oranges and apricots. Propolis, a substance collected by bees from tree bark, is very high in bioflavinoids, and has been used as a natural antibiotic.

Bioflavonoids help activate the healing properties of vitamin C and strengthen the walls of our capillaries. They have been used as a supplement in the treatment of hemorrhoids and varicose veins. Most commercially prepared and "fresh-squeezed" fruit juices lack bioflavonoids because the skins are not ground up in the juice. The fruit or vegetable is just pressed, leaving basically water, some coloring, and some nutrients.

In summary, to be regenerative a diet should include a high percentage of raw food, enzymes, and anti-oxident nutrients. You can look in the back of this book at my chart of the nutrient contents of foods to help in choosing your foods properly.

A LOW-PROTEIN, LOW CALORIE DIET

When I was playing football in college, protein was considered the most important food in our diets. It was easy to consume over 100 grams a day when eating meat at every meal. Then things began to change. Research began to show that a low-protein diet was beneficial. Soon the concentration was on a high complex-carbohydrate intake. Roasted potatoes, pastas, and grains are now served to the athlete. This type of diet supplies the body with highly nutritious foods with an increase of fiber and carbohydrates. (Remember, there is no fiber in meat, eggs, fish, poultry and cheese.) This high carbohydrate diet was initiated into the mainstream because of evidence that a high protein, meat-based diet was linked to colon and rectal cancer.

I began experimenting on my own with a low protein (20 grams daily) low-fat (approximately 8-15%) diet that consisted of 1500-2000 calories a day. I soon found a tremendous advantage in this type of diet: more strength, younger-looking tissues and skin, and weight loss. My theory was that the reason why 2500-3000 calories daily was suggested as the RDA was because the carbohydrates were empty carbohydrates from highly refined foods and sweet desserts. My reasoning was that if one ate highly-nutritious food like whole grains, fruits, potatoes, figs, dates, and sprouted grains for carbohydrates, one would not need so many calories.

I did an interesting experiment with my friend, professional football player, Lou Piccone from the Buffalo Bills. We trained together with a program of running, sprinting, weightlifting, and biking. On just 1500 calories a day we lost weight and remained strong. Our pulse rates and recovery times were better on this diet without meat, fish, eggs, or cheese. Our diet was based on fruits, vegetables, freshly-made fruit and vegetable juices, grains, and enzyme supplementation. We could also train much harder on less sleep.

I have seen the same diet work on sick individuals, or those recovering from illness. Not having a scientific laboratory, I didn't have all the answers as to why this diet was so effective. But I knew it worked. (And I believe that this diet will someday be considered the "anti-aging" diet.) So I started looking for answers. I purchased a book called *The 100-Year-Old Diet* by Dr. Roy Walford[11], and was delighted to see that he scientifically proved my theory that a low-calorie diet was the answer. Walford referred to the "high-low" diet, meaning a diet using high-density nutrient foods and low calorie intake. He stated that, "Calorie for calorie, and especially if you want to restrict fat intake, vegetables are far and away the most nutritious foods." He agreed with me that a diet using 1500-2000 calories a day would supply enough nutrition if the foods used were high-density nutritious ones. He further confirms that this was a superb weight-loss diet. Most weight-loss diets consist of foods that are not the most nutritious, resulting in hunger and overeating, and regaining of the weight that was lost.

One of the major points in this diet is that between 8-13% of the calories come from fat. (Some people use less, like the Pritikin diet, which is about 5% fat.) Vitamins A, D, E and K are fat-soluble vitamins, and require fats in order to be absorbed into the intestine. I suggest using vegetable sources, seeds, nuts, and avocados in their raw state for fat foods. (If you do use seeds and nuts, they should be soaked overnight in distilled water before eating. This helps pre-digest them, raises the enzyme level, and makes them easy to digest. It also releases the enzyme inhibitors. See Appendix B in the back of this book for other suggestions for fat foods.)

A diet using high density, nutritious foods and low calorie foods has been proven to greatly extend the average life-span of animals. Dr. Clyde McCay, at Cornell University[12], fed rats a calorie-restricted diet with the addition of supplements from the time they were weaned. These rats lived significantly longer than the normally fed rats. In 1000 days the normally fed rats died. Most of the calorie-restricted rats were still alive and healthy. The maximum life span of McCay's rats reached 1800 days, equivalent to 150-180 human years. One problem was that the rats on the calorie-restricted diet failed to reach maximum size. This was due to the fact that they were fed this diet from the time of weaning. Wolford points out that a calorie-restricted diet for humans should not start at an early age, but later in life, so as not to affect body size. Furthermore, such a diet should be slowly imposed. Your body needs time to adapt. This is one reason why crash diets don't really work. Also, most crash diets are nutrient-deficient.

McCay also pointed out that the calcification with age (hardening of the arteries) of normal rats was less severe in a rat on a calorie-restricted diet. The pulse rate, which is normally 340 beats per minute, was only 240 beats per minute for the low-calorie rats. There was also less blood-vessel and kidney disease, and less high blood pressure on a calorie-restricted diet. This type of diet lowered the blood pressure and diminished the thickening of the blood vessel walls that usually occurs at old age (arteriosclerosis).

Chronic fatigue, AIDS, and cancer are all auto-immune diseases. With age our normal immune responses decline at least 10-30% of their normal capacity. With AIDS, the self-recognizing immune reactions begin to fail, and the destructive power of the immune system begins to turn on itself, leading to auto-immunity. Dr. Wolford showed that a high-density nutritious food, low carbohydrate diet greatly reduces this negative immune reaction. Anything that strengthens the immune system will help in the anti-aging effect on the body.

Most people consider diseases such as osteoporosis to be "natural" with the aging process. But, as a health practitioner I don't believe this, and have seen it proven false. For example, the parathyroid hormone which normally influences bone and calcium metabolism, increases with age. In animals with significant bone loss, the level of this parathyroid hormone in the blood is always higher than normal. Animals on high density foods and a low calorie diet, however, show no marked increase in this hormone and no bone loss.

Other disease factors are reduced on this type of diet also. Again from Dr. Wolford's book:

> Dr. Earrejo did a very interesting experiment using a high density nutrition, low calorie diet. In his experiment he took 180 men over the age of 65, and divided them into 2 groups. One group was placed on a diet of 2300 calories one day, and the next day, 885 calories. The control group received 2300 calories every day. This was done over a 3-year period. The subjects that received fewer calories spent only 123 days in the infirmary, compared to 219 days from the fully-fed subjects. And their death rate was only one-half the amount of the control group. This shows the effect of the low calorie diet."[13]

Any excess food causes an over-secretion of digestive juices and enzymes. If the body cannot handle the excess, the remainder of the food is unsuitable for the body, and is difficult to evacuate. It does not get digested properly, and ferments in the colon causing a highly toxic, foul-smelling residue. When excess food consumption becomes a habit, evacuation is retarded (constipation). The undigested food attaches itself to the intestinal wall. The bowel then loses its muscle tone, and becomes impacted. Even good food in excess can cause a host of bowel and gastrointestinal difficulties.

Most physiologists now agree that two light meals a day is sufficient to provide all the nutrients necessary for the body to carry on all its function. Of course this is true if one selects the proper high-density, nutritious foods to sustain life. All attempts should be made to eat the best food in proper amounts so as to avoid wasting nerve energy and avoiding overconsumption and malnourishment.

In Sylvester Graham's work[14] on nutrition, he reminds us that debility, sluggishness, constipation, obstructions, and morbid irritability of the alimentary canal have been among the principal roots of both chronic and acute disease in all parts of the world and in all periods of time. The concentrated forms of food, compound preparations, irritating stimuli, and an excess in quantity have been among the principal causes of these difficulties. Also Dr. Tilden, M.D. comments on this subject: "Many people are going to premature graves because they persist in eating more than their system requires, stuffing as long as a morsel can be swallowed or coaxed into going down by the use of relishes." He also says, "Overeating is quickly followed by a constant desire for more food, and the oftener the desire is satisfied, the larger the appetite, and the more uncontrollable it becomes."[15]

EATING FOR USABLE ENERGY

What I am suggesting is to make the body an energy-efficient machine. By this I mean that the calories eaten must be used as energy—i.e., manufacturing proteins, making hormones, and fueling muscular work.

Most people think that if they eat 3000 calories daily, the body uses those 3000 calories daily for energy. This is not so. Actually, on the average, the body is only 33-50% efficient in using calories, and that is if your enzyme level is normal, and you are disease-free. It has been shown that when we decrease calorie intake, the body becomes more energy efficient (closer to 50%). When we increase the calories, the efficiency decreases. A point definitely worth remembering!

Our cells produce ATP (adenosine triphosphate) before the cells can produce energy. ATP is formed by a respiratory process in each cell. It is manufactured from carbohydrates, fats, and proteins. This must be done before our cells can use the food for energy. So, the body doesn't directly use the food as energy. It must be turned into ATP within the cells.

Only 50% of our foods are converted to ATP for energy. When you overeat, less of the foods are used for ATP. When you under-eat, more is used for this cellular metabolic process. At 2500 calories daily, which is the suggested RDA (Recommended Daily Allowances), the efficiency of this process drops to 37%. At 3300 calories a day it drops to 30%[15]. You can see how important it is that every calorie is nutrient-dense. Otherwise your body will become less efficient and put on weight.

CONCLUSION

This chapter has supplied you with the rationale for a significant dietary charge, one that will orient you towards regeneration now, and hopefully for the rest of your life.

It is time to implement the transition with the first action step—the process of detoxification. The next chapter will be your guidebook for this initial part of the ascent.

ACTION STEPS

PART 3

CHAPTER 7

Detoxification

The First Step in Your Transition

> **WARNING:**
> If you are nervous or unsure about changing your diet, or doing a cleaning diet, please see a skilled physician or health practitioner who specializes in these matters. Usually there is no problem in undertaking a cleanse, but it's better to be safe than sorry.

INTRODUCTION

Before you become intuitive about your body's nutritional needs, you must clear the playing field—clean out the body; detoxify it to a certain stage so that it starts giving you dependable feedback. You rarely get this on the everyday, traditional American diet because that diet is always overstimulating the glands. Stimulating foods, spices, drugs, and chemicals build up toxins in the tissues and circulate through the bloodstream. Consequently, you are stimulated to eat more food, and soon even the wrong food feels natural because you are so far away from natural living.

Elimination is an important process, since the removal of waste products and toxins is essential to maintaining health. Whether you are changing to a lighter vegetarian diet, or undertaking a fast, a purification diet will remove much of the surface waste and prepare the body for a better diet and other purification regimes.

During your cleanse a variety of symptoms may manifest. Mucous discharge from the nose, lungs, kidneys, and bowels can result. Skin rashes, headaches, and nauseousness may occur. *These are signs that the cleansing is taking place. They are positive.* Many people get enthusiastic about a purer diet, but give up when they get a little sick, or when the body releases poisons. Understand that it is better to rid the body of these obstructions and experience some acute symptoms now, than to let these poisons remain within the body and develop into a chronic condition later on.

If one takes the proper measures, and uses a cleansing diet, herbal tea, juices, possibly enemas, colonics, proper exercise, warm salt baths, and other cleansing modes, the body will be aided in elimination, and assisted in overcoming some of the adverse symptoms that one may experience during such changes.

One of the main reasons why therapies fail, whether herbal therapy or otherwise, is because the correct use of food is not properly incorporated into the program. This difficulty is easily overcome if one understands the true meaning and use of a cleansing diet, proper food combinations, and a transition diet. A change from a traditional diet to a more vegetarian diet, or raw food diet is a progressive regime, and you must give your body sufficient time to adapt. The bloodstream should receive vitamins, minerals, amino acids, fatty acids, simple sugars, and water, not poisons, from the intestines. When proteins are digested properly, their end product—amino acids—passes from the intestines to the blood. If proteins are improperly combined with other types of food, putrefactive bacteria ferment them into skatols, indols, hydrogen sulfide, and other poisons. When starches and sugars are properly prepared for assimilation by good digestion, their final stage is simple sugars, called monosacchrides, which the body uses without difficulty. But when starches undergo putrefaction from staying in the intestines too long, or are mixed with incompatible substances, they are broken down into acidic acids, alcohol, and carbon dioxide. These byproducts of putrefaction are absorbed into the bloodstream, and affect muscle tissues, joints, organs, glandular ducts, and genetically weak areas, causing pain, arthritis, gout, and acid reaction in the body.

The main objective of dietary therapy is to learn how to adapt to stressful situations and purify your body, particularly the intestinal tract, where large amounts of nutrients can be absorbed. The cleaner you are internally, the more you absorb, and the less you need to eat. The more congested you are, the less you absorb, and the more you must consume. In a pure body, more energy can manifest while eating small amounts of food.

THE CYCLIC NATURE OF THE TRANSITION PROCESS

An amazing thing begins to happen as we start improving our diet. The "worker within" knows the difference between high and low quality food. It immediately begins to use the high quality foods, and eliminate the residues from the past. The intelligence within every cell begins to discard the lower-grade food residues and waste producs from meat, eggs, milk, cheese, dairy, chemicals, drugs, caffeine, nicotine, etc. The body becomes more selective in what foods it begins to metabolize.

For example, if you stop using caffeine the body begins to draw out the caffeine residues from the tissues and the blood. Before the caffeine is completely eliminated from the kidneys, however, while it still circulates through the blood, it can cause uncomfortable symptoms, like headache and fatigue. This is followed by a let-down in energy. Coffee is a stimulant which causes adrenaline secretion, which speeds up the heart and creates a temporary "high." When coffee is omitted from the diet, we no longer feel this stimulant, and the body goes into a resting phase so as to recuperate and regenerate. (Usually the symptoms last from three to ten days.) When the symptoms vanish, the body then becomes stronger, and begins to rebuild using higher quality nutrients.

This natural form of self-cleansing in the body is called *retracing*. If the body could talk, it would say, "Look at all this raw food and freshly made juice. Let's 'retrace' and get rid of all the old bile in the gallbladder. Let's clean the liver, the blood, the joints, clean out all the old debris, clean the veins, the capillaries, so we can rebuild everything with this fresh, live material." Thus the housecleaning and breaking-down process begins. This is known as the catabolic phase (catabolism). Sometimes we experience a fever when the body begins to burn some of this waste. Sometimes the sinuses drip. We might get diarrhea, even a skin rash. Some of the old symptoms that we experienced years ago may reoccur. Recent health problems might reappear. This is all part of the catabolic stage.

When this phase passes, symptoms disappear. Then the body goes into an anabolic stage (anabolism). This stage is a renewing, rebuilding process. It is your reward, and you may feel wonderful. But it might not last long, because as soon as the body builds up its strength, it may start retracing again. This is called the "cyclic power of healing." It would be impossible for the body to eliminate all the poisons that have been accumulating for many years in only three to ten days. It would overburden the lungs, skin, kidneys, and heart, and cause severe degenerative problems.

This brings us to the subject of the "healing crisis," a concept which natural health practitioners understand. Few doctors in the allopathic tradition will acknowledge this, however, so it is important for you to take responsibility to learn about it for yourself.

Keep in mind that not everybody will experience adverse symptoms. Some do, some don't, and most inconveniences will be slight. But remember at all times that your body is becoming stronger, healthier, and more beautiful. So keep going, and you will experience the euphoria of real living.

My book, *Natural Healing With Herbs* (Prescott, AZ: Hohm Press, 1984) gives many suggestions on how to handle these healing crises. It suggests the use of foods, herbs, juices, salt baths, etc. I will give some basic suggestions here, but for more information please refer to that book.

HEALING CRISIS

Webster describes the word *crisis* as "the turning point for better or worse in an acute disease or fever." A healing crisis is known in Naturopathy as "an acute reaction, resulting from the activity of nature's healing forces in overcoming chronic disease conditions."[1]

A crisis is brought about when the body becomes overcrowded with waste and irritating poisons. Cells and tissues begin to throw off the waste which is then carried by the bloodstream to the eliminatory organs—the bowels, kidneys, lungs, skin, nasal passages, ears, throat, bronchi, and genito-urinary organs. These organs then become somewhat irritated and congested, and produce disease symptoms such as colds, boils, kidney and bladder infections, open sores, perspiration, diarrhea, fevers, etc.

These symptoms and the process of elimination are part of the cure. There is nothing to fear, but it is necessary to work *with* them. *Do not* suppress the symptoms with drugs unless absolutely necessary. (In some situations, such as with chronic diseases like cancer, the pain can become severe and drugs may sometimes need to be used.) The drugs themselves accumulate in the body because our organs were not made to handle them. They are stored in fatty tissue and other parts of the body. Tissues imbedded with these foreign elements actually begin a process of degeneration. That is why many natural healers claim that some diseases are in fact "drug diseases," i.e. caused by these inimical elements which only suppress nature's healing forces.

The Naturopathic school of thought distinguishes between a "healing crisis" and a "disease crisis." These may look alike by their outward manifestations, but they are taking place under different conditions.

A "disease crisis" occurs when the body is loaded to its toleration point with toxins and waste products. The body then arouses itself in self-defense and brings forth the acute elimination of toxins in the form of a cold, fever, inflammation, etc. The body is on the defense when it produces a disease crisis.

If the poisons are not adequately eliminated, the body will adapt itself to them and function at a lower energy level. These foreign wastes will continue to accumulate and inhibit the organs from performing their normal functions until finally a chronic disease manifests.

On the other hand, a healing crisis develops because the healing forces are on the *offense*—or ascending, as we say. Through natural living and a balanced, transitional diet, the body will get stronger and automatically start drawing from the tissues and eliminating chronic waste. This will cause the symptoms which we call the *healing crisis*. During a healing crisis, therapy can be used to a much greater extent because the patient already has endurance and can tolerate cleansing herbs, fasting, and advanced water treatments. When people are weaker it is common to recommend energy-building foods, short fasts, and tonic herbs. Once the energy returns, more vigorous cleansing methods can be used.

A healing crisis shows that there is enough energy in the body to eliminate unwanted materials. The crisis can take the form of fevers, excessive menstrual discharge, diarrhea, itching, boils, ulcers, hemorrhages, etc. Reactions will vary according to how seriously ill the person has been, or how much he/she has been abused by the environment.

It is very important to be able to differentiate between a healing crisis and a change for the worse during a disease. Any crisis, if not watched, understood, and properly treated can weaken the individual and last for several days. You will usually see a positive change in a healing crisis after three days. The most severe symptoms begin to decrease, the fever breaks, and the person becomes more relaxed. Psychologically they feel better. If after three days, however, the severe symptoms do not lessen, then a new course of treatment is indicated.

Many times, crises can be avoided if the individual has a strong constitution and properly functioning eliminatory organs. Also, sometimes there are warning symptoms that show that a crisis is coming and the body is trying to eliminate toxins. Dark urine, sluggishness, fevers, coated tongue, sense of irritability and weakness, headaches, and ringing in the ears, are a few warning signs to look for. If therapy is undertaken in these early stages and the body is assisted by the proper use of herbs, enemas, homeopathy, acupuncture, massage, and hydrotherapy, energy blockages that are caused by accumulated waste can often be released. The normal energy flow can be restored to the eliminatory organs and accumulated poisons can be eliminated naturally without a noticeable crisis. Although there is no absolute guarantee that a crisis can be avoided, these natural therapies will always assist nature in reestablishing health and balance.

The body will become stronger after each healing crisis if a better lifestyle is continued. Crises will become farther apart until the day comes when only health is present, and sickness is history. You may still experience slight crises once in a while, but they will usually be brief (one to three days). When they pass they will leave you healthier.

The form the healing crisis takes and how long it lasts depends upon the following:

1. The kind of waste (drugs, mucus, uric acid, etc.) For example, if the mucus is thick, the body will force it out through the mucus membranes producing nasal drip, colds, flu, etc.
2. The condition of the eliminatory organs. For example, if the waste cannot be eliminated through natural pathways, the body will burn it off (fevers) or store it as boils and acne. Nature always picks the best-adapted organs for elimination. Pain in the kidneys, bladder, or bowels might lead us to believe that the painful organ is diseased. On the contrary, it is more likely the strongest eliminative organ in the organism, the one nature is using as an outlet for the unwanted waste.
3. The energy level or vitality of the patient. For example, crises will vary according to how seriously ill the person has been. In a robust individual the toxins are eliminated quickly. A person who is weak, with low vitality, takes a much longer time to eliminate the toxins.

4. The area of congestion in the body. For example, constipation can precede diarrhea; lung congestion can precede a crisis in that area, etc.
5. Climate too plays a great influence on the type of healing crisis. If the weather is cold, the pores of the skin are usually covered and contracted, so the kidneys, bowels, and lungs throw off the excess toxins. In hot climates, the skin can eliminate more acid waste, since people wear lighter clothing and the skin pores are open. Oftentimes, however, when people move to a warmer climate they develop a skin disease. The sun draws out the body's poisons through the open pores. Here they can accumulate and cause skin diseases such as cancer. It is frequently said that "the sun causes skin cancer" or the "hot weather is bad." Of course, too much sun can cause skin problems, but this usually is not the main factor. The poisons are being drawn to the surface for elimination. If the blood was clean, a great percentage of these conditions wouldn't exist.

I have seen serious skin conditions vanish after a thorough cleanse, proper food, rest, exercise, and mental attitude. People then proceed to enjoy sun-bathing after years of not getting the beauty and health-preserving benefits of the sun's rays.

When the healing crisis is over, in both weak and strong persons, toning and strengthening the body is a necessity. Exercise, proper diet, toning herbs, and hydrotherapy can be used.

If you have any questions about the length of an illness or the severity of the problem, consult a qualified physician.

Remember, never go to extremes in dietary changes. Use a slow transition, educate yourself about diet and normal therapeutics, and work with a practitioner who has experience along these lines. Trying to get "too pure too fast" can be destructive and can postpone the achievement of your goal.

In the concluding section of this chapter I will supply you with immediate applications for dealing with the symptoms of healing crises that may be a normal part of your detoxification process. For now, let's begin the purification diet.

THE PURIFICATION DIET FOR INNER CLEANLINESS

PREPARATIONS AND PRECAUTIONS

Duration

The purpose of this diet is to purify and cleanse the body. It may be used for a period of six to fourteen days, or longer if needed. Usually, an individual who has been eating a diet of meat and refined, processed foods, should start with a six-day cleanse. A person who has been on cleansing diets before, or who is eating a vegetarian diet, can use a cleansing diet longer. If adverse symptoms persist over a three to six day period, it usually means the body is extremely toxic, and that shorter cleansing periods can be used for a progressive change in diet, between cleanses, and between your transitional steps. The cleansing diet can be used once every six to ten weeks if necessary. A good maintenance regime is to use a three-day cleanse at the end of every month, while improving your diet between cleanses.

Avoidance of Supplements and Stimulants

While undertaking a cleansing diet, no supplements should be taken. Supplements cause the body to react in a specific manner. Some stimulate the metabolism, some sedate, and some can even change the pH of the intestinal tract. By cleansing your body you will be changing your metabolism, pH, and the physiological reaction of each organ. By having a purer body after the cleanse, your whole supplemental program will usually be different, and supplements may no longer be needed. The goal of *Intuitive Eating* is to have your body be totally reactive by itself. Of course, if you have an illness or a condition that you must support during the cleanse (for example, nervous system, immune system, particular endocrine gland condition, etc.) then use appropriate supplements as necessary. You and your physician will know best.

Nothing should be causing a stimulating or a sedative type of a reaction. That's one reason why no coffee is allowed during the cleanse. You want to intuitively get to know your body the way it really is.

Rest

During a cleansing diet, or actually any diet, try to rest as much as possible. Do some light exercise, like walking, if you feel well enough.

Honor Individual Needs

Skip a meal if the recommended food is too much for you to eat, or if you are not hungry. Remember, everyone is a little different in the amount of solids and liquids that he/she can handle. If a meal is skipped, substitute for it with two cups of freshly made fruit or vegetable juice.

Use Herbs as Necessary

Blood-purifying or laxative herbs can be taken during the cleanse. It is helpful to use the herbs specifically recommended for the areas of the body in need of strengthening or cleansing. A chart and explanation of usage will be found later in this chapter. During acute symptoms, herb tea, tinctures, etc. are usually taken every two hours to strengthen the body. If you have been through cleansing diets before, then usually the diet alone, with juices, vegetable broth, and plenty of liquids, is all that is needed.

Use Acidophilus and Enzymes

During the cleanse, and usually for about three months after, I suggest taking a bacteria culture for the bowel. You can get one from your health food store, but make sure it contains Bifidus and Acidophilus culture.

Most of us seem to have some type of digestive problem, or a difficulty absorbing a particular vitamin or mineral. So sometimes I also suggest taking enzyme supplements before each meal, especially during the cleanse. Purchase an enzyme supplement that has the four major groups of enzymes: amylase, protease, lipase, and cellulase.

The additional enzyme lactase is necessary if you have problems digesting dairy products. So, if you use dairy products buy an enzyme supplement that has all four of the aforementioned enzymes, plus lactase.

Juices

Supplement the body during any clenase by using freshly-made fruit and vegetable juices, a minimum of three times a day between meals. You can choose one from the list in the section on "Dealing With Symptoms" later in this chapter, or make up your own using information in the Chapter 9 on *Juiceology*. If you have a weakness in an organ, or body system, choose the herbs and juices that support that particular system or the organ involved.

Juices will help neutralize toxins in the body, and aid in elimination through the kidneys and liver. Drink one to two cups of freshly-squeezed fruit or vegetable juices between meals. They should be taken one-half hour before, or one hour after, meals. If you are not used to drinking juice it is good to dilute the juices with 25% distilled, purified water, or water that has gone through a reverse-osmosis unit. Usually six to twelve ounces of juice, or juice and water, at a time is suggested. Chew your juices until most of the flavor is gone before swallowing. This is especially true if symptoms of diabetes or hypoglycemia are present. If the juices cause gas or bloating, cut down the amounts taken, or delete them entirely. Vegetable broths, or distilled or purified water can be substituted for juice. Use enemas if gas and bloating are still a problem. (See my book, *Natural Healing With Herbs* for information on enemas.)

Liquid chlorophyll, the juice of green plants, is one of the best blood-purifiers and nutritional supplements. Drink two ounces twice daily mixed with apple, orange or pineapple juice for a tonic.

THE DIET

Breakfast

- One-half hour before eating breakfast mix one heaping teaspoon of psyllium seed powder in eight ounces of orange, pineapple, or apple juice. Drink this immediately or it will thicken. Psyllium seed powder may cause bloating. If this becomes uncomfortable, use an enema or herbal laxatives (cascara sagrada, turkey rhubarb, or a cold infusion of senna tea mixed with a little ginger) for a few days until most of the surface waste clears from the colon.

- For breakfast, eat fresh fruit. Eat at least one-half pound of one type of fruit, or you may mix a fresh fruit salad consisting of two to four types of fruit from among the suggestions below (NO bananas or avocados).
- Fresh, raw fruits, organically grown, and eaten in season whenever possible, may be used. These include: apples, grapes, apricots, cherries, currants, figs, guavas, mangoes, papayas, peaches, pears, ripe pineapples, oranges, grapefruit, plums, persimmons, berries, nectarines, etc. Melons of all kinds are permitted, but should be eaten by themselves, NOT mixed in a salad with other fruits. With dried fruits, use organically grown and unsulphured varieties, and soak to reconstitute. Use: apples, dates, apricots, figs, peaches, prunes, pears, plums, raisins, mangoes, pineapples, and papayas.
- No coffee or tea is permitted. For best digestion, do not drink any liquid with meals.

Lunch

- One-half hour before lunch, mix one heaping teaspoon of psyllium seed powder in eight ounces of orange, pineapple, or apple juice (use fresh juice when possible).
- Fresh Vegetable Salad: Make a chopped salad of fresh, raw vegetables. Use a dressing of cold-pressed olive oil and lemon juice. Oils are not necessary. Use just four of the vegetables listed below. If an individual is not used to raw food, too many different vegetables at a meal can be difficult to digest.
- Use fresh, raw vegetables: artichokes, asparagus, beans, beets, brussel sprouts, carrots, cauliflower, cucumbers, celery, dandelions, endives, eggplants, fresh corn, green peas, green peppers, kale, kohlrabi, lettuce (not iceberg), lotus, okra, onions, parsley, parsnips, pumpkin, radishes, rutabaga, salsify, spinach, sprouts (all kinds), squash (all kinds), swiss chard, tomatoes, and turnips (you may use the leaves or tops also).
- No coffee, tea, milk, or beverages are permitted at lunch. Do not eat dessert.

Dinner

- One-half hour before dinner, drink two cups of vegetable broth. This can be made up in advance and used hot or cold.
- Vegetable Broth: Celery, carrots, beets, zucchini, parsley, onion, green peppers, and one-half-inch thick peelings of potatoes. Chop fine and simmer for one-half hour in distilled water. Strain and drink. You may add fresh garlic to taste when served.
- Fresh Vegetable Salad: Make a salad of fresh, raw vegetables from the lunch list above. Use a dressing of cold-pressed olive oil and lemon.
- Steamed Vegetables: Select two or three vegetables from the lunch list above and steam until tender but still crisp (about five minutes). Season with oregano, basil, dill, rosemary, thyme, or other unprocessed seasonings.
- Bread: One medium slice of whole wheat bread, well toasted, or use unleavened bread. Eat the bread plain.
- No coffee, tea, or desserts are permitted.
- Two hours following dinner, mix one heaping teaspoon psyllium seed powder in eight ounces of orange, pineapple, or apple juice (use fresh juice when possible).

DEALING WITH HEALTH PROBLEMS USING HERBS

This section will be a handy reference for you throughout your detoxification process, your transitional dietary stages, or at any time that symptoms occur due to changes in your diet or eating habits. I will discuss two *major* modalities (herbs and juices) for dealing with symptoms and a wide variety of *minor* or auxiliary approaches.

HERBS

What follows is basically a crash course on the use of herbs. If you'd like more information on how to use herbs, see the back pages for the correspondence course and herbal seminar tapes I have published.

Whatever your symptoms, there are herbs to use that correspond with the body parts affected. Some of these herbs can be put in combinations. Some will be taken in capsule form, while others will be made into an infusion. An infusion is basically a strong tea. To make it, put one ounce of the herb in a stainless steel kettle or pot, add a pint of boiling water, cover, and let steep for twenty minutes. Then, strain out the herbs and you will have approximately three cups of infusion. **The usual dosage is one cup three times a day**. If you are going to use the herb in capsule form (some herbs are bitter and we don't take them in tea form), **the usual suggested dosage is two capsules three times a day between meals.**

Now let's take a look at which herbs correspond to which body parts. For example, if lower back pains present themselves during a cleansing diet, or during one of the transitional diet stages, you would take a tea that would be good for your kidneys, since they are located near the lower back. Excellent teas for this organ would be corn silk or juniper berries. If constipation presents itself, the herb suggested would be cascara sagrada. Two capsules before bed will work like a light laxative.

When the body is purifying itself through the cleansing organs such as the liver, kidneys, bowels, and skin, we will want to assist it—not put excessive stress and strain on the tissues and organs involved. One reason why fasting and cleansing diets don't work is that when the organs are overloaded with mucus and poisons which have been stored in the tissues for years, they become weak, and we experience fatigue. This fatigue will often prolong the cleansing effect of the body unnecessarily.

Here is a list of organs and the corresponding herbs that assist these organs:

ADRENAL GLANDS	LICORICE ROOT • 1-2 capsules 3x day or • 2 cups licorice root tea
BLADDER	BUCHU, NETTLES & PARSLEY CLEAVERS & CORN SILK • All can be taken in tea form: 1 cup 3x day
BLOOD	ALFALFA, BURDOCK, CLEAVERS, DANDELION & RED CLOVER • All can be taken in tea (1 cup 3x day) or capsule form (2 capsules 3x day)
BONES	COMFREY TEA • 1 cup 3x day COMFREY ROOT POWDER • 2 capsules 3x day
BOWELS (constipation)	PSYLLIUM SEED POWDER • 1 tsp. in 8 oz. juice 2-3x day CASCARA SAGRADA • 2 capsules before bed 2-3 nights in a row
CIRCULATION	GINGER ROOT • 1 cup tea 3x day SASSAFRAS, SPEARMINT, YARROW & GINSENG • 1 cup tea 3x day or • 2 capsules 3x day
DIGESTIVE SYSTEM	GENTIAN ROOT • 2 capsules before meals

EYES ***(eyestrain)***	HERBAL EYEBRIGHT • 1 cup tea 3x day or • 2 capsules 3x day FENNEL • 1 cup tea 3x day or • 2 capsules 3x day GOLDENSEAL • 1 cup tea 3x day or • 2 capsules 3x day
GALLBLADDER	DANDELION • 1 cup tea 3x day DANDELION ROOT • 2 capsules 3x day PARSLEY • 1 cup tea 3x day
HEADACHES	WHITE WILLOW BARK • 2 capsules when needed
HEART	HAWTHORNE BERRIES • 2 capsules 3x day
JOINTS	DEVIL'S CLAW COMFREY ROOT • 2 capsules 3x day
KIDNEYS	BURDOCK • 1 cup tea 3x day or • 2 capsules 3x day CLEAVERS • 1 cup tea 3x day DANDELION LEAF • 1 cup tea 3x day

KIDNEYS *(cont.)*	JUNIPER BERRIES • 2 capsules 3x day SHEPHERD'S PURSE • 1 cup tea 3x day or • 2 capsules 3x day
LIVER	BARBERRY • 2 capsules before meals DANDELION LEAF • 1 cup tea 3x day or • 2 capsules 3x day GOLDENSEAL ROOT • 2 capsules 3x day MILK THISTLE • 2 capsules 3x day PARSLEY • 1 cup tea 3x day RED CLOVER • 1 cup tea 3x day or • 2 capsules 3x day
LUNGS	FENUGREEK • 1 cup tea 3x day or • 2 capsules 3x day GARLIC • 2 capsules 3x day MULLEIN • 1 cup tea 3x day or • 2 capsules 3x day LICORICE ROOT • 1 cup tea 3x day or • 2 capsules 3x day

LYMPHATIC SYSTEM	ECHINACEA • tincture, 15 drops in 1/2 cup water 3x day or • 2 capsules 3x day RED CLOVER • 1 cup tea 3x day or • 2 capsules 3x day
MAMMARY GLANDS	LECITHIN THISTLE • 1 cup tea 3x day or • 2 capsules 3x day
MOUTH ***(bad breath)***	CLOVES • chew 3-6 whole cloves as needed SPEARMINT OR PEPPERMINT • 1 cup tea 3x day
MUCUS MEMBRANES ***(sore throat, sinus congestion)***	GOLDENSEAL LEAF • 1 cup tea 3x day GOLDENSEAL ROOT • 2 capsules 3x day SAGE • 1 cup tea 3x day
MUSCLES ***(aching)***	COMFREY ROOT • 2 capsules 3x day COMFREY • 1 cup tea 3x day
NERVOUS SYSTEM	CAMOMILE • 1 cup tea 3x day LADY'S SLIPPER • 1 cup tea 3x day or • 2 capsules 3x day

NERVOUS SYSTEM *(cont.)*	SKULLCAP • 1 cup tea 3x day or • 2 capsules 3x day PLEURISY ROOT • 2 capsules 3x day
PANCREAS	DANDELION LEAF • 1 cup tea 3x day DIGESTIVE ENZYMES • take before meals
PROSTATE	SAW-PALMETTO BERRIES • 2 capsules 3x day PARSLEY ROOT • 2 capsules 3x day PARSLEY LEAF • 1 cup tea 3x day
REPRODUCTIVE SYSTEM ***(female)***	DAMIANA • 1 cup tea 3x day or • 2 capsules 3x day CRAMPBARK *(good herb for cramps)* • 2 capsules 3x day
REPRODUCTIVE SYSTEM ***(male)***	FO-TI • 2 capsules 3x day RED AMERICAN GINSENG • 2 capsules 3x day SAW-PALMETTO BERRIES • 2 capsules 3x day
SINUSES	HORSERADISH • fresh, grate and mix with greens SAGE • 1 cup tea 3x day

SINUSES *(cont.)*	GARLIC • 2 capsules 3x day GOLDENSEAL ROOT • 2 capsules 3x day
SKIN	RED CLOVER • 1 cup tea 3x day
SPLEEN	GOLDENSEAL ROOT • 2 capsules 3x day YELLOW DOCK • 2 capsules 3x day GENTIAN • 2 capsules 3x day
STOMACH	ALFALFA • 1 cup tea 3x day or • 2 capsules 3x day CAMOMILE • 1 cup tea 3x day or • 2 capsules 3x day DANDELION LEAF • 1 cup tea 3x day or • 2 capsules 3x day FENNEL • 1 cup tea 3x day or • 2 capsules 3x day GINGER • 1 cup tea 3x day or • 2 capsules 3x day

For convenience, almost any of these herbs is available in tincture form. (Check your local health food store.) A tincture is a liquid extract of an herb. It is convenient because you can add 25 drops to a cup of water three times a day. You can take the tincture with you in your car, or carry it in your purse or briefcase. *Nature's Way* is one reputable herb company that I recommend.

For those who want more information, please refer to my book, *Natural Healing With Herbs* (Prescott, AZ: Hohm Press, 1984) to find out the exact use of each herb.

THE PROPER USE OF JUICES FOR SYMPTOMS

During your cleanse, or when you're working with specific symptoms, keep in mind that you can use juices in place of or along with the herb teas. For example, if there is liver congestion, you can drink carrot and apple juice, and later on in the day you might want to use an herb called milk thistle, or barberry. You can even drink your glass of juice while taking two capsules of your herb. But it's not necessary that you overdo this supplementation during your cleansing diet. You don't want to overwork a specific organ. If you have questions on this, please refer to a skilled health practitioner who has been using juice and herbs for years. Usually you can ask at your local health food store for names of the practitioners in your area who use these methods.

Here are my recommendations for using juice:

- The usual dosage of juices is eight to ten ounces, three times a day, between meals.
- Juices are drunk one-half hour before meals or one and one-half hours after. If you drink them on an empty stomach they are absorbed very rapidly; usually within five to fifteen minutes they are into the bloodstream.
- It is better to use fruit juices in the morning and during the day, and vegetable juices during the day and in the evening. (I do not suggest using fruit juices after 7 p.m. because the sugars are very stimulating and may cause some sleep disorders.)

- Vegetable juices are your mineral and protein foods (the builders). Fruit juices are your cleansing mineral foods (the cleansers).

Below is a chart that lists the juice combinations to help with symptoms in various organs. If you cannot find all the vegetables and fruits suggested, use some of them, or, go to the chapter on Juiceology that follows, or to J. Kordich's book, *The Power of Juicing*[2]. J. Kordich has been juicing for over 40 years, and his experience is invaluable. His book gives dozens of juice combinations for specific symptoms, organs, and tissues which will be very valuable to you during your stages in diet, or in your daily use of freshly-made fruit and vegetable juices.

Everyday juice combinations that can be used in the home are:

LIVER	CARROT AND APPLE JUICE DANDELION LEAF *(when available)*
KIDNEYS	CARROT, PARSLEY AND APPLE
SKIN	BEET WITH BEET TOPS, CELERY, CUCUMBER, 1/4 POTATO, CARROT AND APPLE
BLOOD	KALE, PARSLEY, GINGER *(small piece)* APPLE AND CARROT
BOWEL	SPINACH, APPLE AND CARROT
GAS	CABBAGE, CARROT AND APPLE
LUNGS	CARROT, PARSLEY, 1/4 POTATO, WATERCRESS, GINGER *(one slice),* MUSTARD GREENS *(when in season)*
ADRENAL	BEET, BEET TOPS, CELERY, ROMAINE
GLANDS	LETTUCE
STOMACH	FENNEL, CABBAGE, CELERY AND APPLE
BLADDER	ALL MELON JUICES AND *(in combination)* CARROT, BEET, CUCUMBER AND PARSLEY
GALLBLADDER	PARSLEY, BEET WITH TOPS, APPLE AND CELERY

OTHER HEALING MODALITIES DURING DETOXIFICATION

- Chiropractors: During detoxification or stages of transition, you can seek out professional help from chiropractors to make sure that the spine and the body are in proper alignment. This is very important during the cleanse and when the body is under stress and there is excess pressure on the organs and tissues.
- Massage is also very good to get the lymphatic system stimulated and help the body cleanse itself.
- Neuromuscular Therapy is excellent for nerve pain, muscle pain, and when the body is misaligned. To find out the name of a neuromuscular therapist in your area, call Paul St. John's Clinic in Largo, Florida (813-541-1800).
- Foot Reflexology is something that everybody can use at home. Working on the feet will take the stress off the internal organs and stimulate circulation in the entire body.
- Straight Fasts are also useful. Fasting is a subject that should be studied before it is attempted. Since it is beyond the scope of this book to discuss fasting in depth I would recommend that you read The Miracle of Fasting, by Paul Brad (Health Science Publishers, 1975.), or find another book on the subject from your health food store. A health practitioner who has the experience in how to guide a person through a fast can be an invaluable resource. I do not suggest long fasts for anybody who is not skilled in fasting.
- A Castor Oil Pack can be very helpful when there is back pain, or liver or gallbladder congestion. The castor oil pack is made with a piece of cotton cloth, usually cut about a foot square. Soak the cloth in castor oil, then place the cloth over the organ in need of healing. Put another cloth on top of the oil-soaked one, and then put a heating pad on top of that. Cover the area with a blanket, or a piece of plastic to keep the heat in. This is one of Edgar Cayce's wonderful remedies. Usually it is done for three consecutive days, for forty-five minutes each day. Wait three days before doing the process again.

- Enemas or colonics can be used during a cleansing diet, between or even during other transitional steps, especially if gas pains, nauseousness, bloating, or a burning feeling is felt throughout the body and intestinal tract. I believe that enemas are very important, even though many people frown on their use. If you don't know how to give yourself an enema, please refer to my book, Natural Healing With Herbs (Prescott, AZ: Hohm Press, 1984) or *Back to Eden*[4] for directions, or, refer to a health professional who can guide you through this process.
  A common enema solution is comprised of two quarts of lukewarm water mixed with one tablespoon of apple cider vinegar. The apple cider vinegar gives it an acid pH, which is very cleansing to the bowel. You can also add four ounces of liquid chlorophyll to two quarts of water for another effective enema solution.
- Skin Brushing: Your skin is called your "third kidney." In other words, if the skin is eliminating properly, this takes the stress off the kidneys. Skin brushing can be used daily for the rest of your life, if need be. It is very refreshing and very cleansing to your body. Start by taking a hot and cold shower, i.e. alternate warm water for 2 minutes with cool water for 2 minutes, back and forth for about 15 minutes. Dry yourself off, and then take a loofa sponge or a light brush and brush the skin. This helps the elimination through the skin.
- Salt Baths And Other Baths: Many symptoms produced by a cleansing diet, as well as headaches, burning feet, fatigue, nauseousness, etc., can be overcome by using warm baths, salt baths, or alternating hot and cold foot baths. When there is a strong body odor or minor skin problem, soak in a tub of warm water for 20-30 minutes with 1-4 pounds of Epsom salts added. This bath will help draw out the poisons from the blood, and take the stress off the liver and kidneys. Dry

yourself and then brush your skin with a natural bristle brush or a loofa to activate the lymphatic flow and circulation. These can be purchased at your local health food store.

Now you have some tools that you can use at home during detoxification or at any point in your transition. You can practice many of these methods on yourself and your children for colds, fevers, flus, or most minor illnesses. These approaches have been used for decades by professionals in clinics around the world, both for chronic disease and acute conditions. With a little effort, you can assist your body to achieve a new level of health.

It is exciting when you realize that you can take part in improving your own life, and that your daily health is your responsibility. Nobody will feed you; nobody will tell you what to do; or do it for you. You must do it yourself. It is important that you take this information, assimilate it, and make it part of your lifestyle. Health is not anything that you can buy. It is something that you personally commit to. This is actually a new way of learning respect for yourself.

CHAPTER 8

The Transitional Diet

STAGE I

CONGRATULATIONS! You are now ready to begin the dietary plan that will move you into a lifestyle of *Intuitive Eating*. It will be a time of new eating adventures, of continued education, and of growing self-awareness. As you progress in this transition your body will become cleaner, your mind will become more alert, and you will feel lighter, stronger, and more in control of your own life and health. You will appreciate what your body knows, and give it what it needs. Best of all, you will start to prefer a healthier diet, thus building a foundation for *Intuitive Eating* as a way of life.

This chapter will give you an overview of the three transitional dietary stages, practical steps for implementing each, and additional nutritional information that will address some common questions about this transition process.

You will learn:

- How to determine your "ideal" weight, and to set a goal to accomplish that.
- How to take your urinary pH so that you can monitor your own acid-alkaline balance throughout the program.
- How to combine foods properly for optimal digestion.

- Where and how to get essential vitamins and minerals from a vegetarian-based diet.

But first, let's take a look at Chart 8.1 and then talk about some general considerations.

CHART 8.1

STAGE ONE	STAGE TWO	STAGE THREE
25 - 40% raw food 20 - 30% total calories as fat	40 - 70% raw food 15 - 25% total calories as fat	75% - 90% raw food 8 - 15% total calories as fat
BEVERAGES	BEVERAGES	BEVERAGES
• limit coffee, tea. Substitute decaffeinated coffee •limit alcohol, carbonated soft drinks. Substitute "natural" soft drinks. Introduce herbal teas. • increase fruit and vegetable juices • introduce freshly made fruit and vegetable juices • eliminate tap water - use distilled, reverse osmosis, or deionized water • cut back on beverages taken with meals	• eliminate caffeinated coffee and tea • use herbal teas, decaf. coffee, coffee substitutes such as Cafix, Postum • limit "natural" soft drinks • increase freshly made fruit and vegetable juices • use distilled, reverse osmosis or deionized water • reduce alcoholic beverages • drink beverages at least 1/2 hr. before meals or 1 1/2 hrs. after meals	• use herbal teas, distilled, reverse osmosis, or deionized water, freshly made fruit and vegetable juices • eliminate decaf coffee and alcoholic beverages • do not drink with meals

STAGE ONE	STAGE TWO	STAGE THREE
CARBOHYDRATES	CARBOHYDRATES	CARBOHYDRATES
Breads:	*Breads:*	*Breads:*
• use whole grain flour and breads without additives or preservatives.	• introduce sprouted whole grain breads, rolls, etc.	• use only sprouted whole grain or Essene breads
Cereals:	*Cereals:*	*Cereals:*
• use whole grain cereals without additives or preservatives • roasted granolas, muesli are fine (no white sugar)	• use whole, raw grains—unroasted	• use organic whole, raw grains - unroasted
Grains:	*Grains:*	*Grains:*
• use whole instead of processed grains	• use organic whole grains	• same as Stage #2
Legumes:	*Legumes*	*Legumes:*
• eliminate processed legumes, substituting fresh dried peas, beans, etc.	• increase use of fresh legumes	• same as Stage #2
Pasta:	*Pasta:*	*Pasta:*
• introduce whole wheat, rice, corn, spinach, artichoke, etc. pastas, eliminating refined, processed white flour pastas	• decrease use of pasta	• eliminate
Sweeteners:	*Sweeteners:*	*Sweeteners:*
• eliminate white sugar using turbinado sugar, Sucanat®, honey, maple syrup, unsulphured molasses instead	• use raw honey, unsulphured molasses, maple syrup, Sucanat® in limited quantities • substitute carob for chocolate	• further limit use of natural sweeteners • use fresh fruits or reconstituted dried fruits to sweeten • water combinations

STAGE ONE	STAGE TWO	STAGE THREE
CONDIMENTS & SEASONINGS	CONDIMENTS & SEASONINGS	CONDIMENTS & SEASONINGS
• eliminate table salt, using sea salt instead • limit use of black pepper • use condiments (catsup, mustard, etc) made without additives or preservatives • use low fat mayonnaise	• eliminate black pepper • limit use of sea salt • use natural herbs and spices and "salt substitues" • limit use of condiments • make your own mayonnaise	• eliminate sea salt • further limit use of condiments • watch for bad combinations
DESSERTS	DESSERTS	DESSERTS
• cut back intake of desserts by one half • use freshly made desserts from natural products • eliminate desserts made with white sugar and white flour	• eliminate use of desserts following meals—unless the dessert is a good combination with the meal	• same as Stage #2 • use as a snack only
FATS AND OILS	FATS AND OILS	FATS AND OILS
• begin to limit intake of butter—use raw unsalted butter • use cold-pressed vegetable oils • eliminate margarine	• further reduce intake of raw butter • use only cold-pressed vegetable oils in dark bottles or cans	• eliminate raw butter • use only cold-pressed vegetable oils in dark bottles or cans

STAGE ONE	STAGE TWO	STAGE THREE
FRUITS	FRUITS	FRUITS
• increase intake of fresh fruit • limit use of canned fruits (packed in their own juices with no sugar or preservatives) • increase use of un-sulphured dried fruits that have been reconstituted in water	• use only fresh fruits and reconstituted, un-sulphured dried fruits	• same as Stage 2
JUICES	JUICES	JUICES
• use bottled, canned, boxed and frozen juices, unsweetened with no additives or preservatives • introduce freshly made fruit and vegetable juices	• reduce use of all pre-packaged juices • increase use of freshly made fruit and vegetable juices	• use only freshly made fruit and vegetable juices

STAGE ONE	STAGE TWO	STAGE THREE
PROTEIN	PROTEIN	PROTEIN
Dairy: • limit use of all dairy products • use certified raw cheese and yogurt when possible—if not available, use nonfat yogurt made without white sugar • use brown fertile eggs • eliminate cow's milk—use soymilk	*Dairy:* • same as Stage #1 • limit use further	*Dairy:* • same as Stage #2 • continue to reduce quantity or eliminate totally
Meat, fish, poultry:	*Meat, fish, poultry:*	*Meat, fish, poultry:*
• eliminate all red meat • use only baked, broiled or roasted fresh fish, chicken or turkey	• reduce use of fish, chicken and turkey • substitute protein alternatives such as tofu, tempeh, TVP (texturized vegetable protein), nuts, seeds, beans, legumes	• eliminate fish, chicken and turkey • use protein alternatives as in Stage #2
Nuts & seeds:	*Nuts & seeds:*	*Nuts & seeds:*
• use unsalted seeds and nuts • limit intake of peanuts, peanut butter - use other seed and nut butters	• use only raw nuts and seeds • begin use of soaked seeds and nuts • limit use of nut butters	• use only soaked seeds and nuts • limit use of nut butters

STAGE ONE	STAGE TWO	STAGE THREE
VEGETABLES	VEGETABLES	VEGETABLES
Salads:	*Salads:*	*Salads:*
• eliminate iceberg lettuce—use romaine, green leaf, red leaf, spinach, etc. • increase the variety of fresh vegetables eaten • limit use of frozen packaged, canned and fried vegetables	• increase salads and varieties of vegetables eaten • increase intake of raw vegetables • eliminate frozen, canned, packaged, fried vegetables	• further increase varieties of fresh vegetables
Salad Dressings:	*Salad Dressings:*	*Salad Dressings:*
• use only natural bottled dressings—no additives, preservatives, etc. • increase use of homemade dressings using cold-pressed oils • reduce size of servings	• eliminate bottled dressings • use freshly made dressings from cold-pressed oils, apple cider vinegar, or lemon juice, fresh herbs and spices • make your own mayonnaise	• same as Stage #2
Soups:	*Soups:*	*Soups:*
• limit use of canned or pre-packaged soups • increase use of homemade soups made with large variety of fresh vegetables, legumes, grains, herbs, seasonings • eliminate soups with red meat	• use only homemade soups—do not overcook • eliminate all poultry and fish • use organic vegetables when available	• same as Stage #2

STAGE ONE	STAGE TWO	STAGE THREE
MISCELLANEOUS	MISCELLANEOUS	MISCELLANEOUS
Candy:	*Candy:*	*Candy:*
• decrease amount of candy • buy health food store varieties	• further decrease amount of health food store candy • increase "home-made candy" made with soaked seeds, nuts and dried fruit	• eliminate store bought candy • use only home-made "candy" as in Stage #2
Ice Cream:	*Ice Cream:*	*Ice Cream:*
• limit use of ice cream—frozen yogurt instead made without white sugar	• eliminate ice cream • use non-dairy frozen desserts such as Rice Dream • use frozen bananas, strawberries, blueberries, etc. blended or put through Champion Juicer	• use non-dairy frozen desserts and frozen fruit creams only as a treat

A LOOK AT THE THREE STAGES

Transition Into Raw Food: As you look over the chart that gives you the overview of the three stages, you'll notice a gradual increase in raw foods. Stage I has 25-40% raw food. Stage II has 40-70%, Stage III 75-90%. Different amounts of raw food are given at each stage to give your body the chance to adapt to this raw food intake. Since raw food is the high energy food that we have spoken about in previous chapters, it forms the basis for the *Intuitive Eating* system.

A New Relationship To Food: Stages are used to give you a chance to slowly develop your relationship with different types of food. One of those basic factors will be learning how and where to shop for the different types of food you will be using in your diet. While many foods can be found in large supermarkets, I recommend that you start exploring your local health food store. Here you will usually find more organic (unsprayed) vegetables, a variety of delightful seasonings that will not rob your food of its nutritional content, and new foods, like sea vegetables, which will add excitement as well as important minerals to your transition diet. Your main consideration is to get food that is nutritionally adequate. High density, nutritious foods, as described in Chapter 6, should be your goal.

Be prepared, in the beginning at least, to take a little more time to shop and to prepare your foods. Recipes may be new, or you may be using foods that you haven't used before. Think of this process as an adventure. Once you get used to eating this way you will take much less time in choice of menus and preparations. To help you through the initial steps, however, I have composed a series of dietary plans, including recipes, which are easy enough for an unskilled cook to prepare. (Dietary Plans for Stage I are included at the end of this chapter.)

You will be encountering the tastes of pure natural foods, perhaps for the first time. Watch the amount of spices or other seasonings you add to your food as these can easily overpower these new tastes. (Many people also develop cravings for the spices instead of for the foods, so use them sparingly.)

How Long At Each Stage: The length of time that you remain at each stage is a matter of your own choice. There is absolutely NO HURRY! It took 20, 30, even 40 years to develop the eating pattern you now have, so have a bit of patience and be confident that you are getting healthier every day. In fact, you may find that you are perfectly content to make the Stage I diet your lifetime plan. It is not necessary to do all three stages in order to become an intuitive eater.

As a helpful guideline, I usually suggest that you work with Stage I and Stage II for 4-6 months each. As with Stage I, once you've moved on to Stage II you may find that this diet is ideal for you, and choose to stay there. Many people design their own diets from a combination of Stage I and Stage II recommendations. I encourage you to be as creative as you wish. Look ahead to the recipes in Stage III even, and use them as you feel inclined.

Observing The Time Of Day For Optimal Digestion: Optimal digestion will generally take place between 10 a.m. and 2 p.m. Yet, I find that I feel better when I eat my meals between noon and 4 p.m. So, I suggest that as you begin this transition into Stage I you experiment to find out what works best for you.

Eating a heavy meal at night is usually not a good idea. The digestive system slows down at night and prepares to go into a cleansing cycle. Therefore, most foods eaten late will remain undigested in the intestinal tract. They ferment, byproducts accumulate, and that produces a breeding ground for viruses and bacteria.

Most people will report feeling heavy, sluggish, or even like they are intoxicated on the morning after eating a big meal late at night. I recommend that the evening meal be the lightest meal, particularly if protein is a part of it. Protein acts as a stimulant, and can disturb your sleeping patterns.

Dealing With Old Habits And Cravings: As you enter each stage you will be giving up certain foods and adding others. Stage I, for instance, decreases the amount of protein and fat—it drops off red meat, preservatives, pork, white sugar, white flour, junk foods. It limits dairy products, coffee, tea, alcohol, carbonated soft drinks, and cuts back on beverages with meals. At the same time it adds freshly-made juices.

During your dietary changes you may experience cravings for some of your old foods, especially those that had emotional value to you—like sweets or pasta, etc. Don't make this a problem. It's normal to have cravings. You are human, and humans need time to adapt. Try to avoid putting a lot of time or energy into resisting your cravings. Instead, put that energy into making one of the dessert recipes included in the meal plans at the end of the chapter. You can even make a whole meal out of this dessert, enough to satisfy any sweet tooth. For quick snacks use figs, dates, or other sweet fruits. If you want a pizza, for instance, make one with a whole-grain crust, and top it with vegetables like peppers, onions, tomatoes, etc. Finally, if nothing else seems to work, eat a small amount of the food you crave, even though it might not be so good for you. If your diet is 90% wholesome, going off a little bit won't hurt you as long as you don't make it a habit.

Using Cleansing And Other Healing Methods To Deal With Any Crises: Since you will be eating more raw food than you may be used to, the added enzymes and nutrients in your new diet will sometimes cause a cleansing effect and may precipitate a health crisis as described in Chapter 7. If you begin to feel sluggish, congested, constipated, or even experience a slight fever or cold, you can begin to use some of the healing modalities suggested in that chapter. These procedures, especially the use of herbs and juices, should be referred to throughout all three stages.

For example: During your first year on a meatless diet it is not uncommon to feel a bit colder than usual—even on days when it's warm and the sun is shining. This is because the circulation is clogged up with waste products that the body is starting to clean out. Once the bloodstream and cells are purified, vitality and health will manifest. Then, even on the coldest days you will be comfortable, and even warm, since your bloodstream will be operating at peak efficiency.

I remember always feeling cold when I was a heavy meat-eater and dairy-user. My bloodstream was laden with mucous and congestion. After many years of cleansing and the use of a vegetarian diet, I noticed that even in those Buffalo, N.Y. winters I stopped getting cold. Hundreds of people who have tested these transitional diets over the years have had a similar experience.

If you do feel the cold more acutely at first, use warm soups, and spices (herbs) such as cayenne, cumin, cardamon, curry, ginseng, and ginger. Drink peppermint or spearmint teas during the day.

A Balanced Diet At Every Stage: One additional factor that makes these transitional stages unique is that daily menus are designed for a nutritional balance. Grams of protein, percentages of total fats, fiber, cholesterol, iron, calcium, potassium, vitamin C, vitamin A, sodium, and phosphorus are all calculated to give you exact amounts which usually will exceed the RDA (Recommended Daily Allowance). So, no need to worry. Plus, with the addition of sea vegetables (explained later in this chapter), and juices (see Chapter 9) your diet will be more than minimally nutritious—it will be moving towards ideal!

SET YOUR WEIGHT GOAL FOR THE TRANSITION

As we begin to design our transition into *Intuitive Eating* it will help to establish an initial weight goal. Look at the chart (8.2) that follows and find out what the suggested weight is for your height. (Usually insurance companies make up these charts.) Reduce that chart-weight by approximately 10-20%. That is your goal—where your body will be most efficient.

Make up your recipes daily so they equal between 1600 and 2000 calories. This is your starting point. If you start gaining weight, decrease the calorie intake by 200-500 calories. If you start losing too fast, increase the calories. Weight loss should be gradual to avoid any metabolic disturbances. As long as you feel good, have high energy, and keep weight loss gradual, you shouldn't experience any difficulty.

HEIGHT AND WEIGHT TABLES

To Make an Approximation of Your Frame Size . . . Extend your arm and bend the forearm upward at a 90 degree angle. Keep fingers straight and turn the inside of your wrist toward your body. If you have a caliper, use it to measure the space between the two prominent bones on either side of your elbow. Without a caliper, place thumb and index finger of your other hand on these two bones. Measure the space between your fingers against a ruler or tape measure. Compare it with these tables that list elbow measurements for medium-framed men and women. Measurements lower than those listed indicate you have a small frame. Higher measurements indicate a large frame.

Height in 1" heels MEN	Elbow Breadth	Height in 1" heels WOMEN	Elbow Breadth
5'2"-5'3"	2 1/2"-2 7/8"	4'10"-4'11"	2 1/4"-2 1/2"
5'4"-5'7"	2 5/8"-2 7/8"	5'0"-5'3"	2 1/4"-2 1/2"
5'8"-5'11"	2 3/4"-3"	5'4"-5'7"	2 3/8"-2 5/8"
6'0"-6'3"	2 3/4"-3 1/8"	5'8"-5'11"	2 3/8"-2 5/8"
6'4"	2 7/8"-3 1/4"	6'0"	2 1/2"-2 3/4"

WOMEN

Height	Small Frame	Medium Frame	Large Frame
4'10"	102-111	109-121	118-131
4'11"	103-113	111-123	120-134
5'0"	104-115	113-126	122-137
5'1"	106-118	115-129	125-140
5'2"	108-121	118-132	128-143
5'3"	111-124	121-135	131-147
5'4"	114-127	124-138	134-151
5'5"	117-130	127-141	137-155
5'6"	120-133	130-144	140-159
5'7"	123-136	133-147	143-163
5'8"	126-139	136-150	146-167
5'9"	129-142	139-153	149-170
5'10"	132-145	142-156	152-173
5'11"	135-148	145-159	155-176
6'0"	138-151	148-162	158-179

Note: Weights at ages 25 to 59 based on lowest mortality. Weight in pounds according to frame (in indoor clothing weighing 3 pounds, shoes with 1-inch heels).

Source: Courtesy of Metropolitan Life Insurance Company Statistical Bulletin, 1983.

MEN

Height	Small Frame	Medium Frame	Large Frame
5'2"	128-134	131-141	138-150
5'3"	130-136	133-143	140-153
5'4"	132-138	135-145	142-156
5'5"	134-140	137-148	144-160
5'6"	136-142	139-151	146-164
5'7"	138-145	142-154	149-168
5'8"	140-148	145-157	152-172
5'9"	142-151	148-160	155-176
5'10"	144-154	151-163	158-180
5'11"	146-157	154-166	161-184
6'0"	149-160	157-170	164-188
6'1"	152-164	160-174	168-192
6'2"	155-168	164-178	172-197
6'3"	158-172	167-182	176-202
6'4"	162-176	171-187	181-207

Note: Weights at ages 25 to 59 based on lowest mortality. Weight in pounds according to frame (in indoor clothing weighing 5 pounds, shoes with 1-inch heels).

Source: Courtesy of Metropolitan Life Insurance Company Statistical Bulletin, 1983.

When you find your best weight, and feel your best, stay at that calorie intake. Sometimes finding your ideal weight may take from one to three years, or longer if you are ill or obese. If you are already at your ideal weight, count your calories and stay at that level. You may find that you will need more calories if you are exercising. Watch the fat intake. The foods that contain fat should be live foods, and they should only be 8-15% of the total calorie intake. Twenty grams of protein is usually all that is necessary. I suggest getting a complete medical exam before undertaking any dietary plan.

BALANCING YOUR pH (Acid-Based Balance)

It is important to check the pH of your urine so as to maintain a normal functioning metabolism, especially while transitioning to a vegetarian-based diet. When we change our food intake, both the quality and quantity, the acid-based balance of the body also may change. Diseased cells find it easier to live in a system where it's either too acid or too alkaline.

Generally, if a diet consists of too many acid foods, like dairy, meat, beans, fats, poultry, cooked grains, and protein, the body will become too acidic. Eating unripe fruit can be acid-forming also because the fruit was not left in the soil long enough to absorb all the alkaline minerals. Most synthetic vitamins are acidifying, especially ascorbic acid, which is not a complete vitamin C supplement. (A good vitamin C supplement is one that contains bioflavinoid.) If we eat too many alkaline foods, like fruits and vegetables, and drink an overabundance of fruit and vegetable juices, we will become too alkaline. Nutritionists have agreed that the diet should be 80% alkaline foods and 20% acid foods. (Consult the chart (8.3) in this section to determine which ones are acid and which are alkaline.) Ultimately, each person must find his/her own balance, which may be a little different from the generic percentages. Also, during times of stress, exercise, or during the menstrual cycle, the pH may vary. So, during these times, it's good to check it. Basically, you only have to check the pH once a week unless you're going through some type of illness where you have to monitor your pH daily.

Digestion is the first line of defense. A person who eats a vegetarian diet which consists of plenty of complex carbohydrates usually has an alkaline urine. If there is acid it means that the digestive system is not properly releasing the alkaline minerals, like calcium, magnesium, potassium, and sodium, from the carbohydrate foods. If proteins (which consist of phosphorous, sulphuric acid, and amino acids) are too heavy in the diet, the urine will be too acid. If a person is eating protein and is not digesting it, the urine can still be too acid from the putrefaction of too much protein in the digestive tract. In all of the above situations there is sometimes a need to take plant enzyme supplements to aid digestion. They are usually taken just before sitting down to eat a meal.

The system of urine testing that I use was taught to me by Dr. Howard Loomis. Collect a large bottle full of urine from several samples over a 24-hour period. Use a dark glass bottle to store the collected urine, and keep the bottle in a brown paper bag in the refrigerator, during the day of collecting. To test it, purchase some pH paper (litmus paper) from your drugstore or health food store. The paper should have a range on it from between 5.5 to 8.0. If you need to order your own litmus paper, contact: Micro Essential Laboratory, Inc., Brooklyn, NY 11210.

To test, dip the paper into the urine. Check the readout based on the instructions that will accompany the paper. It's good to check the pH of your urine once a week for the first month of each transitional stage. Then check it once every two weeks until you get to the dietary stage you wish to remain at. When at that final stage, once a month is all that is necessary.

Usually, a normal pH is between 6.3 and 6.9. Remember that 7.0 is neutral; above 7.0 is alkaline, and below 7.0 is acid. If you are a vegetarian, your urinary pH may be between 6.3 and 7.2. This would be healthy and normal for you, if you feel good. I have seen plenty of healthy vegetarians with a 7.0 to 7.2 urinary pH. But below 6.3 is too acid.

If you are *too acid*, add more vegetable juices, and raw fruits and vegetables to your diet to balance the pH, and decrease the amount of protein and fats in your diet. If this doesn't work, you're probably not digesting your food properly, so you might want to add plant enzymes or consult a physician. Constipation or stress could be the problem.

If you are *too alkaline*, usually above 7.2 for long periods of time, protein digestion may be faulty, or you might not be eating enough protein. In that case, add more protein and digestive enzymes to your diet. One of Paul Bragg's favorite methods of acidifying the urine is to add 1 teaspoon of apple-cider vinegar to a cup of distilled water; drink 1/2 hour before meals, two or three times a day until the pH is normal. You can also use cranberry juice, fermented foods like sauerkraut, or tofu. Make sure you are getting plenty of exercise, since exercise produces lactic acid, which will help acidify the body.

Don't worry if your pH bounces around between 6.3 and 7.0, or is over or under once or twice. If you have a constant acid, or a constant alkaline, urine for three to seven days, then a change would be called for.

Some of the symptoms of being too acid are arthritis, stiffness, headaches, dull mentality, depression, tension in the back of the neck and shoulders, acid stomach, gastritis and canker sores.

An over-alkaline system produces symptoms of nervousness, cramps, spasms, that "spaced-out" feeling, and insomnia.

Once you've found your balance, you will intuitively feel when you are too acid or too alkaline. Use this Acid-Alkaline chart as a handy reference as often as needed.

ALKALINE FORMING FOODS

Dairy Products

Acidophilus, Buttermilk, Milk (Raw), Whey, Yogurt

Nuts

Almonds, Chesnuts, Coconuts

Miscellaneous

Algae, Agar, Alfalfa Product, Baking Soda, Coffee Substitutes, Dried Ginger, Ginseng, Honey, Kelp, Molasses, Salt, Soy Sauce, Teas, Umeboshi, Yeast Cakes

Vegetables

Artichokes, Asparagus, Bamboo Shoots, Beans (all types) Beets and Tops, Broccoli, Cabbage, Carrots, Celery, Cauliflower, Chard, Chicory, Chives, Collars, Cucumber, Dandelion Greens, Dill, Dulse, Eggplant, Endive, Escarole, Garlic, Horseradish, Jerusalem Artichokes, Kale, Kohlrabi, Leeks, Legumes, Lettuce, Mushrooms, Okra, Onions, Parsley, Parsnips, Peppers, Potatoes, Pumpkin, Radish, Rhubarb, Rutabaga, Sauerkraut, Sorrel, Soy Beans, Spinach, Squash, Taro (baked), Turnips, Water Chestnuts, Watercress

Fruits

Apples, Apricots, Avocados, Bananas, Berries (all), Breadfruit, Cactus, Cantaloupe, Carob, Cherries, Citron, Currants, Dates, Figs, Grapes, Grapefruit, Guavas, Kumquats, Lemons, Limes, Mangos, Melons (all), Nectarines, Olives, Oranges, Papayas, Passion Fruit, Peaches, Pears, Persimmons, Pineapple, Pomegranates, Quince, Raisins, Tangerines, Tomatoes

CHART 8.3

ACID FORMING FOODS

All Meat
Poultry, Fish, Beef, Shellfish

Nuts
All Roasted Nuts, Coconut (dried), Peanuts

Miscellaneous
All Alcoholic Beverages, Candy, Cocoa and Chocolate, Coca Cola, Coffee, Dressings, Thick Sauces, Drugs and Aspirin, Jams and Jellies, Flavorings, Marmalade, Mayonnaise, Preservatives (Benzoate, Salt, Smoke, Sulphur, Vinegar), Sago, Soda Water, Tobacco, Vanilla, Vinegar

Whole Grains/Cereals
All Flour Products, Buckwheat, Barley, Breads (all kinds), Cakes, Corn (Cornmeal, Corn Flakes, Hominy), Crackers (all), Doughnuts, Dumplings, Macaroni and Spaghetti, Noodles, Oatmeal, Pies and Pastry, Rice, Rye-Krisp

Neutral Foods
Butter, Lard, Oils, Sugar (white), Ginger

Fruits
All Preserved or Jellied, Canned, Sugared, Dried, Sulphured, Glazed Fruits, Cranberries, Prunes, Plums

Milk
Boiled, Cooked or Pasteurized, Malted, Dried or Canned, Ice Cream, Cream, Cheese (all)

FOOD COMBINING FOR OPTIMAL DIGESTION

Combining foods properly, following nature's laws, is one of the most beneficial things you can do for your health and well-being. The principle behind food combining is that certain classes of food require different enzymes, different rates of digestion, and different pH's for proper digestion. Cooperating with the body's natural digestive processes will help you to optimize digestion, build strength and stamina, conserve energy, and strengthen your immune system.

RULES TO AID DIGESTION

1. Fruits and vegetables should always be eaten at separate meals. Eat only one concentrated protein food or starch at a meal.
2. Drink your fresh vegetable or fruit juices 30 minutes before your meals. Otherwise, avoid drinking liquids 30 minutes before meals, during meals, and for one to two hours following meals as liquids dilute the digestive juices and hinder digestion.
3. Avoid drinking liquids which are too cold (out of the refrigerator or with ice) or too hot (close to the boiling point) since the temperature extremes stress the digestive system and may cause indigestion.
4. Since most dessert items do not combine well with foods eaten at meals, it is best to avoid them or eat the desserts suggested in the recipe section as a full meal.
5. Eat only when hungry.
6. Avoid eating immediately before or after strenuous exercise.
7. Avoid eating when under physical or mental distress.
8. Thoroughly chew all foods and juices.
9. Avoid overeating.
10. Avoid eating three to four hours before retiring to bed. Especially avoid eating fruit or drinking fruit juices at night as it is very stimulating and can cause a wakeful, unpleasant night's sleep.

11. Monitor your digestive efficiency by analyzing your stool after a bowel movement. This may sometimes indicate enzyme deficiency. If your stool is too heavy to float, greasy with undigested fats and other foods, and has a light green color, like okra, this usually means that there is some type of a digestive disturbance, and I suggest using enzymes.

Another important fact is the transit time your food takes from the time you eat it to the time it passes out of the lower colon. To determine this, take 3-5 charcoal tablets (usually a health food store or drug store carries these) with a meal, and check to see what time it is. You should see the charcoal in your stool between 20-25 hours later. If it takes longer or shorter (10-15 hours), your diet is incorrect in some way. You may be using improper food combinations, have a digestive difficulty, lack enough fiber in your diet, or have an enzyme deficiency. Using the food combination chart that follows will remedy many of these conditions. Consult a physician or health-care practitioner if the problems persist.

The chart 8.4 is a food-combining chart to help you prepare the best meals for yourself and your family.

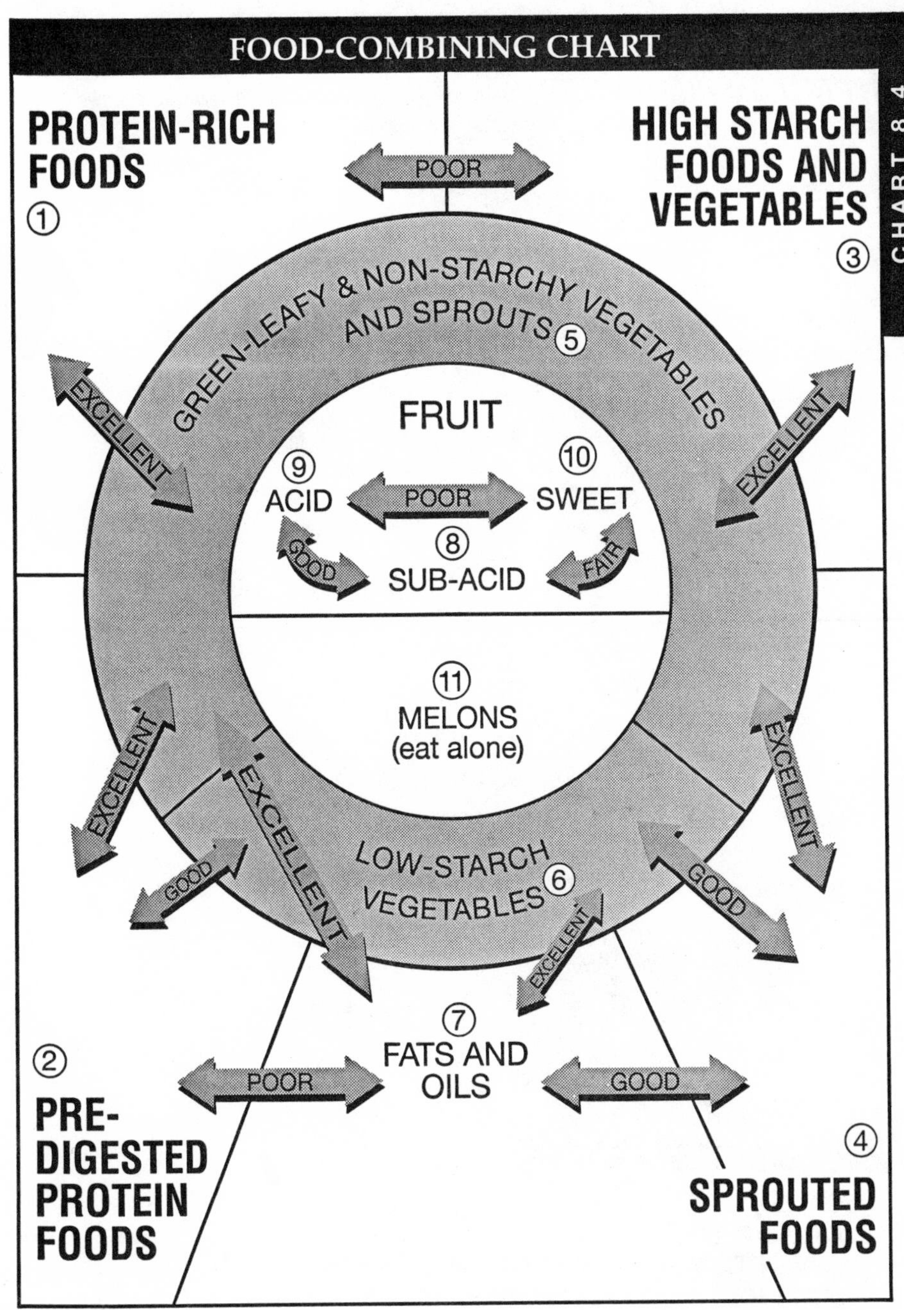
FOOD-COMBINING CHART
CHART 8.4
PROTEIN-RICH FOODS ①
HIGH STARCH FOODS AND VEGETABLES ③
POOR
GREEN-LEAFY & NON-STARCHY VEGETABLES AND SPROUTS ⑤
EXCELLENT
EXCELLENT
FRUIT
⑨ ACID
POOR
⑩ SWEET
GOOD
⑧ SUB-ACID
FAIR
⑪ MELONS (eat alone)
EXCELLENT
EXCELLENT
EXCELLENT
LOW-STARCH VEGETABLES ⑥
GOOD
GOOD
EXCELLENT
⑦ FATS AND OILS
POOR
GOOD
② PRE-DIGESTED PROTEIN FOODS
④ SPROUTED FOODS

CHART 8.4 EXPLANATION

1. PROTEIN-RICH FOODS *(Combines best with leafy green and non-starchy vegetables)*

DAIRY **

EGGS **

FISH **

MEAT *

MILK (COW'S) *

NUTS: *(raw)*

- Acorns
- Almonds
- Beechnuts
- Brazil Nuts
- Butternuts
- Candlenuts
- Cashews
- Chestnuts, dried
- Filberts
- Hazelnuts
- Hickory Nuts (Carya)
- Macadamia Nuts
- Pecans
- Pignolias
- Pine Nuts
- Pistachios
- Walnuts (English & Black)

POULTRY **

SEEDS: *(raw)*

- Chia
- Flaxseed
- Pumpkin
- Sesame
- Sunflower

MISCELLANEOUS:

- Brewer's Yeast **
- Miso
- Nutritional Yeast
- Olives
- Peanuts * (very difficult to digest)
- Soybeans
- Soymilk
- Tempeh
- Tofu
- TVP (texturized vegetable protein)

2. PREDIGESTED PROTEIN

SOAKED NUTS

SOAKED SEEDS

FERMENTED NUT SAUCES, YOGURT, AND CHEESE

FERMENTED SEED SAUCES, YOGURT, AND CHEESE

** Not Recommended*

*** Use in Stages One and Two Only*

CHART 8.4 EXPLANATION

3. HIGH STARCH CONTENT FOODS AND SUGARS

(Combines best with leafy green and non-starchy vegetables)

BREAD

CEREALS AND GRAINS: *(cooked)*

Barley
Buckwheat
Corn
Millet
Oat
Rice, Brown or Wild
Rye
Sorghum
Wheat

DRIED BEANS AND PEAS: *(cooked)*

Azuki Beans
Chick Peas (Garbanzos)
Green Peas
Kidney Beans
Lima Beans
Pinto Beans

PASTAS: **

Artichoke
Corn
Spinach
Whole Wheat
Vegetable

POPCORN

STARCHY VEGETABLES: *(Cooked or Raw)*

Acorn Squash
Banana Squash
Butternut Squash
Corn (fresh, mature)
Hubbard Squash
Potatoes
Pumpkin
Split Peas
Squashes (winter)
Sweet Potatoes
Yams

SYRUPS AND SUGARS: *

Brown Sugar
Candy
Cane Sugar or Syrup
Carob, Roasted or Raw **
Chocolate
Date Sugar
Fructose
Honey, Raw **
Maple Syrup **
Molasses **
White Sugar

MISCELLANEOUS:

Corn Germ **
Wheat Germ **

** Not Recommended*
*** Use in Stages One and Two Only*

CHART 8.4 EXPLANATION

4. SPROUTED STARCH FOODS

CEREALS AND GRAINS: Buckwheat
Rye
Wheat

DRIED BEANS AND PEAS: Adzuki Beans
Chick Peas (Garbanzos)
Green Peas
Kidney Beans
Pinto Beans

LEGUMES: Lentils
Red Lentils

BREADS: Essene Bread
Sprouted Grain Breads

5. GREEN, LEAFY AND NON-STARCHY VEGETABLES

(Combines best with proteins, fats and oils, starches or starchy vegetables)

Cooked or raw:

Asparagus
Bamboo shoots
Beet tops (greens)
Bok choy
Broccoli
Brussel sprouts
Buckwheat lettuce
Cabbage *(white, red Chinese)
Celery
Chives
Collard greens
Corn (fresh and young)
Cucumbers
Dandelion greens
Eggplant
Endive
Escarole
Garlic
Green beans (fresh)
Green peas (fresh)
Jerusalem artichoke
Kale
Kohlrabi
Leafy greens
Leeks
Lettuces:
- Bibb
- Boston
- Leaf
- Romaine

Mint
Mullein
Mushrooms
Mustard greens
Okra
Onions
Parsley
Peppers (red, sweet, green)
Radish greens
Rhubarb
Scallions
Seaweeds:
- Dulse
- Kelp
- Nori
- Wakame, etc.

Sorrel
Spinach
Squashes (summer)
Swiss chard
Turnips
Watercress
Wax beans (yellow)
Wheat grass
Zucchini

SPROUTS: *(do not cook)*

Alfalfa
Cabbage
Fenugreek
Lentil
Mung bean
Mustard seed
Onion
Radish
Red clover
Sunflower greens

** Not Recommended*
*** Use in Stages One and Two Only*

CHART 8.4 EXPLANATION

6. LOW-STARCH VEGETABLES

Artichokes
Beets
Burdock
Carrots
Cauliflower
Corn *(young and sweet)*
Parsnip
Rutabaga
Salsify
Water Chestnut

7. FATS AND OILS

(Combines best with leafy green and non-starchy vegetables)

Avocados

FATS: * Butter
Cream
Fat Meats *
Lard *
Margarine, Vegetable *
Tallow *

Hydrogenated Oils *

OILS: *(cold-pressed oils only)*

Canola oil
Cottonseed oil
Corn oil
Nut oils
Olive oil
Safflower oil
Sesame oil
Soy oil
Sunflower oil

8. SUB-ACID FRUITS

(Combines fairly with acid fruits)

Apples
Apricots
Blackberries
Blueberries
Cherimoyas
Fresh figs
Grapes
Guavas
Huckleberries
Kiwi fruits
Loquat
Mangoes
Mulberries
Nectarines
Papayas
Pears
Prickly pears
Raspberries
Sweet cherries
Sweet peaches
Sweet plums

** Not Recommended*
*** Use in Stages One and Two Only*

heavy protein consumption. Moreover, the high phosphorous content of protein foods causes a lowering of calcium in the blood, and this leads to calcium loss from the bones. (See the food charts in the Appendix to see which foods are high in calcium.) When one starts lowering the protein content and increasing the amounts of vegetables and fruits in the diet, blood calcium normalizes, and calcium loss from bones is diminished.

Another concern for vegetarians has been the effect of oxalates in spinach. It has been thought that oxalates bind with calcium and therefore inhibit its absorption. In one study a group of children ate spinach and other high-oxalate foods, but no evidence was found that these foods caused calcium, vitamin B, or phosphorous difficulties[1].

Phytates, naturally-occuring substances in wheat, rye, oats, and in some seeds and nuts, were also once thought to be a problem. The phytates bind with calcium and inhibit its absorption. In a normally-functioning intestinal tract, however, an enzyme called phytase releases calcium that was bound to phytates, and makes it available for absorption. Another way to eliminate the "phytate problem" is to soak the seeds, nuts, and grains overnight and then wash them thoroughly in the morning. Sprouting foods, which we will discuss in Stage 3, is another excellent way to increase calcium absorption.

ZINC

Phytates may once again be a problem when it comes to zinc absorption. Phytates in grain result in low zinc levels if there is a deficiency in the enzyme *phytase* in the intestinal tract. The key to keeping a normal phytase level is to keep a normally functioning intestinal tract. This is done by using a low protein, low dairy, high fiber, and high fruit and vegetable diet. Such a diet helps keep the bowels regular, and decreases putrefaction and bacteria in the intestines.

During the transition to a vegetable-based diet, it is good to notice what foods are high in zinc, and to capitalize on them through each stage of your dietary change. High zinc foods include: pumpkin seeds, wheat germ, yeast (use small amounts of yeast if you are going to use it), grains such as amaranth, corn, quinoa, and brown rice. Most nuts and legumes contain some zinc, as do vegetables like yams, spinach, parsley, mushrooms, endive and green peas. Sprouting grains eliminates the phytic acid, and can help increase the absorption of zinc.

I suggest that pregnant women, children, athletes, or those experiencing illness pay close attention to using foods high in zinc. Zinc is a crucial element during the healing process. Research verified that using 150 mg. of zinc sulphate daily, healed stomach ulcers in humans twice as fast as placebos did[2]. At UCLA, women who were given zinc supplements for hypertension had less high blood pressure problems and toxemia[3].

Since zinc is involved in all new cell growth, zinc- deficient animals have a reduced ability to heal. In one study a group of older adults was given 220 mg. of zinc sulphate twice daily, over a one-month period. This resulted in an overall increase of disease-resistant factors, such as T-lymphocytes, in their blood.[4]

IRON

To be sure that there is enough iron in your diet, certain measures can be taken. Use foods that are high in iron. Grains such as amaranth, corn meal (whole grain), quinoa, rice; legumes such as aduzi beans, kidney beans, navy beans, lentils; and vegetables such as dandelions, spinach, peas, beans, and green kale are all good sources. Sesame seeds also contain a supply of iron. Proper absorption of iron, however, requires that it be complemented with vitamin C, which is naturally contained in fruits and vegetables. The iron in vegetarian foods was absorbed four times better than the iron in flesh foods, as long as there is at least 65 mg. of vitamin C accompanying the iron. Interestingly enough, most vegetable foods that contain iron also contain adequate amounts of vitamin C.

Dairy products are low in vitamin C, and can inhibit iron absorption. Coffee and tea can decrease iron uptake because the tannic acid in these substances binds with iron. The *American*

Journal of Clinical Nutrition reported that vegetarian women who were regularly menstruating had higher levels of iron than non-vegetarian women of the same age.[5] I believe that anemia is prevalent because our diets contain too much cooked food and too many dairy products, coffee and tea, and not enough raw fruits and vegetables. Dr. Rudolph Balentine's book, *Transition To A Vegetarian Diet*[6], cites a study in which 56 vegetarian women were tested for their iron hemoglobin levels. As I would have suspected, the vegetarian women had much higher hemoglobin levels than did women who followed the "traditional American" diet. Balentine also showed that prolonged use of supplements was not the best solution to a low-iron problem. Progressively higher dosages of iron, when given to pregnant women, resulted in higher levels of iron in the blood, but lower levels of zinc, copper, and selenium. Iron supplements are thought to compete, somehow, with these essential minerals and inhibit their absorption through the intestinal tract.

At first, it is vital to know what foods contain what vitamins and minerals. We can then maintain our health by keeping these foods in our diet. Besides, it is a more scientific way of eating. As you practice *Intuitive Eating* as a way of life, however, you won't have to study a chart to determine what vitamins or minerals you need. Your tastes and feelings will naturally lead you in the right direction.

VITAMIN B12

The question of whether vegetarians get enough B12 is an important one. Symptoms of B12-deficiency are: loss of feeling in the fingers and toes, poor balance, joint pain, constant fatigue and irritability, depression, memory loss, and sometimes even hallucinations. Actually, my research has shown that vegetarians have less to fear about B12-deficiency than do meat-eaters. In fact, meat-eaters have *more* to fear, because of the problems with meat, plus the fact that most of their food is cooked. B12 is heat-sensitive. Research has shown that 24-96% of B12 is destroyed by boiling and baking[7].

Dr. Gabriel Cousens, in his new book *Conscious Eating*, says that vegetarians absorb B12 better than meat-eaters[8]. The meat-eaters might ingest 10 micrograms of B12 daily and yet only absorb 16%, while the vegans (they are people who eat strictly fruits and vegetables and no dairy) might ingest only 1 microgram daily and absorb 70% of the B12.

Past research showing that vegetarians develop B12-deficiencies is incomplete. Cousens' book quotes research from Dr. Immerman[9] showing that the research on this subject in the last 30 years has uncovered no evidence that vegans develop B12-deficiencies. He further states that none of the previous studies used scientific criteria for defining a legitimate B12-deficiency. Since vegans are vegetarians who do not eat dairy products, they should stand more of a chance of a B12-deficiency than natural vegetarians who use dairy, or lacto-oval vegetarians, who use eggs and dairy. But the research doesn't show this.

Dr. Scott, who has been observing vegetarians for 42 years, along with Dr. Gabriel Cousens and myself, all agree that just because meat-eaters have higher levels of B12 in their bodies doesn't mean that the vegetarians with low levels are unhealthy. I would much rather be healthy with a lower level of B12 than run the risk of heart-disease and cancer from meat products just to have a higher level of B12. All in all, the criteria (R.D.A. of B12) for vegetarians should be different from that of meat-eaters. Vegetarians simply don't need as high a level of some nutrients, particularly B12. The metabolism, physiology, and needs of a vegetarian's body are totally different than those of a heavy meat and protein eater. Why should a blood profile from a heavy protein eater be used to determine the criteria for a healthy vegetarian? Looking at this from the other side, vegetarians usually have lower levels of cholesterol and triglycerides than meat eaters. So, if one were to use the vegetarian standards for cholesterol and triglycerides, the meat eaters would be in serious trouble. In fact, they would probably be an endangered species.

We have already considered that a medium-low carbohydrate low-protein diet is healthy. Vegans who live on raw foods, moreover, have less hydrochloric acid and enzymes in the digestive tract because these are not needed to digest heavy proteins, and because the raw food already contains enzymes that help digestion. (See Chapter 5 on Enzymes.)

The body adapts to different diets. So, depending upon what you eat, massive amounts of some nutrients are not always needed. As long as our food is good, we will stay healthy. Vegetarians need not feel threatened any longer by standards that really don't apply to them.

B12 is naturally produced by a bacteria in plants and animals. It is not made by plants and animals, but by a bacteria they contain. Humans have B12 throughout the body—between the teeth, in the gums, tonsils, and saliva. (This is one reason why it's so important not to remove the tonsils of a child.) B12 is produced in the small intestine. It begins its absorption in the stomach when it is split from foods by hydrochloric acid and enzymes. Then it combines with a secretion called "the intrinsic factor for absorption." Stomach secretion must be normal, and all other factors must be right for the B12 absorption. Because of poor eating habits, however, like too much sugar, fruit, protein, alcohol, and coffee, problems can arise. Candida, for instance, is a problem that can upset the B12 balance. (To reestablish good digestion, one must always go back to the proper diet, and sometimes use different cleansing methods or fasting.)

Proper B12 absorption also requires a properly functioning pancreas, because the pancreas secretes enzymes into the small intestine which help digest and aid in the absorption of nutrients. The functioning of the liver and gallbladder will also affect B12 absorption.

Approximately 1 to 10 micrograms of B12 are secreted into the bowel and then into the small intestine daily. We need less than 0.5 micrograms per day. In Dr. Gabriel Cousens' book[10], he reports that 0.2 to 0.25 micrograms daily of B12 is adequate for any individual, and that there is no published research showing that any more is required for health. Cousens also asserts that more B12 is produced in the intestines of vegetarians than in most meat-eaters.

Some of the most popular food sources for B12 are sea vegetables such as nori, wakame, kelp, alaria, and dulse. Other food sources are super blue-green algae, chrorella, nutritional yeast, and plain yogurt. Dr. Scott uses unsalted goat's-milk cheese to help establish B12-evidence in some people. Many practitioners, including Victoras Kulvinskas, author of *Love Your Body*[11], and *Survival Into The 21st Century*[12], Dr. Gabriel Cousens, and myself, have been using super blue-green algae (one gram contains .279 micrograms of B12) to support our B12 intake. This has worked exceptionally well for me.

Additional sea vegetables can easily be added to the diet by putting them in salads, taking them in capsule form, or blending them into juice or smoothies. Also, if you are concerned about B12, iron and/or calcium, seaweeds contain all of the above, plus 56 other minerals. I usually recommend that everybody add sea vegetables to their diet because they contain 20 more minerals than vegetables grown in the soil. Since our soil is so deficient in trace minerals, we must go to the sea to get the added ones. Sea vegetables also protect us from exposure to radioactive elements.

STAGE ONE MENUS

In the pages that follow I suggest a sample dietary plan that you can use to implement Stage I. The plan contains sample recipes as well. Feel free to adapt it to your personal needs. You will find recipes for healthy desserts (treats) in the final pages of Chapter 10. Happy eating!

SEVEN DAY MEAL PLAN FOR STAGE I

• MENU FOR DAY ONE •

BREAKFAST

ORANGE BANANA JUICE*
4 GRAIN CEREAL
BLUEBERRY BANANA MUFFIN

LUNCH

TOMATO COCKTAIL JUICE DRINK
JULIANNA SALAD

LUNCH SNACK

RICE CAKE WITH BLUEBERRY SPREAD*

DINNER

CARROT-SPINACH-APPLE JUICE
TOMATO-CUCUMBER SALAD
DAWN'S BROCCOLI LASAGNA

**indicates no recipe included*

NUTRIENTS	
Protein (gm)	61
Total Fat (gm)	55
Complex Carb (gm)	187
Dietary Fiber (gm)	34
Cholesterol (mg)	110
Sodium (mg)	2462
Potassium (mg)	4149
Vitamin A (RE)	6705
Vitamin C (mg)	174
Iron (mg)	22
Calcium (mg)	1064
Phosphorus (mg)	1443

TOTAL DAILY CALORIES 1674

30% OF CALORIES ARE FROM FAT

RECIPES

4 GRAIN CEREAL

1/2 CUP	BULGUR, DRY
1 CUP	OLD-FASHIONED OATS
1/4 CUP	CORN FLOUR
2 TABLESPOONS	FLAX SEED
1/4 CUP	SEEDLESS RAISINS,
1/2 TEASPOON	GROUND CINNAMON
4 CUPS	WATER
1/4 TEASPOON	SEA SALT
1 CUP	SOYBEAN MILK
4 TABLESPOONS	HONEY

Bring all ingredients except cinnamon to a boil in a 2 quart pot. Cook 7-10 minutes, stirring occasionally. Cover, simmer on low for 15-20 minutes, stirring occasionally. Stir in cinnamon 5 min. before serving. Serve with soy milk and honey or maple syrup to taste. Serves 4.

BLUEBERRY BANANA MUFFINS

3	BANANAS
1	BROWN, FERTILE EGG
1/3 CUP	UNSWEETENED APPLESAUCE
1/3 CUP	PLAIN, NONFAT YOGURT
2/3 CUP	HONEY
1 TEASPOON	PURE VANILLA EXTRACT
3/4 CUP	WHOLE WHEAT FLOUR
1 3/4 CUPS	OATS
2 TEASPOONS	BAKING POWDER
1 TEASPOON	BAKING SODA
1 TEASPOON	GROUND CINNAMON
1/8 TEASPOON	SEA SALT
2 CUPS	BLUEBERRIES, FRESH OR FROZEN

Preheat oven to 375° F. Oil muffin cups (or use muffin liners). Cream first 6 ingredients in blender or food processor. In large bowl, combine dry ingredients. Make a well in center, fold in creamed mixture with spatula until dry ingredients are moistened. Carefully fold in blueberries. Spoon batter into cups; bake about 30 minutes or until toothpick inserted in center comes out clean. Cool on wire rack. Makes 12 muffins. Serves 12.

JULIANNA SALAD

2 CUPS	COARSELY CHOPPED (OR TORN) ROMAINE LETTUCE
2 CUPS	COARSELY CHOPPED (OR TORN) LOOSELEAF LETTUCE
1/2 CUP	SHREDDED CARROTS
1/2 CUP	SLICED CUCUMBER
1	TOMATO, QUARTERED
6 PIECES	SWISS CHEESE, CUT INTO 1" CUBES
6 PIECES	CHEDDAR CHEESE, CUT INTO 1" CUBES
1/2 CUP	TURKEY, COOKED WHITE MEAT WITHOUT SKIN, DICED
1/4 CUP	CHOPPED SCALLIONS
1/2 CUP	PRITIKIN, NO OIL, LOW SODIUM RUSSIAN SALAD DRESSING

Assemble all salad ingredients together, toss with salad dressing. Serves 4.

CARROT-SPINACH-APPLE JUICE

5	CARROTS
1	APPLE
1 CUP	SPINACH LEAVES

Wash produce, remove carrot tops, cut carrots and apple to fit opening of juicer. When juicing spinach, bunch the leaves into a small ball, followed by either a carrot or apple. Serves 2.

TOMATO-CUCUMBER SALAD

4	TOMATOES
2	CUCUMBERS, SLICED
1/2 CUP	CHOPPED ONIONS
2	GARLIC CLOVES, MINCED
1/4 CUP	OLIVE OIL
1/8 CUP	APPLE CIDER VINEGAR
1 TEASPOON	GROUND OREGANO
1 TEASPOON	GROUND BASIL

Quarter tomatoes, then cut each quarter into four pieces. Put in large salad bowl with all other ingredients. Toss well, let marinate for at least one hour. Serves 4.

DAWN'S BROCCOLI LASAGNA

1 PACKAGE	WHOLE WHEAT LASAGNA
1 POUND	SOFT OR FIRM TOFU
2	BROWN FERTILE EGGS
1/2 TEASPOON	SEA SALT
1/2 CUP	CHOPPED PARSLEY
1/4 TEASPOON	BLACK PEPPER
1/2 TEASPOON	GROUND NUTMEG
1/2 TEASPOON	GARLIC POWDER
1 CUP	GRATED PARMESAN CHEESE
10 OUNCES	FROZEN CHOPPED BROCCOLI
1 TABLESPOON	OLIVE OIL
1/2 CUP	CHOPPED ONION
1	SWEET RED PEPPER, DICED
3 CUPS	SLICED MUSHROOMS
4 CUPS	SPAGHETTI SAUCE WITH MUSHROOMS
2 TABLESPOONS	GRATED PARMESAN CHEESE

Prepare lasagna noodles according to package directions for al dente consistency. Drain, rinse under cold water and lay on clean towels. Cover with another towel to prevent drying. To prepare tofu filling, put drained and crumbled tofu in large bowl. Add eggs, salt, parsley, ground pepper, nutmeg, garlic powder, and parmesan cheese. Mix until well blended. Set aside. In large skillet, saute garlic, onions, red pepper, and mushrooms in oil until just tender; add to tofu mixture. Steam broccoli until defrosted. Squeeze well to remove excess water; add to tofu-veggie mixture. Mix well. Preheat oven to 350° F. In a 9x13 inch baking dish, spread 1 1/3 cups of sauce over bottom, put 1 layer lasagna noodles on top of sauce. Cover with one-half of tofu-veggie mixture. Repeat layers of sauce, noodles and tofu mixture once more, ending with layer of noodles and 1 1/3 cups sauce on top. Sprinkle with parmesan cheese. Bake uncovered for 45 minutes, then let sit for 10 minutes before cutting. Serve hot. Serves 16.

• MENU FOR DAY TWO •

BREAKFAST

ORANGE JUICE
AMARANTH CEREAL

LUNCH

TOMATO JUICE
VEGETABLE-BARLEY SOUP

DINNER

CARROT JUICE
CAESAR SALAD
BRAISED CELERY
BAKED STUFFED FISH

**indicates no recipe included*

NUTRIENTS	
Protein (gm)	65
Total Fat (gm)	54
Complex Carb (gm)	213
Dietary Fiber (gm)	33
Cholesterol (mg)	153
Sodium (mg)	2540
Potassium (mg)	6252
Vitamin A (RE)	14616
Vitamin C (mg)	445
Iron (mg)	13
Calcium (mg)	655
Phosphorus (mg)	1425

TOTAL DAILY CALORIES 1662

29% OF CALORIES ARE FROM FAT

RECIPES

AMARANTH CEREAL

1/2 CUP	AMARANTH CRUNCH WITH RAISINS CEREAL
1/2 CUP	SOY MILK

Serve cereal with soy milk. Serves 1.

VEGETABLE-BARLEY SOUP

2	MEDIUM-SIZE POTATOES, CUT IN 1" CUBES
2 CUPS	SLICED ZUCHINNI
3	CARROTS, SLICED
4	TOMATOES, QUARTERED
1 CUP	CHOPPED ONIONS
3 STALKS	CELERY, DICED
1/2 POUND	GREEN BEANS, 1" PIECES
1 1/2 QUARTS	WATER
2 TEASPOONS	GROUND BASIL
1 TEASPOON	CHOPPED PARSLEY
3	GARLIC CLOVES, MINCED
1/3 CUP	BARLEY
1/4 TEASPOON	BLACK PEPPER
1/2 TEASPOON	SEA SALT

Puree tomatoes with garlic in blender. Pour into large pot, add onions. Cook for 5 minutes on medium heat. Add water, potatoes, barley, and spices. Cook until barley is almost done. Add all remaining vegetables, cook on low heat until vegetables are just tender. Garnish with sunflower seeds—serve with whole wheat crackers. Serves 4.

CARROT JUICE

12	CARROTS

Wash carrots, remove tops, cut to fit opening of juicer. Serves 2.

CAESAR SALAD

12 CUPS	ROMAINE LETTUCE
2	GARLIC CLOVES, MINCED
1 TEASPOON	WORCHESTERSHIRE SAUCE
1 TABLESPOON	LEMON JUICE
1/4 CUP	OLIVE OIL
1/8 TEASPOON	BLACK PEPPER
1/4 TEASPOON	SEA SALT
1 TEASPOON	DIJON MUSTARD
1 CUP	SEASONED CROUTONS
1/2 CUP	GRATED PARMESAN CHEESE
1/4 CUP	WATER

Wash, dry, and tear lettuce into medium-sized pieces; chill. In large bowl, put minced garlic, lemon juice, olive oil, and water; mash very well together. Add Worchestershire sauce, salt, pepper, dijon mustard, and optional ingredients; mix together well. Add chilled romaine leaves; toss. Sprinkle with parmesan cheese to taste; toss again. Garnish with croutons. (Optional ingredients: 2 anchovies, mashed, and/or 1 raw egg, beaten—mash with olive oil mixture.) Serves 4.

BRAISED CELERY

2 TABLESPOONS	OLIVE OIL
1/4 CUP	WATER
4 CUPS	DICED CELERY
1/2 TEASPOON	GROUND BASIL
1/4 TEASPOON	PAPRIKA

Put oil, water, celery, and basil in saucepan. Cover and cook 20-25 minutes or until crisp-tender. Sprinkle with paprika. Serve immediately. Serves 4.

BAKED STUFFED FISH

4-6 OUNCES	FISH FILLETS, WHITE
1/4 CUP	CHOPPED ONIONS
3	GARLIC CLOVES, MINCED
2 TABLESPOONS	OLIVE OIL
1/2 TEASPOON	GROUND BASIL
1/2 TEASPOON	DRIED ROSEMARY,
1 SLICE	WHOLE WHEAT BREAD, CRUMBLED
2 TABLESPOONS	TAMARI or BRAGGS AMINOES*
3 TABLESPOONS	WATER
1 TABLESPOON	DRY WHITE WINE
1	BROWN FERTILE EGG
1/2 CUP	WATER
1/2 CUP	DRY WHITE WINE
1/8 TEASPOON	PAPRIKA

Wash fillets, pat dry. Heat oil in a small skillet over low heat; add the onion, garlic, basil, rosemary. Stir while cooking until the mixture turns light brown in color and is very aromatic. Add the bread crumbs and mix well. Now add the tamari, 3 tablespoons water, and 1 teaspoon white wine. Allow to cool. Preheat oven to 400° F. In a small bowl, blend egg with the bread crumb stuffing. Place the fillets on cutting board with tail section towards you. Cut a strip (1/2") of the fillet off the top (neck section) to even out the shape. Mince these fillet strips, and mix well with bread crumb stuffing. Place 1 tablespoon of stuffing on the widest section of fillets, then roll towards the tail, securing with 2 toothpicks, one on each side of center seam line. With a very sharp knife, cut along the seam line. In a shallow baking dish, place the fillets cut side down; add 1/2 cup each water and white wine. Sprinkle with paprika. Bake for 30 minutes Serves 4.

* Bragg's Aminoes are available at most health food stores
or call 1-800-446-1990

• MENU FOR DAY THREE •

BREAKFAST

STRAWBERRY-ORANGE JUICE
WHOLE WHEAT PANCAKES

LUNCH

APPLE JUICE
FRESH FRUIT SALAD
FRUIT DIP OR SPREAD

DINNER

APPLE-CELERY JUICE
BOSTON BIBB SALAD
GARLIC DRESSING
STIR-FRIED CHICKEN AND VEGETABLES

**indicates no recipe included*

NUTRIENTS	
Protein (gm)	50
Total Fat (gm)	56
Complex Carb (gm)	266
Dietary Fiber (gm)	51
Cholesterol (mg)	54
Sodium (mg)	1045
Potassium (mg)	4357
Vitamin A (RE)	1391
Vitamin C (mg)	315
Iron (mg)	14
Calcium (mg)	700
Phosphorus (mg)	1470

TOTAL DAILY CALORIES 1873

27% OF CALORIES ARE FROM FAT

RECIPES

STRAWBERRY-ORANGE JUICE

1 CUP	STRAWBERRIES
2	ORANGES

Peel oranges, leaving as much white as possible. Cut to fit opening of juicer. Wash and rinse strawberries. Feed fruit through juicer. Serves 2.

WHOLE WHEAT PANCAKES

1 1/2 CUPS	WHOLE WHEAT FLOUR
4 TEASPOONS	BAKING POWDER
2 TABLESPOONS	NUTRITIONAL YEAST
1/4 CUP	WHEAT GERM
1 1/2 CUPS	SOY MILK
3 TABLESPOONS	HONEY
2 TABLESPOONS	CORN OIL
2 CUPS	BLUEBERRIES

Heat skillet over medium heat. Mix first four ingredients together. Add liquid ingredients; stir to moisten. Add any one of the following ingredients: mashed bananas, crushed pineapple, raw nuts or seeds, berries, sliced peaches, sliced apples. Stir until mixed. Pour batter by 1/2 cup measure on oiled skillet. When bubbles form, turn and brown on other side. Serve with honey or pure maple syrup. Serves 4.

FRESH FRUIT SALAD

2	BANANAS, SLICED
1 CUP	STRAWBERRIES, SLICED
1	APPLE, CORED, SKINNED AND SLICED
1	PEAR, CORED, SKINNED AND SLICED
20	SEEDLESS GRAPES
1/2 CUP	SEEDLESS RAISINS
1/2 CUP	WALNUTS PIECES

Put all ingredients in a medium sized bowl and toss with Fruit Dip. Serves 2.

FRUIT DIP OR SPREAD

1 CUP	PLAIN, LOWFAT YOGURT
1 CUP	STRAWBERRIES
1/2 CUP	UNBLANCHED ALMONDS
1 TABLESPOON	HONEY

In a blender, process fruit, almonds, and honey until creamy. Mix with yogurt. Use as a dip for fresh fruit or spread thickly on whole wheat toast or whole grain English muffins. Serves 8.

APPLE-CELERY JUICE

6	APPLES
3 STALKS	CELERY

Wash produce. Cut apple to fit opening of juicer. Process. Serves 2.

BOSTON BIBB SALAD

8 LEAVES	BUTTERHEAD LETTUCE, TORN
4 CUPS	CHOPPED SPINACH
1/8 CUP	SLICED RED ONIONS
1 CUP	YELLOW CORN
1 CUP	SHREDDED CARROTS

Assemble all ingredients in salad bowl. Toss with Garlic Dressing. Serves 4.

GARLIC DRESSING

1/4 CUP	OLIVE OIL
2	GARLIC CLOVES, MINCED
2 TABLESPOONS	LEMON JUICE
1 TABLESPOON	ROASTED TAHINI
2 TABLESPOONS	WATER
1 TEASPOON	GROUND OREGANO

Whisk all ingredients in small container. Store covered in refrigerator. Serves 4.

STIR-FRIED CHICKEN AND VEGETABLES

2 CUPS	CHICKEN, WHITE MEAT WITHOUT SKIN
1/4 CUP	CHOPPED ONIONS
2	GARLIC CLOVES, MINCED
1 CUP	CHOPPED CAULIFLOWER
1 CUP	SHREDDED GREEN CABBAGE
1	SWEED RED PEPPER, SLICED
1 CUP	SLICED MUSHROOMS
1 CUP	MUNG BEAN SPROUTS
2 TABLESPOONS	OLIVE OIL
2 TABLESPOONS	TAMARI
2 TABLESPOONS	LEMON JUICE
1/2 TEASPOON	GROUND GINGER
2 TABLESPOONS	WATER

Cut up chicken into bite-sized pieces. Heat oil in large wok or skillet. Saute onion and garlic for 2 minutes.Add the chicken and saute for 2 more minutes. Add the rest of the vegetables, one at a time in the order given, sauteing for one minute after each addition. In small bowl, mix tamari, ginger, vinegar and water and pour over vegetables. Reduce heat, cover and steam 4-5 minutes until done. Uncover, stir and serve immediately. Serves 4.

• MENU FOR DAY FOUR •

BREAKFAST

GUAVA FRUIT JUICE *
WAFFLES

BREAKFAST SNACK

MANGO*

LUNCH

APPLE RASPBERRY JUICE*
BAKED FRENCH ONION SOUP
GREEN BEAN SALAD

LUNCH SNACK

BANANA

DINNER

FRESH CELERY-APPLE-BEET JUICE
GREEK SALAD
STEAMED CABBAGE WITH CARAWAY SEEDS
YAM AND POTATO CASSEROLE

**indicates recipe not included*

NUTRIENTS	
Protein (gm)	37
Total Fat (gm)	48
Complex Carb (gm)	280
Dietary Fiber (gm)	39
Cholesterol (mg)	90
Sodium (mg)	2529
Potassium (mg)	4820
Vitamin A (RE)	1514
Vitamin C (mg)	315
Iron (mg)	15
Calcium (mg)	552
Phosphorus (mg)	1059

TOTAL DAILY CALORIES 1822

24% OF CALORIES ARE FROM FAT

RECIPES

WAFFLES

2 CUPS	WATER
1 TABLESPOON	CORN OIL
2	BROWN FERTILE EGGS
1/2 TEASPOON	SEA SALT
2 CUPS	WHOLE WHEAT FLOUR
4 CUPS	UNSWEETENED APPLESAUCE

In a blender on low speed, blend all ingredients in the order given for 2 minutes. Spoon mixture into hot waffle iron. Cook until golden brown and crispy. Serve with unsalted butter and maple syrup or honey, or topped with your favorite pureed fresh fruit (strawberries and blueberries are excellent.)

Serves 4.

BAKED FRENCH ONION SOUP

1 1/2 CUPS	SLICED ONIONS (IN ROUNDS)
1 TABLESPOON	OLIVE OIL
2 TABLESPOONS	WATER
1 1/2 QUARTS	PRITIKIN READY-TO-SERVE CHICKEN BROTH
1/4 CUP	CHEDDAR CHEESE, SHREDDED
6 SLICES	WHOLE WHEAT BREAD

Sauté onions in 1 tablespoon oil and water. Add bouillon, salt, and pepper. Simmer 30 minutes. Pour into a casserole dish or soup tureen. Sprinkle grated cheddar cheese over slices of toasted bread. Place under broiler for cheese to melt. Float on soup. Sprinkle with grated parmesan cheese, if desired. Serves 4.

GREEN BEAN SALAD

1/2 POUND	GREEN BEANS
1/2 CUP	CHOPPED ONIONS
2 TABLESPOONS	WATER
2 TABLESPOONS	OLIVE OIL
1/4 TEASPOON	SESAME OIL
1 TEASPOON	RED WINE VINEGAR
1 TEASPOON	HONEY
1 TABLESPOON	TAMARI OR BRAGG'S AMINOES
1 TABLESPOON	LEMON JUICE
1/4 TEASPOON	GROUND GINGER
2 TABLESPOONS	SESAME SEEDS
1/8 TEASPOON	BLACK PEPPER
1 CUP	SHREDDED CARROTS

Snap ends from beans, cut in half crosswise. Place in boiling water for about 4 minutes or until crisp tender. Drain, immerse in cold water, then drain again. Pat dry. Thinly slice the onion, saute in 2 tablespoons water briefly. Combine olive oil and next 6 ingredients with whisk. Add green beans, onion, and shredded carrots. Toss well, then sprinkle with sesame seeds and pepper to taste. Chill 30 minutes before serving. Serves 2.

FRESH CELERY-APPLE-BEET JUICE

2 STALKS	CELERY
1	APPLE
1/2	SMALL BEET

Wash produce well. Cut apple to fit size of opening of juicer. Cut 2 slices from beet. Process through juicer. Serves 1.

GREEK SALAD

3 CUPS	SPINACH LEAVES
12	ROMAINE LETTUCE LEAVES
8	LARGE BLACK OLIVES, SLICED
1/2 CUP	FETA CHEESE
1	SWEET RED PEPPER (CUT INTO ROUNDS)
1	SWEET GREEN PEPPER (CUT INTO ROUNDS)
1/4 CUP	RED ONION ROUNDS
4 TABLESPOONS	OLIVE OIL
2 TABLESPOONS	LEMON JUICE
1/8 TABLESPOON	WORCHESTERSHIRE SAUCE
1/2 TEASPOON	DIJON MUSTARD
1/4	TOMATO
1 TABLESPOON	FETA CHEESE
3 TABLESPOONS	WATER
1 TEASPOON	SEA SALT
1/8 TEASPOON	BLACK PEPPER
1/2 TEASPOON	GROUND BASIL
1 TABLESPOON	CHOPPED ONIONS
1/2 TEASPOON	RED WINE VINEGAR

In large salad bowl, tear lettuce and spinach into bite-sized pieces. Add olives, feta, peppers, and red onion rounds. Blend the rest of the ingredients in a blender until smooth and add to salad. Toss well. Serves 4.

STEAMED CABBAGE WITH CARAWAY SEEDS

4 CUPS	COARSELY CHOPPED GREEN CABBAGE
1 TEASPOON	CARAWAY SEEDS
1 CUP	WATER
1/2 CUP	PRITKIN, NO OIL, NO SODIUM ITALIAN SALAD DRESSING

In a large skillet, bring water and cabbage to a boil. Reduce heat, steam with cover on until tender, about 10 minutes. Put cabbage in a large bowl, add caraway seeds and dressing. Toss and serve immediately. Serves 4.

YAM AND POTATO CASSEROLE

2 CUPS	SLICED YAMS
4	POTATOES, SLICED
1/2 CUP	CHOPPED ONIONS
2	GARLIC CLOVES, MINCED
2 TABLESPOONS	WATER
1/2 TEASPOON	GROUND OREGANO
2 TABLESPOONS	TAHINI
1 TABLESPOON	TAMARI OR BRAGG'S AMINOES
1/2 CUP	WATER

Preheat oven to 350° F. Saute garlic and onion in water over medium heat for 1 minute. Stir in the yams, potatoes, and continue cooking for 5 minutes. Add the oregano, saute for 2 minutes more. Combine tahini, tamari, water—blend well. Transfer vegetables to lightly oiled 2 quart casserole dish, cover with sauce. Cover dish, bake 35-40 minutes. Serves 4.

• MENU FOR DAY FIVE •

BREAKFAST

FRESH PINEAPPLE-ORANGE JUICE
BANANA FRENCH TOAST

LUNCH

V-8 COCKTAIL JUICE
COUSCOUS SALAD
CARROT-CELERY-CUCUMBER-GREEN PEPPER GARNISH

LUNCH SNACK

APPLESAUCE/YOGURT SNACK

DINNER

CARROT-APPLE JUICE
FRENCH ONION SOUP
STEAMED BROCCOLI PARMESAN
**indicates no recipe included*

NUTRIENTS	
Protein (gm)	54
Total Fat (gm)	37
Complex Carb (gm)	262
Dietary Fiber (gm)	32
Cholesterol (mg)	154
Sodium (mg)	1936
Potassium (mg)	4942
Vitamin A (RE)	7632
Vitamin C (mg)	454
Iron (mg)	14
Calcium (mg)	1235
Phosphorus (mg)	1415

TOTAL DAILY CALORIES 1762

19% OF CALORIES ARE FROM FAT

FRESH PINEAPPLE-ORANGE JUICE

2 CUPS	PINEAPPLE
2	ORANGES

Peel oranges, leaving as much white on as possible. Twist off top of pineapple. Cut 2 -1" slices of pineapple, remove skin, cut into strips to juice. Process. Serves 2.

BANANA FRENCH TOAST

3	BROWN, FERTILE EGGS
3	BANANAS
1 1/2 TEASPOONS	GROUND CINNAMON
1 TEASPOON	PURE VANILLA EXTRACT
12 SLICES	WHOLE WHEAT BREAD
4 CUPS	SLICED STRAWBERRIES
4 TABLESPOONS	MAPLE SYRUP
1/4 CUP	WATER

Put first 4 ingredients in blender and puree. Dip both sides of bread in liquid. Saute over low heat in non-stick pan until lightly browned on both sides or bake in 400° F. oven for 8 minutes on each side or until lightly browned. Serve with strawberries pureed with maple syrup and water. Serves 4.

COUSCOUS SALAD

3 CUPS	WATER
1 1/2 CUPS	COUSCOUS
1	SWEET RED PEPPER, SLICED
1	CARROT, SHREDDED
1/4 CUP	CHOPPED PARSLEY
3 TABLESPOONS	CHOPPED ONIONS
1/2 CUP	SLIVERED ALMONDS
2 TABLESPOONS	OLIVE OIL
4 TABLESPOONS	WATER
2 TABLESPOONS	CIDER VINEGAR
2 TEASPOONS	HONEY
1 TEASPOON	DIJON MUSTARD
1/2 TEASPOON	SEA SALT

Bring water to boil. Stir in couscous, cover pot, remove from heat. Let sit 5 min., fluff with fork, turn into large mixing bowl to cool. Add next 5 ingredients. In a separate small bowl, mix the last 7 ingredients together to make the dressing. Stir dressing into salad. Serves 4.

CARROT-CELERY-CUCUMBER-GREEN PEPPER GARNISH

2	CARROTS, SLICED INTO STICKS
2 STALKS	CELERY, SLICED INTO STICKS
1	SLICED CUCUMBER, SLICED
1	SWEET GREEN PEPPER (CUT INTO ROUNDS)

Arrange around couscous salad. Serves 4.

APPLESAUCE/YOGURT SNACK

1 CUP	UNSWEETENED APPLESAUCE
1 CUP	LOWFAT VANILLA YOGURT

Mix applesauce and yogurt together for a quick snack. Serves 1.

CARROT-APPLE JUICE

8	CARROTS
2	APPLES

Wash produce, remove carrot tops, cut to fit juicer. Serves 2.

FRENCH ONION SOUP

1 1/2 POUNDS	ONIONS, SLICED INTO ROUNDS
2 TABLESPOONS	WHOLE WHEAT FLOUR
2 QUARTS	WATER
2 TABLESPOONS	OLIVE OIL
1/4 CUP	GRATED PARMESAN CHEESE
4 TABLESPOONS	JENSEN'S BROTH & SEASONING (VEGEX OR BOUILLON)

Heat oil in large saucepan under medium-high heat. Add onions, stir often to coat. Reduce heat so onions brown gently (don't allow to burn). Stir in flour and allow to brown (4-5 minutes) Remove from heat and slowly add warm water to which bouillon, Jensen's Broth & Seasoning* or vegex has been dissolved. Bring to boil, allow to simmer with cover for 20-25 minutes or until done. Serve with croutons or parmesan cheese. Serves 4.

*Jensen's Broth and Seasoning is available at most health food stores or call 1-619-755-4027

STEAMED BROCCOLI PARMESAN

1 1/2 POUNDS	BROCCOLI, CUT INTO FLOWERETTES
1/4 CUP	WATER
1	GARLIC CLOVE, MINCED
1/2 CUP	SLICED MUSHROOMS
1/2 CUP	DICED CHICKEN OR TURKEY (WHITE MEAT WITHOUT SKIN)
1/4 CUP	GRATED PARMESAN CHEESE
1/8 TEASPOON	BLACK PEPPER

Place broccoli into medium-sized saucepan with 1 inch boiling water. Cook, uncovered, for 5 minutes. Cover, simmer 5 more minutes. Drain, saving liquid for later. Saute garlic and mushrooms in a little water in large skillet. Add broccoli, chicken or turkey, and saute 4-6 minutes until hot. If pan dries, add broccoli water. Sprinkle with parmesan cheese and black pepper. Serve immediately. Serves 4.

• MENU FOR DAY SIX •

BREAKFAST

GRAPE JUICE*
OATMEAL

LUNCH

CLAMATO JUICE*
STUFFED BAKED TOMATOES

LUNCH SNACK

BAKED APPLE

DINNER

CARROT-PARSLEY-APPLE JUICE
SIMPLE SPINACH SALAD
NEWBERG-STYLE CARROTS
GRILLED CHICKEN BREASTS
**indicates no recipe given*

NUTRIENTS	
Protein (gm)	65
Total Fat (gm)	46
Complex Carb (gm)	236
Dietary Fiber (gm)	30
Cholesterol (mg)	350
Sodium (mg)	2476
Potassium (mg)	4339
Vitamin A (RE)	10275
Vitamin C (mg)	160
Iron (mg)	21
Calcium (mg)	558
Phosphorus (mg)	1137

TOTAL DAILY CALORIES 1797

23% OF CALORIES ARE FROM FAT

RECIPES

OATMEAL

1 1/2 CUPS	OLD-FASHIONED OATS
4 CUPS	WATER
1/4 TEASPOON	SEA SALT
1 CUP	SOY MILK
4 TABLESPOONS	HONEY
4 SLICES	WHOLE WHEAT BREAD
4 TABLESPOONS	APPLE BUTTER

Combine oats and water in 2 quart saucepan, bring to boil. Cover pan, reduce heat, simmer for 10-15 minutes. Stir often. Variations: (1) Add 1/2 teaspoon cinnamon, 1/2 cup raisins, chopped dates or figs. (2) Add 1 sliced banana 5 minutes before done - stir. Serve oatmeal garnished with 1 tablespoons sunflower seeds. Add soymilk and honey to taste. Serve with whole wheat toast with apple butter. Serves 4.

STUFFED BAKED TOMATOES

6	TOMATOES
1/2 CUP	CHOPPED ONIONS
1/2 CUP	CHOPPED SCALLION
2 TABLESPOONS	TOMATO SAUCE
1/2 POUND	TOFU, FIRM, CRUMBLED
1 CUP	BROWN RICE, COOKED
1/4 CUP	CHOPPED PARSLEY
1 TEASPOON	GROUND BASIL
1/8 TEASPOON	RED OR CAYENNE PEPPER

Wash tomatoes, scoop hollow on stem end, remove pulp with spoon (reserve), leaving shell. Saute over medium heat the next 4 ingredients. Combine last four ingredients with tofu mixture. Stuff tomatoes, place in lightly oiled baking pan. Bake 20-25 minutes at 375° F. Variations: Add 1/2 cup parmesan cheese or sprinkle with seasoned bread crumbs. Serves 6.

BAKED APPLE

1 1/2 CUPS	APPLE JUICE
1 CUP	SEEDLESS RAISINS
4	APPLES
1/2 TEASPOON	GROUND CINNAMON

Soak raisins in apple juice. Preheat oven to 350° F. Wash and core apples. Set apples in casserole dish. Place raisins in core of each apple, drizzle apple juice soak water over apples and pour rest in bottom of baking dish. Sprinkle with cinnamon. Cover and bake for 30 minutes. Serves 4.

CARROT-PARSLEY-APPLE JUICE

10	CARROTS
1 CUP	PARSLEY
1	APPLE

Wash produce, remove carrot tops, cut carrots and apple to fit opening of juicer. Bunch parsley to process, followed by carrot or apple. Serves 2.

SIMPLE SPINACH SALAD

8 CUPS	SPINACH LEAVES
10	MUSHROOMS, SLICED
4	HARD-BOILED EGGS, QUARTERED
1	AVOCADO, SLICED
1 CUP	SEASONED CROUTONS
1/4 CUP	OLIVE OIL
1/2 CUP	RED WINE VINEGAR
2 TABLESPOONS	DIJON MUSTARD
2 TABLESPOONS	LEMON JUICE
2 TABLESPOONS	HONEY

Wash, dry, and tear spinach leaves into salad bowl. Add sliced mushrooms. Whisk olive oil, vinegar, mustard, lemon juice, and honey in small bowl; pour onto salad. Toss well. Add croutons. Top with quartered hard-boiled eggs and sliced avocado. Serves 4.

NEWBERG-STYLE CARROTS

4 CUPS	SLICED CARROTS
1 TEASPOON	SEA SALT
1 TEASPOON	HONEY
2 TABLESPOONS	OLIVE OIL
2 TABLESPOONS	WHOLE WHEAT FLOUR
3/4 CUP	WATER
1/4 CUP	SOY MILK
1/2 TEASPOON	CHOPPED PARSLEY
2 TEASPOON	CHOPPED ONIONS
2 TEASPOON	CHOPPED SWEET GREEN PEPPERS

Place carrots, honey, and salt into 1 inch boiling water in a medium sized saucepan. Cover, cook 12-15 minutes or till just crisp tender. Put oil (or butter) in another pan. Blend in flour. Add stock or water, soymilk, parsley, onion, green pepper. Stir, cook 5 minutes or till thickened. Add carrots, serve hot. Serves 4.

GRILLED CHICKEN BREASTS

4	BONELESS CHICKEN BREASTS
1 CUP	PRITIKIN, NO OIL, NO SODIUM CREAMY ITALIAN SALAD DRESSING

Marinate chicken breasts in dressing for 1 hour. Fire up grill to medium heat and grill on one side for 5-6 minutes, brush with more marinade, turn over, and grill for about 5 minutes more or until done. Serve immediately. Serves 4.

• MENU FOR DAY SEVEN •

BREAKFAST

STRAWBERRY-BANANA SMOOTHIE

LUNCH

V-8 JUICE*
MUSHROOM-OAT BURGERS

LUNCH SNACK

FROZEN YOGURT

DINNER

CARROT-CELERY JUICE
COLE SLAW
VEGETABLE-RICE BAKE

**indicates no recipe included*

NUTRIENTS	
Protein (gm)	41
Total Fat (gm)	32
Complex Carb (gm)	247
Dietary Fiber (gm)	30
Cholesterol (mg)	13
Sodium (mg)	1479
Potassium (mg)	4897
Vitamin A (RE)	13598
Vitamin C (mg)	218
Iron (mg)	17
Calcium (mg)	758
Phosphorus (mg)	1266

TOTAL DAILY CALORIES 1580

18% OF CALORIES ARE FROM FAT

RECIPES

STRAWBERRY-BANANA SMOOTHIE

1 CUP	STRAWBERRIES
4	BANANAS
4	APPLES

Make fresh apple juice and add to blender. Add fresh or frozen bananas, strawberries and blend. Variation: Use peaches instead of strawberries. Serves 2.

MUSHROOM-OAT BURGERS

1 TABLESPOON	OLIVE OIL
1 1/2 CUPS	CHOPPED ONIONS
1/2 CUP	SHREDDED CARROTS
1/4 CUP	DICED CELERY
1 CUP	CHOPPED MUSHROOMS
4 CUPS	WATER
1/4 CUP	TAMARI
1/3 CUP	GRATED PARMESAN CHEESE
2	GARLIC CLOVES, MINCED
1 TEASPOON	GROUND OREGANO
5 CUPS	OLD-FASHIONED OATS, UNCOOKED
2	TOMATOES, SLICED
20	ROMAINE LETTUCE LEAVES
10	WHOLE WHEAT BUNS
10 TABLESPOONS	CATSUP

Saute first 5 ingredients in non-stick pan until soft. Meanwhile, in 4 quart pan, bring water to boil. Add vegetables to water with next 4 ingredients. Slowly add oats one cup at a time, stirring well. Cook for 5 minutes until thick. Cover and let sit 15 minutes. Let cool and shape into patties. Put on oiled baking sheet, bake 20 minutes at 350° F. Turn over and bake an extra 25 minutes. Serve hot or cold with whole wheat buns and trimmings. Serves 10.

CARROT-CELERY JUICE

12	CARROTS
4 STALKS	CELERY

Wash carrots and celery, remove tops, cut to fit opening of juicer and process.

Serves 2.

COLE SLAW

1 1/2 CUPS	SHREDDED GREEN CABBAGE
1 CUP	SHREDDED RED CABBAGE
1/2 CUP	CHOPPED ONIONS
1/2 CUP	SWEET GREEN PEPPERS, CHOPPED
2 TEASPOONS	HONEY
1 TABLESPOON	LEMON JUICE
2 TABLESPOONS	CIDER VINEGAR
1/4 CUP	SOY MAYONNAISE

Toss all ingredients together in a large bowl until well mixed. Chill 1/2 hour in refrigerator before serving. Serves 4.

VEGETABLE-RICE BAKE

1 1/2 CUPS	LONG GRAIN BROWN RICE
1 CUP	BULGUR
2 1/2 CUPS	WATER
1 CUP	FIRM TOFU, MASHED
1 TABLESPOON	SAFFLOWER OIL
1/2 TEASPOON	GROUND SAGE
2 STALKS	CELERY, CHOPPED
1 CUP	GREEN CABBAGE, SHREDDED
2	CARROTS, SLICED
1 CUP	SLICED ZUCCHINI
1/2 CUP	GREEN PEAS
1/2 CUP	SLICED MUSHROOMS
1/2 CUP	CHOPPED ONIONS
2 SLICES	WHOLE WHEAT BREAD, CRUMBLED
2 TEASPOONS	BUTTER
2 TABLESPOONS	SAFFLOWER OIL
2 TABLESPOONS	WHOLE WHEAT FLOUR
1 1/2 CUPS	SOY MILK
1 TABLESPOON	MISO
1 TABLESPOON	TAMARI
1/2 TEASPOON	GROUND BASIL

For crust, boil water and add rice and bulgar. Cook in heavy, covered pan until liquid is absorbed and rice is tender. Set aside, keeping cover on pan to fluff and cool. Then add tofu, sage, and oil to rice mixture, mix well, and pat into oiled casserole dish. Preheat oven to 350° F.For filling, steam fresh or frozen vegetables to fill casserole dish. Cover with sauce. Sprinkle with bread crumbs that have been tossed with melted butter. For sauce: heat oil, stir in flour until brown, add soy milk and seasonings, mix well. Stir over med. heat until thick. Pour over vegetables. For bread crumbs: melt 1 tablespoons. butter or oil and toss with bread crumbs. Cover casserole. Place in 350° F. oven for 30 minutes. Serves 6.

CHAPTER 9

The Health Benefits of Juicing

As you are well aware by now, juicing is one of the foundations of the *Intuitive Eating* system. While there is much information about nutrition, and some even refer to the use of juices, few sources, if any, teach you how to make up your own juice formulas and juice combinations for specific health needs. That is one of the reasons why this book is unique.

For many years now I have tested the effects of juice through kinesiology and advanced physiology. I have even computerized everything and used electro-magnetics (EAV) to find out precisely how different juices work on the various organs of the body.

The result is a simple system, which I call "Directional Juicing," and this chapter will explain that approach. As you progress through the Transitional Stages you will be encouraged more and more to use fresh fruit and vegetable juice, so it is important that you understand why juice is recommended, when to use juice, and what juices work best for what problems or conditions.

WHY JUICE?

Juice is a food — the easiest form of food to digest. It contains vitamins, enormous amounts of alkaline minerals, and enzymes in liquid form, which means that it can be immediately assimilated. Within a few minutes after drinking a glass of juice, nutrients are entering your bloodstream and producing the energy you need for work or play.

Solid food, on the other hand, takes hours to digest and this process can steal much of your body's energy. This is why I strongly recommend juices for people who are older or those recovering from illness. Using juice three times a day between meals would greatly improve the recuperative powers of almost any patient, yet few traditional doctors will ever suggest such a simple approach. Using juice is such a safe and effective way to rebalance the body, no matter what the condition. Juices cleanse the system, rebuild it, and balance it.

The use of juices between meals is one of the most effective ways to cut down on cravings for unhealthy or unnecessary foods. We start to feel nourished by the juice in a way we haven't experienced before. Soon we are choosing to eat in a way that supports this new form of nourishment.

For children, juicing can be a real boon. Juices feed a child with instant energy, strengthen the immune system, and help to inhibit cravings for unnatural junk foods. Because of its highly concentrated nutritive value, juices can also start to replace some of the heavy food that was normally eaten at mealtimes. Eating several big meals a day makes the organism dull, and diminishes creativity. Freeing up the energy used for digestion provides us a greater storehouse of healing potential and intellectual activity.

I want to stress that juicing is not a therapy. Actually, I believe that juice is the foundation of all therapies. Some people can't take heavy supplements or drugs. Others can't radically change their eating habits, but almost everybody can start drinking juice. No matter what types of treatment you are using for any health problem, no matter what kind of a diet you are following for weight control, no matter how old you are (or young), the easiest, fastest, and most efficient way to get nutrients and enzymes into your body is through juices.

JUICE FOR ENZYMES

Many of the degenerative diseases of our times — like diabetes, certain types of cancer, and hypoglycemia — are related to the degenerative state of our diets. Over the years we have greatly increased our use of preserved, processed, and overcooked foods. After only a few months on this type of diet, animals begin to show changes in organ weight and corresponding glandular imbalances. This is the result of enzyme deficiency.

Take a look at Chart 9.1 which compares the organ weights of rats that were fed a variety of diets. You need to know that when a part of the body gets overworked and becomes enzyme deficient, it swells up. The brain, the pancreas, the liver — all act this way. Now notice that on a raw meat diet the body weight of the rat, in grams, was 124.4 and that the percentage weight of the pancreas was .175, the liver 6.51, the kidneys 1.10, and the heart .546.

CHART 9.1

ORGAN WEIGHT OF RATS ON RAW OR COOKED DIET ONE GRAM PER 100 GRAMS OF BODY WEIGHT

Authority & Diet	Year	Body Weight grams	Pancreas %	Liver %	Kidneys %	Heart %
H. Brieger, raw meat diet	1937	124.4	0.175	6.51	1.10	0.456
H. Brieger, raw vegetable	1937	125.0	0.159	5.82	0.738	0.403
H. Brieger, raw mixed diet	1937	126.0	0.161	6.45	0.984	0.406
H. Brieger, average of above	1937	125.1	0.165	6.26	0.941	0.422
H.H. Donaldson, random diet	1924	125.4	0.521	5.68	0.913	0.447

From: Enzyme Nutrition *by Dr. Edward Howell, published by Avery Publishing Group, Inc., Garden City Park, N.Y. Reprinted by permission.*

Look down to the next line. On a raw vegetable diet the rat weighed almost exactly the same, 125 grams. Yet the percentange weight of the organs was significantly lower — the pancreas, for example, was now .159 instead of .175. The liver was 5.82 instead of 6.51, and so on. Why is that? Because it hasn't been overworked — that's why! The body doesn't have to overwork to handle excess protein, and the raw vegetables contain the necessary enzymes which make digestion easy. So the organ stays smaller.

Go on to the next line — the mixed food diet, meaning raw and cooked food. Here the percentage weight of the pancreas is more than that of the raw vegetable diet, and less than that of the raw meat diet. This is an indicator of what cooked food does — it also causes the organs to swell up and become heavier.

Finally, look at the weight of the pancreas on the bottom line, The H.H. Donaldson study, using a random diet, fed the rats essentially cooked food. Here the pancreas weight measures three times larger than on a raw vegetable diet. Amazing? I think so. It is also sad when you realize that this happens to us.

Some of our hormones are made out of amino acids, which come from proteins. *Protease* is the enzyme that digests protein, and is therefore extremely important in this hormone-creation process. For many of us this enzyme is not present in sufficient amount or strength to accomplish adequate protein digestion. That is one reason why I sometimes suggest enzyme supplements for my clients, and why I stress the use of juicing to supply large amounts of enzymes. We need the hormones! PMS, diabetes, hypoglycemia, cancer — these are all conditions related to glandular imbalance. Once again, diet needs to become our first line of defense against disease, and our first line of offense in building strength and balance throughout the whole body.

HOW MUCH JUICE?

Years ago when people would ask me how much juice they should drink I would say, "Stand up straight, tip to your right, and if the juice comes out your ear you've had enough." But seriously, while a daily maintenance dosage of juice is usually three eight-ounce glasses, you can always drink more. If you are under the care of a physician or health practitioner who uses juice as a foundation for his/her therapies he/she will probably recommend more.

Since sensitivities and tastes vary greatly, you may want to dilute your juices with purified water. When you are juicing for children under five years of age, I recommend diluting the juices about 25-50% with water. The only real warning with drinking large amounts of juice is to watch your urinary pH. (Read how to do this in Chapter 8.) Juicing can keep the body very alkaline, and you want to keep your urinary pH between 6.3 and 7.0.

Remember that juicing is not a therapy, but the *foundation* of all therapies, so don't neglect your other forms of treatment. Besides, we can't always count on fruits and vegetables alone having all the proper nutrients in them because the soil has been so depleted and many of our foods have been shipped in from far away so that they do not ripen properly on the tree or vine.

WHICH JUICES, AND WHEN

Fruit juices are the cleansers, and vegetable juices are the toners and builders. Fruit juices are more cleasing than vegetable juices. Sometimes a three-day juice fast is an excellent way to help clean out the body. Vegetable juices are good cleansers too, but are also heavier in proteins. They are the body's building and toning foods.

Either fruit or vegetable juices can be used to clean the body. Which you choose will depend upon your needs and sensitivities. Some people cannot tolerate much fruit sugar, so vegetable juices would be more appropriate for them. Some people choose to use both — fruit juice in the morning and vegetable juices in the afternoon.

If you are trying to tone certain organs you will use the corresponding juices for that particular organ (see the chart that follows in the section on *Directional Juicing*).

Never drink fruit juices at night. They are high in sugar and can keep you awake. At night the body goes into a cleansing cycle, so it needs a rest. During the day your body will be in a digestive cycle and will more easily handle the heavier and/or more stimulating foods. Keep these cycles normal. If you eat too much at night you throw your body into a digestive cycle and then it doesn't get to purify itself. So, do your light eating at night. Juice your cucumbers, parsley, celery, or other light vegetables that will help to relax you. As you eat with your body's preferred cycle, you will find that you feel more balanced. It's a wonderful feeling. So, honor your body.

Usually juice about a half-hour before your meals. Don't juice 15 minutes before you eat. It takes about 25 minutes for that juice to get out of the stomach, sometimes a little longer. (If you burp and still "feel" your juice you're probably bloated. Then don't eat for a while.) If you are in good shape, and your pH is normal, the juice will probably be out of your stomach in 25 minutes.

Dilute all beet and green drinks. Anytime you use beet juice or green drinks (spinach, parsley, kale, etc.) always dilute them with some apple, carrot, or other type of juice. All green juices are very strong, so you don't need a lot of them. They also contain some acids that could irritate the stomach, which is another reason to dilute them.

Maximize the use of cruciferous vegetables. The anti-cancer effects of cruciferous vegetables are well known by the American Cancer Society.[1] These vegetables, which include: cabbage, cauliflower, kale, mustard greens, rutabaga, broccoli, brussel sprouts, collard leaves, radishes, and turnips — contain a variety of nitrogen compounds called *indols.* Indols are involved in many health-promoting activities in the body. For example, they stimulate the production of certain enzymes that may detoxify potential carcinogens. In the *Journal of the National Cancer Institute*[2] it was reported than when animals were given indols there was a significant increase in the rate at which the active form of estrogen, which may trigger the growth of breast tumors, was converted to a safer, inactive hormone. Many recent studies have also indicated that cruciferous vegetables may be protective against other cancers as well.

Support your bioflavonoids. (Flavonoids.) You have already read about the regenerative quality of bioflavonoids in Chapter 6. Bioflavonoids (or Flavonoids) are the plant pigments that provide remarkable protection against free-radical damage. They also help the body to modify its allergens, viruses, and carcinogens, while supporting the activity of the immune system. Bioflavonoids also act as anti-inflammatory agents in the body, and help to strengthen capillary walls and to fight infections.

Most of the foods that contains bioflavonoids can be easily juiced. The chart (9.2) that follows shows which foods are rich in flavonoids.

DIRECTIONAL JUICING FOR SPECIFIC HEALTH PROBLEMS

In the U.S. when we think of nutrition we think of eating, digestion, and the distribution of the nutrients through the glands. In China, however, nutrition is considered in terms of energy — Does the food have enough energy in it to activate the energy systems of the body? So, Eastern and Western nutritional approaches are a bit different. I have combined these two systems in a very practical way. Using advanced technology, kinesiology, and magnetics I have determined exactly what foods and juices are good for what parts of the body, and for what conditions.

In herbology and juiceology, as in Chinese acupuncture, if you are working with the kidneys you always work with the bladder too. If you work with the lungs you also work with the large intestine. These are *coupled organs* — i.e. they are on similar energy pathways within the body. Another way to say this is that the energy from one flows in the direction of the other. That's why I call this system "Directional Juicing." These coupled organs (see Chart 9.3.) always work together. The liver works with the

CHART 9.2

FLAVONOID CONTENT OF SELECTED FOODS

Milligrams (mg) per 100 grams edible portion (100 grams = 3.5 oz.)

FOODS	4-Oxo-flavonoids[1]	Anthocyanins	Catechins[2]	Biflavans
Fruits				
Grapefruit	50			
Grapefruit juice	20			
Oranges, Valencia	50-100			
Orange juice	20-40			
Apples	3-16	1-2	20-75	50-90
Apple juice				15
Apricots	10-18		25	
Pears	1-5		5-20	1-3
Peaches		1-12	10-20	90-120
Tomatoes	85-130			
Blueberries		130-250	10-20	
Cherries, sour		45		25
Cherries, sweet			6-7	15
Cranberries	5	60-200	20	100
Cowberries		100	25	100-150
Currants, black	20-400	130-400	15	50
Currant juice		75-100		
Grapes, red		65-140	5-30	50
Plums, yellow		2-10		
Plums, blue		10-25	200	
Raspberries, black		300-400		
Rasperries, red		30-35		
Strawberries	20-100	15-35	30-40	
Hawthorn berries			200-800	
Vegetables				
Cabbage, red		25		
Onions	100-2,000	0.25		
Parsley	1,400			
Rhubarb		200		
Miscellaneous				
Beans, dry		10-1,000		
Sage	1,000-1,500			
Tea	5-50		10-500	100-200
Wine, red	2-4	50-120	100-150	100-250

1 4-Oxo-flavonoids: flavanones, flavones and flavanols (including quercetin)

2 Catechins include proanthocyanidins

Source: "Nutritive Value of American Foods in Common Units," U.S.D.A. Agriculture Handbook No. 456 gall bladder. The spleen works with the pancreas and the stomach. So, if you are going to work with the stomach you also need to work with the spleen and pancreas, and so on.

Chart 9.4 will show you what foods will relate with what organs. These are the foods you will use to make juices.

The simple rules of *Directional Juicing* are:

1. Use four foods to make a juice combination, but no more. About 70% of the juice should be from foods that affect the primary organ of consideration.
2. Always try to work with the coupled organs. Include about 30% of the juice from a food that affects that coupled organ.
3. Never work with more than two organs at one time unless they are each in the same Direction.

Let's say I want to put a combination together for the kidneys. Perhaps I have lower backache, or maybe a history of kidney problems. Because the kidney is coupled with the bladder I will also want to work with the bladder. So, to make a balanced juice combination I would want about 70% of the combination to be from juices that are going to affect the kidney (or the main organ in consideration) and about 30% from a juice that affects the coupled organ, in this case the bladder. I would choose three foods from the kidney chart and one from the bladder chart and juice them.

Sometimes you will find that one food is common to both organs, so *definitely* use that one. Then you only have to use a total of three foods to make your combination. (The fewer the better.) Parsley, for example, is common for both the kidneys and the bladder, so in this case parsley would be included for sure.

Following this simple series of instructions is all you need to use juicing to move you into the realm of *Intuitive Eating*.

COUPLED ORGANS/MERIDIANS

Kidney/Bladder | Liver/Gall Bladder

Stomach/Spleen/Pancreas | Lungs/Small Intestine/Large Intestine

Heart/Circulation/Thyroid/Adrenals

CHART 9.3

CHART 9.4

JUICES RELATED TO COUPLED ORGANS
(Meridians)

Kidney	Bladder	Liver	Gall Bladder
Green pepper	Romaine	Carrot	Bok Choy
Parsley	Onion	Lettuce	Beet Greens
Ginger	Mustard	Tomato	Watercress
Watermelon	Greens	Spinach	Dandelion
Endive	Broccoli	Watercress	Endive
Dandelion	Spinach	Grapefruit	Strawberry
Grapefruit	Blueberry	Parsley	Radish
Beet	Parsley	Endive	Kale
Zucchini	Red Grapes	Dandelion	Mustard Greens
	Lemon		Plum
	Lettuce		Beets
	Turnips		Green Beans
	Orange		Sweet Potato
	Celery		

Heart	Circulation (heart)	Thyroid/Adrenals
Green Beans	Red Pepper	Kale
Cilantro	Strawberry	Bok Choy
Green Grape	Cucumber	Apple
Dandelion	Ginger	Ginger
Lime	Red Cabbage	Parsley
	Romaine	Turnips
	Radishes	Strawberry
	Beets	Garlic
	Acorn Squash	

Stomach	Spleen	Pancreas
Parsley	Radish	Romaine
Red Cabbage	Watercress	Zucchini
Grapefruit	Beets	Watercress
Radish	Beet Greens	Radish
Pear	Red Pepper	Acorn Squash
Kiwi	Red Cabbage	Parsley
Green Cabbage	Parsley	Sweet Potato
	Cranberry	String Beans
	Apple	Turnip
	Tomato	Cucumber
	Lettuce	Spinach
	Garlic	Celery

Lungs	Small Intestine	Large Intestine
Garlic		Garlic
White Potato	Romaine	Spinach
Red Potato	Green Grape	Cherry
Cilantro	Zucchini	Butternut Squash
Green Grape	Kale	Watercress
Strawberry	Pear	Bok Choy
Carrot	Nectarine	Mustard Greens
Spinach	Spinach	Tomato
Ginger		
Romaine		
Lime		
Radish		
Pineapple		

CHAPTER 10

The Transitional Diet

STAGE II

THE OVERVIEW

You are now ready to begin a very important phase of eating. By this time, your weight will have begun to stabilize. If you still need to lose more weight it will probably happen during this phase because raw food is increased to 40-70%. The high-density nutritious food, and the fiber content of this diet will give you that full, satisfied feeling. Your taste buds and your eating habits have probably changed significantly, and hopefully you are adapting well to this new type of eating routine.

Most people stay at this stage for 4-6 months before entering Stage III. Some of you may decide to stay at Stage II but use some of the recipes from Stage III. That's fine. Your transition into Stage III will be easier than you think if you have remained in Stage II for six months. Your intuition may tell you precisely when to move into Stage III.

If you have problems digesting larger percentages of raw food, find the percentage of raw food you're comfortable with. Try to stay within the 40-70% raw food range. If you have digestive problems, add plant digestive enzymes before meals. Consult your health practitioner if necessary.

STAGE TWO

40 - 70% raw food

BEVERAGES
• eliminate caffeinated coffee and tea
• use herbal teas, decaf. coffee, coffee substitutes such as Cafix, Postum
• limit "natural" soft drinks
• increase freshly made fruit and vegetable juices
• use distilled, reverse osmosis or deionized water
• reduce alcoholic beverages
• drink beverages at least 1/2 hr. before meals or 1 1/2 hrs. after meals

CARBOHYDRATES
Breads:
• introduce sprouted whole grain breads, rolls, etc.
Cereals:
• use whole, raw grains—unroasted
Grains:
• use organic whole grains
Legumes
• increase use of fresh legumes
Pasta:
• decrease use of pasta
Sweeteners:
• use raw honey, unsulphured molasses, maple syrup, Sucanat® in limited quantities
• substitute carob for chocolate

CONDIMENTS & SEASONINGS
• eliminate black pepper
• limit use of sea salt
• use natural herbs and spices and "salt substitutes"
• limit use of condiments
• make your own mayonnaise

DESSERTS
• eliminate use of desserts following meals—unless the dessert is a good combination with the meal

FATS AND OILS
• further reduce intake of raw butter
• use only cold-pressed vegetable oils in dark bottles or cans

FRUITS
• use only fresh fruits and reconstituted, un-sulphured dried fruits

JUICES
• reduce use of all pre-packaged juices
• increase use of freshly made fruit and vegetable juices

STAGE TWO

40 - 70% raw food

PROTEIN

Dairy:

- same as Stage #1
- limit use further

Meat, fish, poultry:

- reduce use of fish, chicken and turkey
- substitute protein alternatives such as tofu, tempeh, TVP (texturized vegetable protein), nuts, seeds, beans, legumes

Nuts & seeds:

- use only raw nuts and seeds
- begin use of soaked seeds and nuts
- limit use of nut butters

VEGETABLES

Salads:

- increase salads and varieties of vegetables eaten
- increase intake of raw vegetables
- eliminate frozen, canned, packaged, fried vegetables

Salad Dressings:

- eliminate bottled dressings
- use freshly made dr0essings from cold-pressed oils, apple cider vinegar, or lemon juice, fresh herbs and spices
- make your own mayonnaise

Soups:

- use only homemade soups—do not overcook
- eliminate all poultry and fish
- use organic vegetables when available

MISCELLANEOUS

Candy:

- further decrease amount of health food store candy
- increase "homemade candy" made with soaked seeds, nuts and dried fruit

Ice Cream:

- eliminate ice cream
- use non-dairy frozen desserts such as Rice Dream
- use frozen bananas, strawberries, blueberries, etc. blended or put through Champion Juicer

More freshly-made fruit and vegetable juices are used in this stage. Juices should be drunk between meals, or one-half hour before you eat. Caffeinated coffee and tea are omitted, and herbal teas and distilled water, or water that has been purified with a reverse osmosis unit, complement this stage.

You may feel bouts of fatigue because you miss the stimulating effects of coffee or tea. This will be temporary. Your body will rebuild itself and soon energy and vitality will be a permanent part of your life without the need for stimulants.

Drinking fluids before meals is also omitted. You may have a little water with meals if necessary, but remember, too much liquid with meals dilutes digestive juices and will weaken your digestion. Many people experience gas and bloating because of this habit. Your body will not need as much fluid intake because your diet contains more fluid—from the intake of juices as well as from the fruits and vegetables. The diet alone will help hydrate your body.

Fat and protein are reduced in Stage II. You will be amazed to know that most fruits and vegetables are complete proteins, and that protein intake really isn't a problem. You will be getting enough protein just by following our recipes.

What is nice about this stage is that more non-meat substitutes—like tofu, tempeh, textured vegetable protein (TVP)—are used. They are not only easier to digest than meat, but they don't put the digestive strain on the body and deplete energy. These foods help preserve energy so it can be used for other metabolic processes and healing.

Desserts should be used as a meal, not before or after. This should not be a problem because you will naturally be eating less food and these desserts will be filling. You may find out, as I did, that one regular meal a day plus one dessert meal will be enough food for you. The raw juices alone will supply a large percentage of your nutrients.

Fish and poultry will be kept to a minimum at first. As you increase your raw food through this stage, poultry will be eliminated altogether. You will see that legumes, seeds, nuts, and grains will take the place of poultry. These are much better sources of protein. Fish can be used as long as you want it, or at least until you learn what fats and proteins to use in your diet. For an example, fish contains eicosapentacoic acid (EPA) which is a derivative of linolenic acid (omega -3). (Fatty acids are thoroughly covered in Chapter 4.) Diets high in EPA protect against heart disease, strokes, and peripheral vascular diseases. EPA also decreases cholesterol and triglycerides.

A substitute for fish oils, and a much better source for EPA, is flax seed. Flax seed is higher in omega -3 than all other oils, and this cuts blood cholesterol by 25% and triglycerides by 65%. Your body will make EPA from linolenic acid. (Soak 3 tsp. of flax seed overnight, and, in the morning, blend into juices. You can also blend it with water, honey, and bananas. Grind flax seed in a coffee grinder and sprinkle it on salads and soups.) Flax seed or flax seed oil can be taken daily. Ask at your local health food store about a company called *Omega Nutrition,* my choice for the best source of flax seed oil. Two to three teaspoons of the oil can be taken daily in juice or blends. Please re-read the section in Chapter 4 on Fats and Oils for more information.

If you need to use recipes from Stage I, it's okay to do so, especially if you prefer some of those recipes, or if you choose to keep some of those foods in your diet generally.

Sprouted grains and breads are introduced at this stage. They are easier to digest than the whole grains because one digestive stage is already done outside the body. In other words, they are predigested. The proteins are broken down to amino acids, fats to fatty acids, and carbohydrates to simpler sugars. This digestive process, which would otherwise have to be done by the body, is done by sprouting. It has been estimated that it takes 40-80% of the body's energy to digest a 100% cooked food meal. This is a waste of energy. Sprouted food preserves a great deal of that energy, which is then available for other metabolic processs. Sprouts can be purchased from health food stores and even from some large supermarkets. Flour-less, sprouted-grain bread is also available from health food stores. To sprout your own grains read the directions given in Stage III, Chapter 11.

Please remember to use proper food combining as explained in Chapter 8, and the methods suggested for dealing with a healing crisis (Chapter 7).

SEVEN DAY MEAL PLAN FOR STAGE 2

• MENU FOR DAY ONE •

BREAKFAST

SEED/NUT MILK RECIPE

LUNCH

CARROT-APPLE-CHARD-GINGERROOT JUICE
SPROUT SALAD WITH MISO-MUSTARD DRESSING
VEGGIE-TOFU SANDWICH

DINNER

CARROT-CUCUMBER-BEET JUICE
MIXED VEGETABLE SALAD
FRENCH DRESSING
STEAMED ASPARAGUS
QUINOA

NUTRIENTS	
Protein (gm)	52
Total Fat (gm)	44
Complex Carb (gm)	227
Dietary Fiber (gm)	53
Cholesterol (mg)	0
Sodium (mg)	1463
Potassium (mg)	5598
Vitamin A (RE)	21117
Vitamin C (mg)	267
Iron (mg)	29
Calcium (mg)	731
Phosphorus (mg)	1514
TOTAL DAILY CALORIES	**1611**

25% OF CALORIES ARE FROM FAT

RECIPES

SEED/NUT MILK

2 TABLESPOONS	ALMONDS
2 TABLESPOONS	SESAME SEEDS
2 TABLESPOONS	SUNFLOWER SEEDS
2 TABLESPOONS	PUMPKIN SEEDS
2	BANANAS
1 TEASPOON	PURE VANILLA EXTRACT
1 TABLESPOON	HONEY

Soak seeds and nuts in one pint of pure water overnight. Rinse and drain water from mixture. Throw soaking water away. Put mixture into blender with one cup of water. Blend until smooth, then add rest of water. Blend again. Strain mixture through a stainless steel strainer or cheese-cloth. Throw pulp away. Put 1/2 seed/nut liquid into clean blender. Add bananas, vanilla and honey to taste. Blend. Add other 1/2 of liquid to blended mixture. Serve. Makes (3) 8-oz. glasses. Serves 3.

SPROUT SALAD WITH MISO-MUSTARD DRESSING

4 CUPS	ALFALFA SPROUTS
2 CUPS	MUNG BEAN SPROUTS
1	SWEET RED PEPPER, SLICED
1/2 CUP	ZUCCHINI SQUASH, SLICED
1	SCALLION, SLICED
2 TABLESPOONS	MISO
2 TABLESPOONS	DIJON MUSTARD
1 TABLESPOON	LEMON JUICE
3 TABLESPOONS	OLIVE OIL
2	GARLIC CLOVES, MINCED

Assemble all ingredients in large salad bowl. In separate bowl, mix together miso and mustard. Add lemon juice, oil, garlic and beat with a whisk until well blended. Pour over salad and toss gently. Serves 4.

VEGGIE-TOFU SANDWICH

8 OUNCES	FIRM TOFU
1/2	CUCUMBER, CHOPPED
1/2	SWEET GREEN PEPPER, CHOPPED
1/4 CUP	CHOPPED ONIONS
1 TEASPOON	CHOPPED PARSLEY
1 TEASPOON	BRAGG'S AMINOES
1 CUP	ALFALFA SPROUTS
8 SLICES	WHOLE WHEAT BREAD

Mash the tofu in a bowl. Add the rest of the ingredients and blend until mixture is creamy. Spread thickly on toasted bread; add sprouts; top with second slice of toasted bread or serve open face. Serves 4.

CARROT-CUCUMBER-BEET JUICE

10	CARROTS
1	CUCUMBER
1/4	BEET

Wash and prepare all produce. Remove carrot tops, cut to fit juicer opening. Serves 2.

MIXED VEGETABLE SALAD

2 CUPS	ROMAINE LETTUCE, COARSELY CHOPPED (OR TORN)
1 CUP	ALFALFA SPROUTS
1	SWEET GREEN PEPPER, SLICED
1/2	CUCUMBER, SLICED
1/2 CUP	RED CABBAGE, SHREDDED
1/2 CUP	BROCCOLI, CHOPPED
1/2 CUP	CAULIFLOWER, CHOPPED
1/2 CUP	CARROTS, SHREDDED
2 STALKS	CELERY, CHOPPED
1	GARLIC CLOVE, MINCED

Wash and prepare vegetables. Assemble in large salad bowl. Toss gently with French Dressing and serve. Serves 4.

FRENCH DRESSING

2/3 CUP	NATURAL CATSUP
1 TEASPOON	CELERY SEED
1 TEASPOON	CHOPPED ONIONS
1/3 CUP	CIDER VINEGAR
1/4 CUP	HONEY
2/3 CUP	WATER
1/2 CUP	OLIVE OIL

Place all ingredients in a blender and process until smooth. Serves 12.

STEAMED ASPARAGUS

1 1/2 POUNDS	ASPARAGUS
1/2 TABLESPOON	PRITIKIN, NO OIL, NO SODIUM ITALIAN SALAD DRESSING

Wash asparagus, snap off tough ends. Bring water to boil in pot, add asparagus in steamer basket and steam for 5 minutes. Remove to serving dish, drizzle on dressing. Serves 4.

QUINOA

6 CUPS	WATER
2 2/3 CUPS	QUINOA, DRY
2 TABLESPOONS	BRAGG'S AMINOES

Rinse quinoa thoroughly by using a fine mesh strainer or by running fresh water over the quinoa in a pot and draining. Place quinoa and water in a sauce pan and bring to a boil. Reduce to a simmer, cover and cook until all of water is absorbed (10-15 minutes). Add Bragg's Aminoes or tamari at end of cooking time. Serves 4.

• MENU FOR DAY TWO •

BREAKFAST

SMOOTHIE

BREAKFAST SNACK

APPLE WITH RAISINS

LUNCH

CARROT-CELERY-CUCUMBER JUICE
SPROUT SALAD
DIJON-MISO DRESSING
SCRAMBLED TOFU WITH VEGETABLES

DINNER

CARROT SUPREME JUICE
BARLEY-VEGETABLE SOUP
SHREDDED CARROT-CABBAGE SALAD
CORNBREAD

NUTRIENTS	
Protein (gm)	47
Total Fat (gm)	46
Complex Carb (gm)	268
Dietary Fiber (gm)	58
Sugar (gm)	14
Cholesterol (mg)	0
Sodium (mg)	504
Potassium (mg)	6280
Vitamin A (RE)	19589
Vitamin C (mg)	313
Iron (mg)	38
Calcium (mg)	1115
Phosphorus (mg)	1244

TOTAL DAILY CALORIES 1776

23% OF CALORIES ARE FROM FAT

RECIPES

SMOOTHIE

4	APPLES
2	BANANAS
2 TEASPOONS	GROUND CINNAMON
1 TABLESPOON	HONEY
2 TEASPOONS	PURE VANILLA EXTRACT

Prepare fresh apple juice by washing, cutting, and feeding apple through juicer. May also use soaked almond milk instead of apple juice. Add apple juice to blender along with frozen or fresh banana and rest of ingredients. Blend well and serve. Variation: use fruit in season for a delightful change.

Serves 2.

APPLE WITH RAISINS

1	APPLE
1/4 CUP	SEEDLESS RAISINS

Core and slice apples. Sprinkle with raisins. Serves 1.

CARROT-CELERY-CUCUMBER JUICE

8	CARROTS
2 STALKS	CELERY
1	CUCUMBER
1	APPLE

Wash, dry and prepare vegetables for juicing. Serves 2.

SPROUT SALAD

2 CUPS	ALFALFA SPROUTS
1 CUP	MUNG BEAN SPROUTS
2 TABLESPOONS	SESAME SEEDS
2	TOMATOES, QUARTERED

Assemble ingredients and mix with Dijon-Miso dressing. Serves 2.

DIJON-MISO DRESSING

2 TABLESPOONS	MISO
2 TEASPOONS	DIJON MUSTARD
2 TABLESPOONS	LEMON JUICE
1/4 CUP	OLIVE OIL
2	GARLIC CLOVES, MINCED

By hand, in a small container, mix miso and mustard. Add lemon juice, olive oil, and garlic. Whip until well blended. Store in refrigerator in a small covered container. Serves 4.

SCRAMBLED TOFU WITH VEGETABLES

1/2 CUP	CHOPPED ONIONS
2	GARLIC CLOVES, MINCED
1/2 CUP	SWEET GREEN PEPPERS, CHOPPED
1/2 CUP	BROCCOLI FLOWERETTES
1/2 TEASPOON	GROUND OREGANO
1/2 TEASPOON	GROUND BASIL
1/2 TEASPOON	CUMIN SEED
1/4 CUP	TOMATO PASTE
1 1/2 CUPS	FIRM TOFU

Saute onion, garlic, green pepper, and other vegetables in a small amount of water briefly over medium heat. Add seasonings and tomato paste and stir in. Add mashed tofu and continue to saute until done (2-3 minutes).

Serves 2.

CARROT SUPREME JUICE

8	CARROTS
1	APPLE
1 CUP	KALE, CHOPPED
1 CUP	PARSLEY, CHOPPED
1	GINGER ROOT

Wash and dry produce. Cut top off carrots. Cut a 1/2" knob of gingerrot. Cut apple and carrots to fit juicer's opening. Bunch parsley into a ball to feed through juicer. Follow parsley and kale with carrot. Serves 2.

BARLEY-VEGETABLE SOUP

1/3 CUP	BARLEY, RAW
5 CUPS	WATER
1	BAY LEAF
1/4 TEASPOON	GROUND SAGE
1/4 TEASPOON	GROUND OREGANO
1/2 CUP	CHOPPED ONIONS
1 CUP	CARROTS, SLICED
1/2 CUP	CELERY, CHOPPED
1/2 CUP	ZUCCHINI SQUASH, SLICED
1 TEASPOON	JENSEN'S BROTH AND SEASONING

Bring water to boil in large soup pot, add barley, bay leaf, Jensen's and herbs and let simmer. In a separate pan, add a small amount of water to saute vegetables. You may add Bragg's Aminoes to the water. Add onion and stir for 1-2 minutes, then add carrot and celery and stir a few more minutes. Add zucchini and stir once more. Reduce heat and simmer until al dente (10 minutes). Add more water if needed. Add vegetables to soup pot, simmer until done. Serves 4.

CORNBREAD

1 1/2 CUPS	WHOLEGRAIN YELLOW CORNMEAL
1/4 CUP	WHOLE WHEAT FLOUR
1/4 CUP	SOYBEAN FLOUR
1 TEASPOON	BAKING POWDER
3 TABLESPOONS	SAFFLOWER OIL
3 TABLESPOONS	BLACKSTRAP MOLASSES
1 CUP	WATER
1	EGG REPLACER EQUIVALENT (available at health food store)

Measure and add dry ingredients to a large mixing bowl. Measure liquid ingredients in a separate measuring cup. Add liquid ingredients to dry ingredients and mix just enough to make flour disappear. Pour into oiled 8"x8" baking pan and bake about 30 minutes at 350° F. or until toothpick comes out cleanly. Serves 9.

• MENU FOR DAY THREE •

BREAKFAST

BANANA-PINEAPPLE SMOOTHIE

LUNCH

CARROT-PARSLEY-GARLIC JUICE
SLOPPY JOE TEMPEH
STEAMED CORN ON COB WITH OLIVE OIL

DINNER

CARROT-BROCCOLI JUICE
BASIL TOMATOES
PASTA VEGETABLE SALAD

NUTRIENTS	
Protein (gm)	48
Total Fat (gm)	48
Complex Carb (gm)	304
Dietary Fiber (gm)	71
Cholesterol (mg)	0
Sodium (mg)	2565
Potassium (mg)	7029
Vitamin A (RE)	22304
Vitamin C (mg)	441
Iron (mg)	24
Calcium (mg)	690
Phosphorus (mg)	1361
TOTAL CALORIES	**1919**

23% OF CALORIES ARE FROM FAT

RECIPES

BANANA-PINEAPPLE SMOOTHIE

4 CUPS	PINEAPPLE
2	BANANAS, FROZEN

Prepare pineapple for juicing and process through juicer. Pour juice into blender to which you may add fresh or (better yet) frozen bananas. Blend well and serve. Serves 2.

CARROT-PARSLEY-GARLIC JUICE

10	CARROTS
1	APPLE
1 STALKS	CELERY
1 CUP	PARSLEY
2	GARLIC CLOVES

Wash and prepare produce for juicing. Remove carrot tops. Process through juicer, following parsley with carrot or apple. Wrap garlic inside parsley to process. Serves 2.

SLOPPY JOE TEMPEH

1/2 CUP	CHOPPED ONIONS
1 TABLESPOON	OLIVE OIL
2 CUPS	TOMATO SAUCE
1/4 TEASPOON	CHILI POWDER
1/4 TEASPOON	GROUND CUMIN SEED
8 OUNCES	TEMPEH (available at health food stores)
2 SLICES	WHOLE WHEAT BREAD
1/2 CUP	PARSLEY, CHOPPED

Cut tempeh into 1/2" cubes and steam for 20 minutes. Saute onion in olive oil until translucent. Add rest of ingredients and simmer for 20 minutes. Serve over rice or wholegrain bread and garnish with fresh parsley. Serves 2.

STEAMED CORN ON COB WITH OLIVE OIL

2 EARS	CORN, WHITE OR YELLOW
1 TABLESPOON	OLIVE OIL
1/2 TEASPOON	JENSEN'S BROTH AND SEASONING*

Bring water to a boil in a pot with steamer basket. Add corn and steam for 15 minutes. Remove from basket and brush with olive oil and Jensen's seasoning. Serves 2.

CARROT-BROCCOLI JUICE

10	CARROTS
1	APPLE
1 CUP	BROCCOLI
1 STALK	CELERY

Wash and prepare produce for juicing. Remove carrot tops. Cut produce to fit size of opening and process. Serves 2.

BASIL TOMATOES

8	TOMATOES
1 TABLESPOON	GROUND BASIL
1/4 CUP	OLIVE OIL
1 TABLESPOON	LEMON JUICE

Quarter tomatoes. Depending on size, you may want to cut the quarters again. Whip dressing ingredients together, drizzle over tomatoes and gently toss. Serves 4.

*Jensen's Broth and Seasoning is available at most health food stores, or call 1-619-755-4027

PASTA VEGETABLE SALAD

2 CUPS	WHOLE WHEAT ELBOW MACARONI
1/2 CUP	CHOPPED ONIONS
1/2 CUP	CELERY, DICED
1 CUP	CARROTS, SLICED
1 CUP	BROCCOLI, CHOPPED
1 CUP	CAULIFLOWER, CHOPPED
1/2 CUP	CUCUMBER, SLICED
1	SWEET GREEN PEPPER, SLICED
1/2 CUP	PARSLEY, CHOPPED
2 TABLESPOONS	LEMON JUICE
1 TABLESPOON	HONEY
2 TABLESPOONS	BRAGG'S AMINOES
1 TEASPOON	GROUND BASIL
1 TEASPOON	GROUND DILL
1/2 TEASPOON	MUSTARD SEED
3 TABLESPOONS	OLIVE OIL

Add pasta to a pot of boiling water. Cook uncovered for 12-15 minutes. Drain and rinse. Meanwhile, steam coarsely chopped vegetables (except cucumber, green pepper and parsley) until al dente. Remove from heat and allow to cool. Assemble ingredients and pour on marinade, tossing gently. You may serve this warm in the winter as well. Combine all marinade ingredients separately by hand. Mix and add to salad. Toss gently. Serves 4.

• MENU FOR DAY FOUR •

BREAKFAST

PINEAPPLE-GRAPEFRUIT-APPLE JUICE
DATE-APRICOT SAUCE OVER BANANAS

LUNCH

CARROT-CELERY-PARSLEY JUICE
CELEBRATION SALAD

DINNER

CARROT-SPINACH-KALE-GINGER JUICE
GARDEN POTATO SALAD
GREENS AND COMPANY

NUTRIENTS	
Protein (gm)	32
Total Fat (gm)	45
Complex Carb (gm)	336
Dietary Fiber (gm)	62
Cholesterol (mg)	0
Sodium (mg)	484
Potassium (mg)	7447
Vitamin A (RE)	22241
Vitamin C (mg)	423
Iron (mg)	24
Calcium (mg)	737
Phosphorus (mg)	1232

TOTAL DAILY CALORIES 1925

21% OF CALORIES ARE FROM FAT

RECIPES

PINEAPPLE-GRAPEFRUIT-APPLE JUICE

4	PINEAPPLE SLICES, 1" THICK
1	GRAPEFRUIT, PINK OR RED
2	APPLES

Peel grapefruit leaving as much white on as possible. Skin pineapple and wash apples. Cut each to fit opening of juicer. Serves 2.

DATE-APRICOT SAUCE OVER BANANAS

1 CUP	WATER
10	NATURAL, WHOLE, PITTED DATES
20	DRIED APRICOTS
2 TABLESPOONS	FLAX SEED
2	BANANAS, SLICED

Soak dates, apricots, flax seeds overnight in pure water to cover. Place soaked fruit, seeds, and water in blender and puree. Serve over sliced bananas. Serves 2.

CARROT-CELERY-PARSLEY JUICE

10	CARROTS
4 STALKS	CELERY
1 CUP	PARSLEY

Wash all produce and cut to fit opening of juicer. Serves 2.

CELEBRATION SALAD

1 CUP	PARSLEY, CHOPPED
1 CUP	CARROTS, SHREDDED
1/4 CUP	CHOPPED ONIONS
1/2 CUP	SUNFLOWER SEEDS
2 CUPS	COOKED BROWN RICE
2 TABLESPOONS	LEMON JUICE
3 TABLESPOONS	SESAME OIL
1/2 TEASPOON	GROUND OREGANO
1/2 TEASPOON	GROUND BASIL
1/2 TEASPOON	GARLIC POWDER
4	ROMAINE LETTUCE LEAVES
1	TOMATO, CUT IN WEDGES
1/2 CUP	CUCUMBER, SLICED
1/4 TEASPOON	PAPRIKA
1/2 TEASPOON	JENSEN'S BROTH AND SEASONING

Mix parsley, carrot, onion and sunflower seeds together. Toss lightly with rice and 1 tablespoon of lemon juice. Whisk rest of lemon juice with oil, herbs and Jensen's and mix with vegetable-rice mixture. Marinate for at least one-half hour in refrigerator. Arrange each plate with 2 lettuce leaves, 4 tomato wedges, and 5 cucumber slices. Put mound of rice mixture in center. Sprinkle with paprika. Serves 2.

CARROT-SPINACH-KALE-GINGER JUICE

8	CARROTS
1 CUP	SPINACH, CHOPPED
1 CUP	KALE, CHOPPED
1	GINGER ROOT

Wash all produce, remove carrot tops, cut 1/4" knob of gingerroot. Process through juicer. Serves 2.

GARDEN POTATO SALAD

1 CUP	CHOPPED ONIONS
2 STALKS	CELERY, CHOPPED
1/2 CUP	PARSLEY, CHOPPED
2	GARLIC CLOVES, MINCED
1 TABLESPOON	OLIVE OIL
2 TABLESPOONS	RED WINE VINEGAR
1/2 TEASPOON EACH	OREGANO AND BASIL
3 CUPS	GREEN SNAP BEANS
2 CUPS	YELLOW SNAP BEANS
5	POTATOES
8	BUTTERHEAD LETTUCE LEAVES
3	TOMATOES
1 TEASPOON	JENSEN'S BROTH AND SEASONING

Combine onions, celery, parsley, garlic, olive oil, vinegar, basil, oregano in a dish. Allow to marinate while rest of salad is prepared. Trim beans, slice on diagonal; steam until crisp tender. Quarter potatoes; steam until tender. An hour before serving, combine beans and potatoes with marinated vegetables. Add Jensen's and more vinegar to taste. Serve on bed of lettuce and garnish with tomatoes. Serves 6.

GREENS AND COMPANY

8	LETTUCE LEAVES, TORN
2 CUPS	SPINACH, CHOPPED
1 CUP	CARROTS, SHREDDED
1 CUP	BEETS, GRATED
2 CUPS	ALFALFA SPROUTS
1	SWEET GREEN PEPPER, SLICED
1 CUP	BROCCOLI, CHOPPED
1 CUP	PRITIKIN, NO OIL, NO SODIUM, CREAMY ITALIAN SALAD DRESSING

Prepare and assemble all salad ingredients. Serve with dressing. Serves 4.

• MENU FOR DAY FIVE •

BREAKFAST

APPLE JUICE
HOT BREAKFAST RICE

LUNCH

CARROT-SPINACH-CELERY JUICE
ZUCCHINI SALAD
CORN AND TOMATO SAUTE

LUNCH SNACK

HOMEMADE SESAME CANDY

DINNER

ENDIVE SUPREME
ENDIVE SALAD
CUCUMBER DRESSING
EGGPLANT-ZUCCHINI MEDLEY

NUTRIENTS	
Protein (gm)	38
Total Fat (gm)	37
Complex Carb (gm)	302
Dietary Fiber (gm)	72
Cholesterol (mg)	0
Sodium (mg)	1087
Potassium (mg)	7049
Vitamin A (RE)	16552
Vitamin C (mg)	294
Iron (mg)	27
Calcium (mg)	877
Phosphorus (mg)	1288

TOTAL DAILY CALORIES 1857

18% OF CALORIES ARE FROM FAT

RECIPES

APPLE JUICE

3	APPLES

Wash fruit. Cut to fit opening. Serves 1.

HOT BREAKFAST RICE

3 CUPS	COOKED BROWN RICE
1 CUP	SEEDLESS RAISINS
1/4 CUP	DRIED ALMONDS, SLICED OR DICED
1/8 TEASPOON	GROUND NUTMEG
1 CUP	APPLE JUICE
1 CUP	WATER
2 TABLESPOONS	TAHINI SESAME BUTTER
1 TEASPOON	PURE VANILLA EXTRACT
1 TEASPOON	GROUND CINNAMON
1 TEASPOON	LEMON PEEL, GRATED
1	BANANA, SLICED
2 TABLESPOONS	SESAME SEEDS

Mix rice, raisins, almonds, and nutmeg together. Add rest of ingredients. Turn into oiled casserole. Arrange sliced banana on top and sprinkle with toasted sesame seeds. Bake uncovered at 350° F. for 30 minutes. Or for a ready-made hot breakfast, turn into crockpot before retiring, turn on low, and have ready-made breakfast in the morning. Serves 6.

CARROT-SPINACH-CELERY JUICE

8	CARROTS
1	APPLE
1/2 CUP	CHOPPED SPINACH
1 STALK	CELERY

Wash produce. Cut off carrot tops. Cut to fit size of opening and process. Serves 2.

ZUCCHINI SALAD

4 CUPS	SLICED ZUCCHINI
1 CUP	SHREDDED RED CABBAGE
1 CUP	SHREDDED GREEN CABBAGE
1/2 CUP	DICED CELERY
1/4 CUP	CHOPPED ONIONS
1/4 CUP	HONEY
1/4 CUP	CIDER VINEGAR
2 TEASPOONS	CELERY SEED
1/4 TEASPOON	SEA SALT

Have zucchini, cabbage, celery, and onion ready in bowl. Cook honey, vinegar, celery seed, and salt in a small pan for just 1 minute. Pour dressing over vegetables, toss and serve. Serves 4.

CORN AND TOMATO SAUTE

4 CUPS	YELLOW CORN, CUT OFF COB
1 1/2 CUPS	TOMATOES, CHOPPED
1/4 TABLESPOON	OLIVE OIL
1/2 TABLESPOON	HONEY
1/2 TEASPOON	OREGANO
1/8 TEASPOON	BLACK PEPPER

Combine all ingredients in a medium skillet or 1 quart saucepan. Saute for 7-10 minutes or until corn is tender, stirring often. Serve hot. Serves 4.

HOMEMADE SESAME CANDY

1/2 CUP	TAHINI SESAME BUTTER
1/4 CUP	DATES, CHOPPED
1 TABLESPOON	CAROB POWDER
2 TABLESPOONS	HONEY
2 TABLESPOONS	SESAME SEEDS
2 TABLESPOONS	DRIED, UNSWEETENED, SHREDDED COCONUT MEAT

Stir first 5 ingredients together; form into balls. Dip each ball in coconut and refrigerate. Makes about 18 balls. Serves 6.

ENDIVE SUPREME

8	CARROTS
1	APPLE
1/2 CUP	ENDIVE
1/2 CUP	PARSLEY
1/2 CUP	KALE

Wash and dry all vegetables and apple. Cut tops off carrot. Cut vegetables to fit opening of juicer. Serves 2.

ENDIVE SALAD

4 CUPS	COARSELY CHOPPED ENDIVE
1 CUP	CHOPPED PARSLEY
4	TOMATOES, SLICED
2	SCALLIONS, DICED
1	AVOCADO, SLICED
8 OUNCES	FIRM TOFU, CUBED

Wash greens and vegetables, trim endive. Cut or tear greens into bite-size segments and arrange in salad serving bowl. Add sliced tomatoes, sliced scallions, chopped parsley, avocado and tofu. Pour on cucumber dressing and toss to mix. Serves 4.

CUCUMBER DRESSING

1	CUCUMBER
1/4 CUP	CHOPPED ONIONS
1	GARLIC CLOVE, MINCED
1 TABLESPOON	LEMON JUICE
2 TABLESPOONS	WHITE WINE VINEGAR
2 TABLESPOONS	HONEY
1 TABLESPOON	TAHINI SESAME BUTTER
1 TABLESPOON	DILL
3/4 CUP	SOYMILK

Place all ingredients except soymilk and dill in blender and process briefly. Add soymilk and dill and process briefly again. Store in small air-tight container. Serves 4.

EGGPLANT-ZUCCHINI MEDLEY

1/2 CUP	CHOPPED ONIONS
1	GARLIC CLOVE, MINCED
2 CUPS	SLICED ZUCCHINI
2 CUPS	GREEN SNAP BEANS, CUT IN 1" PIECES
1	EGGPLANT, CUT IN 1/2" CUBES
4	TOMATOES
1 TABLESPOON	BASIL
1 TEASPOON	OREGANO
6 OUNCES	TOMATO PASTE
2 TABLESPOONS	BRAGG'S AMINOES
1 TEASPOON	JENSEN'S BROTH AND SEASONING

Saute garlic and onion in 2 tablespoons of water for 2 minutes. Add herbs, zucchini, green beans, eggplant, and tomatoes in succession, sauteing briefly between each addition. Add a little water as needed to prevent sticking. Mix in tomato paste. Cover and simmer over medium heat, stirring occasionally, for 20 minutes or until vegetables are soft. Add Bragg's Aminoes and Jensen's Broth and Seasoning to taste. Serve immediately. Serves 4.

• MENU FOR DAY SIX •

BREAKFAST

APPLE-KIWI-STRAWBERRY JUICE
BANANA-GRAPE-PEACH FRUIT SALAD

LUNCH

CARROT-CELERY-PARSLEY JUICE
CABBAGE-CUCUMBER SALAD
SOY BURGERS

DINNER

CARROT-APPLE-CAULIFLOWER JUICE
BROCCOLI MEDLEY
MILLET CASSEROLE

NUTRIENTS	
Protein (gm)	55
Total Fat (gm)	34
Complex Carb (gm)	370
Dietary Fiber (gm)	68
Cholesterol (mg)	6
Sodium (mg)	1552
Potassium (mg)	6857
Vitamin A (RE)	23232
Vitamin C (mg)	421
Iron (mg)	37
Calcium (mg)	853
Phosphorus (mg)	1556

TOTAL DAILY CALORIES 2062

18% OF CALORIES ARE FROM FAT

RECIPES

APPLE-KIWI-STRAWBERRY JUICE

4	APPLES
2	KIWIFRUIT
1 CUP	STRAWBERRIES

Wash all fruit, cut to fit opening of juicer. Process. Serves 2.

BANANA-GRAPE-PEACH FRUIT SALAD

2	BANANAS, SLICED
40	SEEDLESS GRAPES
4	PEACHES, SLICED
1 TABLESPOON	LEMON JUICE

Wash all fruit, peel the bananas, remove grapes from stem, remove pit and skin from peaches. Assemble sliced bananas, grapes and sliced peaches in serving bowls and drizzle with lemon juice. Serves 2.

CARROT-CELERY-PARSLEY JUICE

10	CARROTS
2 STALKS	CELERY
1 CUP	PARSLEY

Wash produce, remove carrot tops, cut to fit opening of juicer. Bunch parsley to process, followed by carrot. Serves 2.

CABBAGE-CUCUMBER SALAD

2 1/2 CUPS	SHREDDED GREEN CABBAGE
1 CUP	SLICED CUCUMBER
1/2 CUP	DICED CELERY
1/4 CUP	CHOPPED ONIONS
3 TABLESPOONS	SOY MAYONNAISE
1/4 TEASPOON	GROUND BASIL
1/4 TEASPOON	BLACK PEPPER

Combine all ingredients and toss lightly. Serve immediately. Serves 4.

SOY BURGERS

1 3/4 CUPS	FIRM TOFU, MASHED
1/2 CUP	SHREDDED CARROTS
2 TABLESPOONS	ALMOND BUTTER
2	GARLIC CLOVES, MINCED
3 TABLESPOONS	CHOPPED PARSLEY
1/4 CUP	CHOPPED ONIONS
1/2 TEASPOON	GROUND THYME
1/2 TEASPOON	GROUND SAGE
2 TABLESPOONS	TAMARI
2	TOMATOES, SLICED
2 CUPS	ALFALFA SPROUTS
8 SLICES	WHOLE WHEAT BREAD, TOASTED

Mix all ingredients in large bowl. Shape into 8 or more patties that are about 1/2" thick. Press patties firmly between hands to make sure they hold well. Bake on baking sheet in oven at 350° F. for 20 minutes. Serve with tomato slices and sprouts on toasted wholegrain bread. Serves 4.

CARROT-APPLE-CAULIFLOWER JUICE

10	CARROTS
1	APPLE
1 CUP	CAULIFLOWER

Wash produce, remove carrot tops, cut all produce to fit juicer opening. Serves 2.

BROCCOLI MEDLEY

1/4 CUP	WATER
2 TABLESPOONS	BRAGG'S AMINOES
1 1/2 CUPS	COARSELY CHOPPED BROCCOLI
4	CARROTS, SLICED
1/2 CUP	CHOPPED ONIONS
2	GARLIC CLOVES, MINCED
1 CUP	SLICED ZUCCHINI
1 TABLESPOON	TAMARI
1/2 TEASPOON	JENSEN'S BROTH AND SEASONING*

Wash and prepare vegetables. In a large saute pan, add 1/4 cup of water and 2 tablespoons of Bragg's Aminoes to cover the bottom of pan. Add garlic and onion and saute briefly. Then add rest of vegetables, cover, and saute until al dente, stirring occasionally and adding water if necessary to prevent burning. Remove to serving dish, add Jensen's Broth and tamari; toss gently. Serves 4.

MILLET CASSEROLE

2 CUPS	WHOLE-GRAIN MILLET
1/2 CUP	CHOPPED ONIONS
2	GARLIC CLOVES, MINCED
1 TABLESPOON	OLIVE OIL
1/2	SWEET RED PEPPER, SLICED
3 STALKS	CELERY, DICED
6 CUPS	WATER

Dry roast millet in a skillet, stirring constantly until the millet becomes fragrant. Remove from heat. Heat the oil in a 3-quart saucepan over medium heat, saute the onion and garlic for 2-3 minutes. Add chopped red pepper and celery, stirring well. Add millet, water and salt and bring to boil. Reduce heat, cover, simmer 40 minutes or until done. Serve in casserole dish, garnished with red pepper rings. Serves 4.

*Jensen's Broth and Seasoning is available at most health food stores or call 1-619-755-4027

• MENU FOR DAY SEVEN •

BREAKFAST

STRAWBERRY SUMMER SOUP
MILLET BREAKFAST MUFFINS

BREAKFAST SNACK

4 FIGS, FRESH OR DRIED

LUNCH

CARROT-APPLE-BEET JUICE
BIBB LETTUCE WITH BASIL
SUMMER RICE SALAD

DINNER

CARROT-APPLE-SPROUT-CELERY JUICE
FRESH CORN PEPPER SALAD
TOMATO-ZUCCHINI SAUTE
ARTICHOKE SURPRISE

** indicates recipe not included*

NUTRIENTS	
Protein (gm)	35
Total Fat (gm)	34
Complex Carb (gm)	318
Dietary Fiber (gm)	71
Cholesterol (mg)	1
Sodium (mg)	714
Potassium (mg)	6961
Vitamin A (RE)	17520
Vitamin C (mg)	442
Iron (mg)	20
Calcium (mg)	857
Phosphorus (mg)	1463
TOTAL DAILY CALORIES	**1813**

17% OF CALORIES ARE FROM FAT

RECIPES

STRAWBERRY SUMMER SOUP

4 CUPS	STRAWBERRIES
1	APPLE
1	PEAR
1 CUP	BLUEBERRIES
2	BANANAS, SLICED
2 TEASPOONS	GROUND CINNAMON
8 SLICES	WHOLE WHEAT ESSENE BREAD

Soak raisins overnight in pure water. Wash and prepare fruit. Core and dice apple and pear. Peel banana. Put 3 cups of strawberries in blender and puree. (May have to do in batches.) Add apple, pear, drained raisins (reserve liquid for later use), half of blueberries and cinnamon. Blend well. Pour into large deep bottomed dish or pot. Add rest of sliced fruit. Serve with sprouted wheat or Essene bread. Serves 4.

MILLET BREAKFAST MUFFINS

1 1/2 CUPS	WHOLE WHEAT FLOUR
3 TEASPOONS	BAKING POWDER
2/3 CUP	WHOLE-GRAIN MILLET, COOKED
1 CUP	WATER
1/2 CUP	SEEDLESS RAISINS
1/3 CUP	PLAIN, NONFAT YOGURT
2 TABLESPOONS	HONEY

Preheat oven to 400° F. Place paper liners in muffin tins. Mix dry ingredients together. In separate bowl, mix wet ingredients and raisins together. Combine wet ingredients with dry. Spoon into muffin tins. Bake for 20 minutes. Serves 12.

CARROT-APPLE-BEET JUICE

8	CARROTS
1	APPLE
1/2 CUP	BEET GREENS
1/2	BEET

Wash and prepare produce. Cut off carrot tops. Cut to fit juicer opening. Serves 2.

BIBB LETTUCE WITH BASIL

12	BIBB LETTUCE LEAVES
4 CUPS	ALFALFA SPROUTS
1 TEASPOON	GROUND BASIL
4	TOMATOES, QUARTERED
1/2 CUP	PRITIKIN NO OIL, LOW SODIUM RUSSIAN SALAD DRESSING

Wash and dry the lettuce. Tear into pieces and put into salad bowl along with sprouts, basil, and quartered tomatoes. Add dressing. Serves 4.

SUMMER RICE SALAD

6 CUPS	WATER
3 CUPS	LONG GRAIN BROWN RICE
1	CARROT, FINELY MINCED
3	SCALLIONS, MINCED
1	SWEET RED PEPPER, MINCED
1	SWEET GREEN PEPPER, MINCED
10	RADISHES, MINCED
1 CUP	PARSLEY, FINELY CHOPPED
1/4 CUP	LEMON JUICE
1/4 CUP	RED WINE VINEGAR
1/4 CUP	OLIVE OIL
1/4 CUP	WATER
2	GARLIC CLOVES, MINCED
2 TABLESPOONS	HONEY
1 TEASPOON	CURRY POWDER

To six cups of boiling water add brown rice. Cover pot and cook over medium heat until done (about 45 minutes - 1 hour) Fluff with fork, set aside and let cool. Prepare vegetables by finely mincing the carrots, onions, peppers, radishes, and parsley. Combine marinade ingredients in separate container. Add vegetables and marinade to rice. Stir to mingle flavors and chill before serving at least two hours. Serves 6.

CARROT-APPLE-SPROUT-CELERY JUICE

8	CARROTS
1	APPLE
2 CUPS	ALFALFA SPROUTS
2 STALKS	CELERY

Wash and prepare produce, remove carrot tops. Bunch sprouts when juicing and follow with carrot. Serves 2.

FRESH CORN PEPPER SALAD

2	SWEET RED PEPPERS, CUT INTO STRIPS
2	SWEET GREEN PEPPERS, CUT INTO STRIPS
2 CUPS	YELLOW SQUASH, SLICED
2 CUPS	ZUCCHINI SQUASH, SLICED
8	ROMAINE LETTUCE LEAVES
1 CUP	YELLOW CORN, FRESH OFF COB
1 CUP	PLAIN NONFAT YOGURT
1 TABLESPOON	OLIVE OIL
1 TABLESPOON	LEMON JUICE
1	GARLIC CLOVE, MINCED
1 TEASPOON	GROUND BASIL

Remove seeds from peppers and cut into strips. Blanch squash, zucchini, and eggplant for 2 minutes; set aside. Tear lettuce leaves into pieces and mix these plus dressing with all ingredients by hand. You may add a few chopped walnuts when you serve it. For dressing: whisk yogurt, oil, lemon juice, garlic and basil together. Serves 4.

TOMATO-ZUCCHINI SAUTÉ

4 CUPS	SLICED ZUCCHINI
4	TOMATOES, CHOPPED
2	GARLIC CLOVES, MINCED
1/2 CUP	CHOPPED ONIONS
1 TABLESPOON	OLIVE OIL
1/2 TEASPOON	GROUND BASIL
1/2 TEASPOON	GROUND OREGANO

Saute garlic and onion in olive oil in large skillet over low heat until transparent. Turn heat to medium, add zucchini, tomatoes, and seasonings and simmer 12-15 min. until vegetables are cooked but not too soft. Add parmesan cheese if desired. Stir and serve. Serves 4.

ARTICHOKE SURPRISE

4	ARTICHOKES
2 TABLESPOONS	LEMON JUICE
1/4 CUP	OLIVE OIL
1/2 TEASPOON	GARLIC POWDER
1 TEASPOON	JENSEN'S BROTH AND SEASONING

Trim artichoke leaves and wash. Steam artichokes for 45 to 50 minutes. Remove from steamer. Remove leaves from artichokes, chop up the heart and place in bowl. In a separate bowl, whisk together the lemon juice, olive oil, garlic powder and Jensen's. Pour over artichoke leaves and toss well. Serve warm. Serves 4.

HEALTHY TREATS FOR STAGES I AND II

STRAWBERRY SHORTCAKE

8 CUPS	STRAWBERRIES, SLICED
1/4 CUP	HONEY
2 CUPS	WHOLE WHEAT FLOUR
2 TABLESPOONS	HONEY
1 TABLESPOON	BAKING POWDER
1/2 TEASPOON	SEA SALT
1/4 CUP	RAW BUTTER
1	BROWN FERTILE EGG
3/4 CUP	SOY MILK
1 1/2 CUPS	VANILLA LOWFAT YOGURT

Preheat oven to 450° F. Stir together strawberries and 1/4 cup honey. Set aside. For biscuits, stir together flour, baking powder and salt in a large mixing bowl. Cut in butter until mixture resembles coarse crumbs. In a small bowl combine egg, honey and soymilk. Add to dry ingredients and stir to moisten. Drop by heaping spoonfuls onto ungreased baking sheet and bake 10-12 min. or until golden. Split biscuits, fill and top with fruit and yogurt. Serves 6.

BLUEBERRY (OR PEACH) SHORTCAKE

For blueberry shortcake, prepare as in strawberry shortcake recipe except omit the strawberries and the honey. Mash 2 cups whole blueberries, stir in 1/4 cup honey. Then stir in 2 cups whole blueberries. Set aside. Spoon berry mixture and yogurt over top of biscuits. For peach shortcake, prepare as above, except omit the berries and honey. Stir together 4 cups peeled sliced peaches and 1/3 cup honey. Set aside and serve as above. Serves 6.

EASY STRAWBERRY YOGURT BREAD

1 1/2 CUPS	WHOLE WHEAT FLOUR
1 1/2 CUPS	ALL-PURPOSE, UNBLEACHED FLOUR
1 1/2 TEASPOONS	BAKING SODA
1 TEASPOON	BAKING POWDER
1 TEASPOON	SEA SALT
1/4 TEASPOON	GROUND NUTMEG
2	BROWN FERTILE EGGS
1 TEASPOON	PURE VANILLA EXTRACT VANILLA
1/2 CUP	HONEY
2 CUPS	STRAWBERRY, LOWFAT YOGURT
1/3 CUP	SAFFLOWER OIL

Preheat oven to 350° F. Lightly oil and flour an 8 1/2 x 4 1/2 inch loaf pan. Set aside. Combine first 5 ingredients in a large bowl until well blended. In another large bowl, beat the wet ingredients well. Add the flour mixture to the egg mixture and beat just until blended and almost smooth. Turn batter into prepared pan. Bake for 45 to 50 minutes. Cool 5 minutes in pan, remove and finish cooling on rack. Makes 2 loaves. Serves 16.

ALMOND BUTTER COOKIES

1/4 CUP	SAFFLOWER OIL (OR RAW BUTTER, SOFTENED)
1/2 CUP	MAPLE SYRUP
2/3 CUP	ALMOND BUTTER
1/4 TEASPOON	SEA SALT
1 1/2 CUPS	WHOLE WHEAT FLOUR
1/2 CUP	CHOPPED ALMONDS

Preheat oven to 350° F. Beat together oil (or butter) and maple syrup. Mix in almond butter. Combine dry ingredients except nuts and mix into wet ingredients. Mix in chopped almonds reserving enough to sprinkle on top of cookies. Drop by teaspoonful onto oiled cookie sheet. Make a small well in the center of each cookie and sprinkle chopped almonds in the indentation. Bake for 12 to 15 min. Cool on wire rack. Makes approximately 2 dozen. Serves 8.

WHOLE WHEAT BANANA BREAD

1 1/4 CUPS	ALL-PURPOSE, UNBLEACHED FLOUR
1/2 CUP	WHOLE WHEAT FLOUR
1 TEASPOON	BAKING SODA
1/4 TEASPOON	SEA SALT
1/4 CUP	SAFFLOWER OIL
1	BROWN, FERTILE EGG
1 CUP	BANANAS, MASHED
1 TEASPOON	PURE VANILLA EXTRACT

Preheat oven to 350° F. Combine first 4 ingredients in a small bowl. Stir well, set aside. Combine honey and oil in a medium bowl; beat until well blended. Add egg; beat until light. With electric mixer running a low speed, add flour mixture alternately with banana, beginning and ending with flour mixture. Stir in vanilla. Pour batter into an oiled and floured 8x4x2-inch loaf pan. Bake for 45-50 minutes. Cool 15 minutes in pan, remove to wire rack. Serves 16.

COCONUT ALMOND CARROT CAKE

1 CUP	WHOLE WHEAT FLOUR
1/2 CUP	ALL-PURPOSE, UNBLEACHED FLOUR
1/2 TEASPOON	SEA SALT
1 TEASPOON	GROUND CINNAMON
1 CUP	HONEY
2	BROWN, FERTILE EGGS
1 CUP	CARROTS
1/2 CUP	CHOPPED ALMONDS
1/2 CUP	SEEDLESS RAISINS
1 CUP	UNSWEETENED FLAKED COCONUT

Preheat oven to 350° F. Mix first 5 ingredients; set aside. Beat honey and oil at medium speed of electric mixer until well mixed. Stir in flour mixture. Add eggs, one at a time, beating after each addition. Stir in carrots, nuts, raisins, and 2/3 cup coconut. Pour into oiled and floured 9-inch Bundt pan. Bake for 35 minutes. Cool in pan 15 minutes. Remove from pan and finish cooling on rack. Frost with Almond Glaze. Serves 16.

ALMOND GLAZE

2 CUPS	APPLE JUICE
4 TEASPOONS	ARROWROOT POWDER
2 TABLESPOONS	HONEY
1/8 TEASPOON	SEA SALT
2 TEASPOONS	ALMOND EXTRACT

Dissolve arrowroot with juice in saucepan. Heat over low flame, stirring constantly until juice bubbles, thickens and becomes clear. Stir in honey and almond extract. Drizzle over cake or cool and "frost" cake. Variations: Substitute orange, strawberry, or other juice for apple juice. Add vanilla extract or grated lemon peel. Serves 16.

WHOLE WHEAT BLUEBERRY MUFFINS

1 1/3 CUPS	WHOLE WHEAT FLOUR
1 CUP	OLD-FASHIONED OATS
1/4 CUP	HONEY
1 TABLESPOON	BAKING POWDER
1/2 TEASPOON	CINNAMON
1 CUP	SOY MILK
1	BROWN, FERTILE EGG
3 TABLESPOONS	SAFFLOWER OIL
1 1/2 CUPS	BLUEBERRIES

Preheat oven to 425° F. Line muffin cups with paper baking cups. Combine dry ingredients. Add soymilk, egg and oil; stir just until dry ingredients are moistened. Fold in blueberries; fill prepared muffin cups 2/3 full. Bake 25 to 30 minutes or until light golden brown. Makes one dozen muffins. Serves 12.

APPLE-NUT MUFFINS

2 CUPS	WHOLE WHEAT FLOUR
1 CUP	ALL-PURPOSE, UNBLEACHED FLOUR
1 TABLESPOON	BAKING POWDER
1 TEASPOON	GROUND CINNAMON
1/8 TEASPOON	SEA SALT
1/2 CUP	MAPLE SYRUP
1/2 CUP	CORN OIL
1 TEASPOON	PURE VANILLA EXTRACT
3/4 CUP	WATER
4 OUNCES	FIRM TOFU
2	APPLES, PEELED, CORED, CHOPPED
1/2 CUP	CHOPPED WALNUTS

Preheat oven to 375° F. Sift dry ingredients into a large bowl. Puree maple syrup, oil, vanilla, water and tofu in a blender until smooth. Add wet to dry ingredients, mix until just moistened. Gently fold in apple and walnuts. Put paper muffin cups into muffin tin. Pour batter into cups 2/3 full and bake for 20 minutes or until golden brown. Makes 12 muffins. Serves 12.

GLAZED PINEAPPLE COUSCOUS CAKE

6 CUPS	APPLE JUICE
1/8 TEASPOON	SEA SALT
1 TABLESPOON	LEMON JUICE
2 CUPS	COUSCOUS
5 CUPS	CRUSHED AND DRAINED PINEAPPLE
1/8 TEASPOON	SEA SALT
2 TABLESPOONS	ARROWROOT POWDER
2 TABLESPOONS	WATER

Bring 5 cups apple juice and sea salt to a boil in saucepan; add lemon rind and juice. Add couscous and reduce heat; stir till almost thick. Remove from stove; stir in 2 cups pineapple. Pour cake into 9" x 13" glass baking dish. Allow to cool; cut into squares. Glaze: Bring 1 cup apple juice to a boil. Add 3 cups pineapple and salt; bring to a boil. Cover; simmer 15 minutes. Dilute arrowroot in water; add to cooked fruit; simmer 5 minutes; stir until thick. Drizzle over squares. Serves 12.

CAROB BROWNIE FROZEN YOGURT CAKE

1/2 CUP	RAW BUTTER
1/3 CUP	HONEY
1/3 CUP	TURBINADO (RAW) SUGAR
1	BROWN, FERTILE EGG
1/2 TEASPOON	SEA SALT
1 TEASPOON	PURE VANILLA EXTRACT
1/2 CUP	CAROB POWDER
1 TABLESPOON	CORN OIL
2/3 CUP	WHOLE WHEAT FLOUR
1 TEASPOON	BAKING POWDER
1 CUP	CHOPPED WALNUTS
1/2 GALLON	NONFAT, FROZEN YOGURT (VANILLA OR OTHER FLAVOR)

Cream butter, honey and sugar until fluffy. Beat in egg, salt and vanilla. Beat together carob powder and oil then add to butter mixture. Mix flour and baking powder then add to carob mixture. Add nuts. Spread very thin in a 9x13 inch pan. Bake at 350° F. for 25 to 30 minutes. Cool. Spread vanilla (or other flavor) frozen yogurt over top. Cover with plastic wrap and freeze overnight. Serves 16.

CHAPTER 11

The Transitional Diet

STAGE III

STAGE III is what I call the *ultimate diet*. At least it is ultimate for most of us. Decaffeinated coffee, dairy products, fish, and poultry are totally omitted at this stage. Natural sweeteners and oils are used sparingly, and your raw food intake is increased to 75-90% of the diet.

What makes this stage unique is that it puts more emphasis on sprouted, predigested foods. These are foods that are easy to digest. Fruit is already a predigested food. This means that the proteins are broken down to amino acids, fats down to fatty acids, and carbohydrates down to simple sugars. This saves on the body's digestive juices and enzymes because one whole digestive step has been done outside the body. These predigested foods not only save on the body's total enzyme level, but also take less energy to digest. Many people, however, do not realize how valuable these savings are. You only have so much energy in your body for healing, digestion, thinking, and all other metabolic processes. If you can save a percentage of energy daily by eating predigested foods, think of the effect it will have on healing and longevity. Predigested foods, the use of enzymes, and raw juices

STAGE 3

75% - 90% raw food

BEVERAGES
- use herbal teas, distilled, reverse osmosis, or deionized water, freshly made fruit and vegetable juices
- eliminate decaf coffee and alcoholic beverages
- do not drink with meals

CARBOHYDRATES

Breads:
- use only sprouted whole grain or Essene breads

Cereals:
- use organic whole, raw grains - unroasted

Grains:
- same as Stage #2

Legumes:
- same as Stage #2

Pasta:
- eliminate

Sweeteners:
- further limit use of natural sweeteners
- use fresh fruits or reconstituted dried fruits to sweeten
- water combinations

CONDIMENTS & SEASONINGS
- eliminate sea salt
- further limit use of condiments
- watch for bad combinations

DESSERTS
- same as Stage #2
- use as a snack only

FATS AND OILS
- eliminate raw butter
- use only cold-pressed vegetable oils in dark bottles or cans

FRUITS
- same as Stage 2

JUICES
- use only freshly made fruit and vegetable juices

STAGE 3 75% - 90% raw food	
PROTEIN *Dairy:* • same as Stage #2 • continue to reduce quantity or eliminate totally *Meat, fish, poultry:* • eliminate fish, chicken and turkey • use protein alternatives as in Stage #2 *Nuts & seeds:* • use only soaked seeds and nuts • limit use of nut butters VEGETABLES *Salads:* • further increase varieties of fresh vegetables *Salad Dressings:* • same as Stage #2 *Soups:* • same as Stage #2	MISCELLANEOUS *Candy:* • eliminate store bought candy • use only homemade "candy" as in Stage #2 *Ice Cream:* • use non-dairy frozen desserts and frozen fruit creams only as a treat

are definitely a prerequisite to longevity. How can anybody think that eating cookies, meat, processed foods, refined grains, and the use of mega-vitamins will increase life span? Obviously, the preferred choice is to give the body the best raw material available out of which it can reconstitute tissue, blood, and hormones.

CHART 11.1

SPROUTING CHART

SEED	Soaking time (hours)	rinse (times/ day)	ready in (days)	sprouting equipment	description (at harvest)
aduki	8-12	3	5	bag/jar	bean & tail
alfalfa	8	3	7	basket/jar	green leaf
barley	8	3	3-5	bag/jar	grain & sprout tail
beans	8-12	3	3-5	bag/jar	bean & sprout tail
chick peas	8	4	4	bag/jar	bean & sprout tail
buckwheat	8	3	2-3	bag/jar	grain & tail
buckwheat *(for lettuce)*	8	3	9	basket/tray	green leaf
cabbage	8	3	5	basket/jar	green leaf
clover	8	3	6	basket/jar	green leaf
fenugreek	8	3	8	basket/jar	green leaf
lentil	8	3	5	bag/jar	bean & tail
millet	8	3	3	bag/jar	seed & tail
mungbean	8	3	5	basket/bag/jar	bean & tail
pea	8	3	5	bag/jar	bean & tail
radish	8	3	5	basket/jar	green leaf
rye	8	3	2	bag/jar	grain & tail
soybean	8	4-5	3	bag/jar	bean & tail
sunflower, shelled	8	2	2	bag/jar	seed & tail
sunflower, whole *(for greens)*	8	3	9	basket/tray	green leaf
wheat, hard *(for breads)*	8-15	2	2	bag/jar	grain & tail (1/4" tail)
wheat hard *(for wheat grass) for juicing*	8-15	2-3	12-14	basket/tray	wheatgrass 3" high
wheat, soft *(for snacks, cookies, crackers)*	8-15	2	2	bag/jar	grain & tail (1/4" tail)

NOTES:

1. For sprouts that develop green leaves - their peak nutritional value comes at the time when the sprout throws off its hull and splits into its first pair of leaves.
2. Sprouting equipment - methods including jar with cheesecloth or netting secured on top, sprouting basket, sprouting bag, tray with soil.
3. For more information on sprouting contact: The Sprout House, 40 Railroad Street, Great Barrington, MA 01230

CHART 11.2

VITAMIN CONTENT (MICROGRAMS PER GRAM) OF DRY SEEDS AND OF SEEDS GERMINATED FOR 5 DAYS IN SAND CULTURES

KIND OF SEED	Riboflavin dry	Riboflavin germinated	Niacin dry	Niacin germinated	Thiamine dry	Thiamine germinated	Biotin dry	Biotin germinated
barley	1.3	8.3	7.2	12.9	-	7.9	0.4	1.2
corn	1.2	3.0	17	40	6.2	5.5	0.3	0.7
oats	0.6	12.4	11	48	10.0	11.5	1.2	1.8
soybeans	2.0	9.1	27	49	10.7	9.6	1.1	3.5
lima (large)	1.0	2.0	15	29	6.7	5.0	0.1	0.1
lima (small)	0.9	4.0	11	41	4.5	6.2	0.1	0.4
green eye pea	1.8	9.7	20	60	11.0	12.0	0.4	1.1
mungbean	1.2	10.0	26	70	8.8	10.3	0.2	1.0
pea	0.7	7.3	31	32	7.2	9.2	-	0.5

From: Sprout for the Love of Everybody *by Victor P. Kulvinskas. Used with permission.*

Sprouting is very simple. Even children can learn to do it, and most children love to. Any glass jar or stainless steel pot can be turned into a "sprouter." Health food stores carry sprouting supplies, and most food co-ops carry sprouting seeds. Chart 11.1 gives you directions on how to sprout—i.e. soaking time, how many times to rinse your seeds, and how many days before harvesting.

One of the major advantages of eating sprouted food, besides its being predigested, is its nutritional profile. Look at Chart 11.2 which describes how sprouting increases the nutritional contents. For instance, barley, dry, has 1.3 micrograms per gram of Riboflavin. After it is germinated (sprouted) for 5 days, it increases to 8.3 micrograms, a sixfold increase. The rest of the chart is self-explanatory.

Sprouting makes proteins, carbohydrates, and fats more digestible, and in most cases more nutrient rich. The total fat content of corn is reduced by oxidation after sprouting for 120 hours. The fat is actually broken down and the glycerol part of the fat molecule becomes part of the carbohydrate metabolism of the seed. Very small amounts of the fat accumulate in the seed itself, which is one reason why predigested fat does not accumulate in our arteries. With sprouting, soluble carbohydrates are broken down to glucose for easy assimilation and digestion. Protein is broken down to total amino acids in 120 hours.

At the same time, sprouting increases the enzyme content of foods. For example, when peas are sprouted their amylase activity begins to increase after only two days. After 96 hours the amylase activity is four times greater. So, sprouted (germinated) food increases in both nutrients and enzymes and is much easier to digest. Here we have the ultimate food, one of the main components of longevity. That's why I call Stage III the *ultimate diet*.

You will recall, in the chapter on enzymes, that Dr. Edward Howell refers to the pre-digestive stomach in animals and humans. What this means is that the food sits in our cardiac (upper part of our stomach), or pre-digestive, stomach for 30-60 minutes before enzymes are secreted to it. If the food is raw, the enzymes already contained in the food can actually digest a percentage of the food within this part of the stomach. This takes the stress off the pancreas. The pancreas will not have to produce and secrete as many enzymes to digest the whole food because it is partially digested. This saves the pancreas from enzyme exhaustion and strengthens the immune system.

Now let's take this concept a little further, which is what this whole book has been leading up to. If the food eaten is not only raw but also sprouted (which not only makes the food predigested but increases its enzyme content and nutrients), we have the ultimate food. The food is easy to digest, nutrients are easy to assimilate, and the enzyme-secreting organs are *preserved*. Some enzymes are actually re-absorbed back into the body which can further aid the metabolic processes. This is the real Fountain of Youth, make no mistake about it! A pre-digested food diet, in my opinion, should be used for elderly people and folks who are trying to recover from illness.

Sprouts, germinated seeds and nuts, grains, leafy green vegetables, and freshly-made juices, with the addition of sea vegetables, are the ultimate foods. If you adopt this diet, you will know what I mean by *Intuitive Eating*. You will honor your body's intelligence and your mind will work at a higher level. Your weight will stabilize, and your body will take its natural shape. Exercise will be a pleasure. You will know by how you feel that this evolutionary dietary path was the right direction for you.

As they approach Stage III many people think that their social eating habits will have to change completely, and that they can no longer go to restaurants with their friends. This is an old concept and is totally untrue. Most restaurants now have meals for vegetarians, and you can bring your own spices and order romaine lettuce for your salads. (In other words, a Caesar salad without dressing.) Then you can add your own dressing. You can get soups and baked potatoes at almost any restaurant. Also, if you decide to slip off your diet for awhile, this would be the time to do it. Sometimes when I eat out with friends I will order a whole-grain pasta dish and salad. It doesn't hurt me a bit, especially since I know my diet is 95% correct. Besides, I don't backslide too far or do it often. For me, the use of dairy and meat are out of the question, so I might have a salad, with a baked potato smothered in freshly-chopped parsley and grated raw onion.

There is nothing wrong with being a little different and a little original. At this stage in eating you won't care what others think because you will know what is right for you. If other people want to poison themselves, that's their problem, not yours. An opinion from an uneducated standpoint should mean little to those who know what they want from life and stand strong in their conviction. A vegetarian diet is not new, and almost everybody knows what causes heart disease and hardening of the arteries. If people refuse to listen, they are effectively refusing to live in a way that maximizes their health and well-being.

SEVEN DAY MEAL PLAN FOR STAGE III

• MENU FOR DAY ONE •

BREAKFAST

GRAPEFRUIT-APPLE JUICE
BANANA FIG PUDDING

LUNCH

CARROT-KALE PLUS JUICE
SPINACH-MUSHROOM SALAD
TOMATO DRESSING
SAUTEED TOFU

LUNCH SNACK

STRAWBERRIES*

DINNER

BLENDED SALAD
VEGETABLE PLATTER
TOMATO AND BASIL DIP
SCALLOPED POTATOES WITH ONIONS
COOKED GREEN PEAS

**indicates no recipe included*

NUTRIENTS	
Protein (gm)	40
Total Fat (gm)	29
Complex Carb (gm)	297
Dietary Fiber (gm)	44
Cholesterol (mg)	0
Sodium (mg)	1464
Potassium (mg)	6878
Vitamin A (RE)	13517
Vitamin C (mg)	551
Iron (mg)	26
Calcium (mg)	758
Phosphorus (mg)	1129
TOTAL DAILY CALORIES	**1681**

15% OF CALORIES ARE FROM FAT

RECIPES

GRAPEFRUIT-APPLE JUICE

2	PINK GRAPEFRUIT
2	APPLES

Peel grapefruit leaving as much white on as possible. Wash apple and cut to fit opening. Cut grapefruit to fit opening. Feed through opening and juice. Drink immediately. Serves 2.

BANANA FIG PUDDING

5	DRIED FIGS
2 TABLESPOONS	FLAX SEEDS
1 CUP	WATER
3	BANANAS
1/4 CUP	SEEDLESS RAISINS

Soak 5 dried figs and flax seeds overnight in pure water to cover. Pour figs, seeds, and water in blender in morning to which you add 3 ripe bananas and blend well. As a pudding, you may serve this alone or add a handful of raisins to pudding after blending. Serves 2.

CARROT-KALE PLUS JUICE

10	CARROTS
1	APPLE
1 SLICE	GINGER ROOT, 1/8" THICK
1 STALK	CELERY
1 CUP	KALE, CHOPPED

Wash and prepare produce. Cut to fit juicer opening. Feed through opening. Serves 2.

SPINACH-MUSHROOM SALAD

4 CUPS	SPINACH, CHOPPED
1/2 CUP	MUSHROOMS, SLICED
1/2	AVOCADO, SLICED

Wash, dry and prepare greens and vegetables for salad. Assemble ingredients in medium size serving bowl. Add Tomato Dressing. Serves 2.

TOMATO DRESSING

1 CUP	FRESH TOMATO JUICE
1 CUP	TOMATO SAUCE
1/3 CUP	CIDER VINEGAR
1/4 TEASPOON	LEMON JUICE
1/2 TEASPOON	BASIL
1/2 TEASPOON	OREGANO
1/2 TEASPOON	THYME

Mix all ingredients together in a large jar. Serves 8.

SAUTÉED TOFU

4 OUNCES	FIRM TOFU
1	GARLIC CLOVE, MINCED
1 TABLESPOON	BRAGG'S AMINOES*
2 TABLESPOONS	WATER

Drain tofu. Cut into 1/2" cubes. In a medium saute pan, add one clove minced garlic to one tablespoon of water. Saute briefly, then add cubed tofu and one tablespoon of Bragg's Aminoes. Stir. Saute for 5 minutes, stirring occasionally. Add to salad still warm. Serves 2.

*Bragg's Aminoes are available at most health food stores or call 1-800-446-1990

BLENDED SALAD

8	ROMAINE LETTUCE LEAVES
2	TOMATOES
1	CUCUMBER
1	SWEET GREEN PEPPER
2 STALKS	CELERY
2 TABLESPOONS	LEMON JUICE

Wash and dry all produce and cut into large pieces. Add tomato to blender first, followed by cucumber, pepper, lettuce, lemon juice, and celery. You can use celery stalk as a pusher. Blend well and pour into serving bowls. Serves 4.

VEGETABLE PLATTER

4	CARROTS
2	SWEET GREEN PEPPERS
1	CUCUMBER
2 STALKS	CELERY
1 CUP	ZUCCHINI SQUASH, SLICED
1	SWEET RED PEPPER
1 CUP	CAULIFLOWER

Wash vegetables and cut into finger size pieces. Arrange on a platter around dip. Serves 4.

TOMATO AND BASIL DIP

2 TABLESPOONS	LEMON JUICE
2 TABLESPOONS	BRAGG'S AMINOES
2 TABLESPOONS	HONEY
2 OUNCES	FIRM TOFU
1/2	TOMATO
1 TEASPOON	BASIL
1	SCALLION
1 TEASPOON	JENSEN'S BROTH AND SEASONING*

Combine all ingredients in a blender and process until smooth. Add one teaspoon Jensen's Broth and Seasoning. Serves 4.

*Jensen's Broth and Seasoning is available at most health food stores or call 1-619-755-4027

SCALLOPED POTATOES WITH ONIONS

4	POTATOES
1 CUP	ONIONS
3 TABLESPOONS	WHOLE WHEAT FLOUR
3 TABLESPOONS	OLIVE OIL
1 CUP	SOY MILK, PLAIN

Thinly slice onions and potatoes (with skins on). Put one layer of potatoes, onions, and one tablespoon each olive oil and flour in a 1-1/2 quart casserole dish. Then continue layering ingredients until casserole is full. Pour plain soymilk over top. Bake uncovered for one hour at 350° F. or until lightly brown on top. Variation: Add grated parmesan cheese before baking (Diets I and II). Serves 8.

• MENU FOR DAY TWO •

BREAKFAST

PINEAPPLE JUICE
APPLE-BANANA SALAD
SOAKED SEED/NUT SAUCE OVER FRUIT

LUNCH

CARROT-GINGER-BEET JUICE
BROWN RICE WITH VEGETABLES

LUNCH SNACK

CANTALOUPE*

DINNER

CARROT-APPLE-PARSLEY JUICE
GREEN DUO SALAD
STEAMED BROCCOLI WITH OLIVE OIL AND LEMON JUICE

**indicates no recipe included*

NUTRIENTS	
Protein (gm)	32
Total Fat (gm)	30
Complex Carb (gm)	332
Dietary Fiber (gm)	32
Cholesterol (mg)	0
Sodium (mg)	2401
Potassium (mg)	6212
Vitamin A (RE)	23899
Vitamin C (mg)	477
Iron (mg)	16
Calcium (mg)	773
Phosphorus (mg)	1070

TOTAL DAILY CALORIES 1834

15% OF CALORIES ARE FROM FAT

RECIPES

PINEAPPLE JUICE

3 RINGS PINEAPPLE, CUT INTO 1" SLICES

For 8 oz. of juice - take 3 one inch rings of pineapple, cut to size and run through juicer. Serves 1.

APPLE-BANANA SALAD

2 APPLES
2 BANANAS

Wash, core and cut apple into 1/2" cubes. Peel and slice banana. Add both to serving bowl and mix. Pour Soaked Seed/Nut Sauce over fruit.

Serves 2.

SOAKED SEED/NUT SAUCE OVER FRUIT

1 TABLESPOON SUNFLOWER SEEDS
1 TABLESPOON ALMONDS
4 DRIED FIGS
1 TABLESPOON ROASTED TAHINI
1 TABLESPOON FLAX SEEDS
1 TABLESPOON HONEY

Soak nuts and figs in water to cover overnight. In morning, use hand blender if possible or regular blender with sparing amounts of water and blend soaked nuts and figs. Add honey and tahini and blend well. Pour over diced fruit in season such as chopped or grated apples, pears, bananas, nectarines, peaches, blueberries, etc. Serves 2.

CARROT-GINGER-BEET JUICE

10 CARROTS
1/4 BEET
1 APPLE
1 SLICE GINGER ROOT, 1/2" THICK

Wash vegetables and fruit. Cut vegetables and fruit to fit opening of juicer. Feed through juicer. Serves 2.

BROWN RICE WITH VEGETABLES

3 CUPS	WATER
1 1/2 CUPS	BROWN RICE
1/2 CUP	CHOPPED ONIONS
2 CUPS	BROCCOLI FLOWERETTES
1 CUP	CARROTS, SLICED
1 CUP	CAULIFLOWER, CHOPPED
4 TABLESPOONS	BRAGG'S AMINOES

Bring 3 cups of water to boil in a large pan. Add brown rice and reduce temperature to medium heat. Cook until rice has absorbed all water and is tender. Meanwhile saute vegetables in another large frying pan using water instead of oil to gently saute the vegetables until al dente. When rice is done and vegetables are ready, add vegetables to rice, add herbs and seasonings. Toss gently and serve warm. Serves 2.

CARROT-APPLE-PARSLEY JUICE

10	CARROTS
1	APPLE
1/2 CUP	PARSLEY

Wash produce, remove carrot tops. Cut to fit opening of juicer. Juice. Serves 2.

GREEN DUO SALAD

8	ROMAINE LETTUCE LEAVES
8	LOOSELEAF LETTUCE LEAVES
4 CUPS	ALFALFA SPROUTS
1/2 CUP	RED CABBAGE, SHREDDED
1/2 CUP	CARROTS, SHREDDED
2 TABLESPOONS	LEMON JUICE
2 TABLESPOONS	OLIVE OIL
2 TABLESPOONS	HONEY

Prepare lettuce greens by washing, drying, and then tearing into bite-sized pieces. Clean and prepare rest of salad fixings and put in salad bowl. Mix dressing ingredients; toss with salad. Serves 4.

STEAMED BROCCOLI WITH OLIVE OIL AND LEMON JUICE

4	BROCCOLI SPEARS
3 TABLESPOONS	OLIVE OIL
1 1/2 TABLESPOONS	LEMON JUICE

Wash broccoli and cut into 1/2" flowerettes and the stalk into 1/2" cubes (cut off any tough sections). Place into a vegetable steamer and cook until al dente. Remove from heat and place on serving platter. Drizzle olive oil and lemon juice on top. Serve. Serves 4.

• MENU FOR DAY THREE •

BREAKFAST

APPLE-STRAWBERRY JUICE
BANANA MILLET BREAKFAST

LUNCH

CARROT-APPLE-SPINACH-PARSLEY JUICE
CAULI SANDWICH
VEGETABLE MARINADE

DINNER

V-6 JUICE
BOK CHOY STIR FRY

NUTRIENTS	
Protein (gm)	47
Total Fat (gm)	31
Complex Carb (gm)	349
Dietary Fiber (gm)	37
Cholesterol (mg)	8
Sodium (mg)	1359
Potassium (mg)	6121
Vitamin A (RE)	13918
Vitamin C (mg)	484
Iron (mg)	26
Calcium (mg)	757
Phosphorus (mg)	1403

TOTAL DAILY CALORIES 1915

15% OF CALORIES ARE FROM FAT

RECIPES

APPLE-STRAWBERRY JUICE

2 CUPS STRAWBERRIES
4 APPLES

Wash fruit and cut to fit opening of juicer and process. Serves 2.

BANANA MILLET BREAKFAST

1/2 CUP MILLET
2 BANANAS
1 1/2 CUPS WATER

Soak millet overnight in pure water. In morning, blend ingredients together. Cook over low flame for 5 minutes. A very nice alkaline dish. Serves 2.

CARROT-APPLE-SPINACH-PARSLEY JUICE

10 CARROTS
1 APPLE
1 CUP SPINACH, CHOPPED
1 CUP PARSLEY, CHOPPED

Wash produce well. Cut carrot tops off. Cut produce to fit size of opening on juicer. Serves 2.

CAULI SANDWICH

2 CUPS	CAULIFLOWER
2 TEASPOONS	LEMON JUICE
1/2 TEASPOON	GROUND CUMIN
1/4 TEASPOON	OREGANO
1/4 TEASPOON	CORIANDER SEED
1/8 TEASPOON	MUSTARD SEED
1/4 CUP	SOY MAYONNAISE
4	WHOLE WHEAT PITA BREAD
2	TOMATOES
2 CUPS	ALFALFA SPROUTS

Cook cauliflower until soft. Mash cauliflower and then add lemon juice, seasonings, and mayonnaise. Cut pitas in half. Spread mixture inside each half of the pita and add tomato and sprouts. Serves 4.

VEGETABLE MARINADE

1 1/2 CUPS	CAULIFLOWER, COARSELY CHOPPED
1 1/2 CUPS	BROCCOLI, CHOPPED
1 CUP	CROOKNECK SUMMER SQUASH, SLICED
1 CUP	ZUCCHINI SQUASH, SLICED
1	SCALLION, SLICED
1	SWEET GREEN PEPPER, SLICED
1	SWEET RED PEPPER, SLICED
1/2 POUND	MUSHROOMS, SLICED
1 CUP	GREEN SNAP BEANS, SNIPPED AND CUT
1/4 CUP	OLIVE OIL
3 TABLESPOONS	LEMON JUICE
1 TEASPOON	GARLIC POWDER
1/4 CUP	WATER
4 TABLESPOONS	BRAGG'S AMINOES

Wash and prepare all vegetables. Combine in large bowl. Combine all marinade ingredients in separate container and then pour over vegetables. Let stand for at least 2 hours. Toss lightly. Drain marinade before serving and save for other use. Serves 6.

V-6 JUICE

4	TOMATOES
2 STALKS	CELERY
1	SWEET GREEN PEPPER
2	CARROTS
1	SMALL ONION
1	GARLIC CLOVE

Wash all vegetables and cut to fit opening of juicer. Juice and garnish each glass with one celery stalk. Serves 2.

BOK CHOY STIR FRY

2 TABLESPOONS	MISO
1 TABLESPOON	HONEY
5 PIECES	GINGER ROOT (1" DIAMETER X 1/8" THICK)
3/4 CUP	WATER
1/2 CUP	BROCCOLI, CHOPPED
1	CARROT, SLICED
1 STALKS	CELERY, DICED
1/2 CUP	SLICED ONION
1/2 CUP	CAULIFLOWER, CHOPPED
1 TEASPOON	OLIVE OIL
3 CUPS	CHINESE CABBAGE, PAK-CHOI OR BOK CHOY,SHREDDED
1/2 CUP	FIRM TOFU, CUBED
1 TABLESPOON	SESAME SEEDS
6 CUPS	COOKED BROWN RICE

Mix miso, honey, ginger and water. Set aside. Wash and prepare vegetables. Stir-fry vegetables with oil in wok or heavy frying pan. After 5 minutes, add greens and stir 1 minute. Add miso mixture and tofu. Stir and cover. Steam over reduced heat another 5 minutes or until cooked to taste. May serve over brown rice or as is. Serves 4.

• MENU FOR DAY FOUR •

BREAKFAST

FRESH ORANGE JUICE
DATE APPLE BREAKFAST

LUNCH

CARROT-APPLE-RADISH-BEET JUICE
GAZPACHO SOUP

DINNER

CARROT-PARSLEY-KALE-APPLE JUICE
BROCCOLI SLAW
ADZUKI BEAN SQUASH CASSEROLE

NUTRIENTS	
Protein (gm)	40
Total Fat (gm)	26
Complex Carb (gm)	299
Dietary Fibern (gm)	36
Cholesterol (mg)	0
Sodium (mg)	713
Potassium (mg)	6634
Vitamin A (RE)	19705
Vitamin C (mg)	491
Iron (mg)	19
Calcium (mg)	703
Phosphorus (mg)	1079

TOTAL DAILY CALORIES 1627

15% OF CALORIES ARE FROM FAT

RECIPES

FRESH ORANGE JUICE

6 VALENCIA ORANGES

Peel oranges, leaving as much outer white as possible. Cut to fit opening of juicer. Serves 2.

DATE APPLE BREAKFAST

1/3 CUP	ALMONDS
1 1/2 CUPS	WATER
2	APPLES
1 CUP	DRY DATES, CHOPPED

Soak dates and almonds overnight in pure water to cover. Blend dates and almonds into a thick paste. Mix shredded apple with mixture, topped with a sprinkle of cinnamon. Serves 2.

CARROT-APPLE-RADISH-BEET JUICE

8	CARROTS
1	APPLE
3	RADISHES
1/4	BEET
1 SLICE	GINGER ROOT, 1/8" THICK
1	SWEET GREEN PEPPER

Wash and prepare produce. Remove carrot and radish tops, cut to fit opening of juicer. Process. Serves 2.

GAZPACHO SOUP

6 CUPS	TOMATOES, CHOPPED
1	SWEET GREEN PEPPER
1/2 CUP	CHOPPED ONIONS
1	CUCUMBER
3 TABLESPOONS	LEMON JUICE
2 TABLESPOONS	BRAGG'S AMINOES

Puree half of the tomatoes in a blender. Add coarsely chopped pepper, onions, cucumber and blend. Add rest of tomatoes, seasonings, lemon juice and blend briefly. Chill before serving for a refreshing summer treat. Serves 5.

CARROT-PARSLEY-KALE-APPLE JUICE

10	CARROTS
1/2 CUP	PARSLEY
1 CUP	KALE, CHOPPED
1	APPLE

Wash all produce, remove carrot tops, cut to fit opening of juicer and process. Serves 2.

BROCCOLI SLAW

1 1/2 CUPS	BROCCOLI, CHOPPED
1 1/2 CUPS	RED CABBAGE, SHREDDED
3	SCALLIONS
3 TABLESPOONS	OLIVE OIL
1 1/2 TABLESPOONS	LEMON JUICE

Prepare vegetables (use food processor for cabbage) and assemble in salad bowl. Toss gently with lemon juice and olive oil. Serves 4.

ADZUKI BEAN SQUASH CASSEROLE

2 CUPS	ADZUKI BEANS, DRY
2 CUPS	HUBBARD WINTER SQUASH, PEELED AND CUBED
1/2 CUP	CHOPPED ONIONS
3 TABLESPOONS	BARLEY MISO

Soak adzuki beans overnight in pure water to cover. Rinse and cover with fresh pure water; cook until tender (1 hour). Peel, seed the squash, cut into 1/2" cubes. Steam cubed squash and onions until tender. Combine adzuki beans and vegetables in large pot, adding a little water if needed to prevent sticking. Cook over medium heat for 20-30 minutes, stirring occasionally. Remove from heat. Add miso dissolved in a little water to mixture. Serves 4.

• MENU FOR DAY FIVE •

BREAKFAST

CANTALOUPE JUICE
DATE WHIP

LUNCH

CARROT-CUCUMBER-CELERY-APPLE JUICE
MARINATED CAULIFLOWER-VEGETABLE SALAD

LUNCH SNACK

CASABA MELON*

DINNER

CARROT-CABBAGE-CELERY-GINGER JUICE
GREEN SALAD
DIJON DRESSING
BAKED BUTTERNUT SQUASH
WHEAT RICE

**indicates no recipe included*

NUTRIENTS	
Protein (gm)	37
Total Fat (gm)	25
Complex Carb (gm)	352
Dietary Fiber (gm)	41
Cholesterol (mg)	0
Sodium (mg)	885
Potassium (mg)	7572
Vitamin A (RE)	24324
Vitamin C (mg)	493
Iron (mg)	21
Calcium (mg)	716
Phosphorus (mg)	1371

TOTAL DAILY CALORIES 1835

13% OF CALORIES ARE FROM FAT

RECIPES

CANTALOUPE JUICE

1 CANTALOUPE MELON

Wash outside of melon thoroughly. Cut strips to fit size of juicer opening and process. Serves 2.

DATE WHIP

10 WHOLE NATURAL DRY DATES, PITTED
2 TABLESPOONS FLAX SEEDS
6 DRIED UNCOOKED PRUNES, PITTED
1 CUP WATER
3 BANANAS

Soak dried fruit and flax seed overnight in pure water to cover. Blend soaked fruit with water and bananas in blender. Garnish with slices of banana or raisins. Serves 2.

CARROT-CUCUMBER-CELERY-APPLE JUICE

10 CARROTS
1/2 CUCUMBER
2 STALKS CELERY
1 APPLE

Wash and prepare all produce for juicing. Process. Serves 2.

MARINATED CAULIFLOWER-VEGETABLE SALAD

1 1/2 POUNDS	CAULIFLOWER
1/2 CUP	CIDER VINEGAR
3 TABLESPOONS	OLIVE OIL
1 TABLESPOONS	LEMON JUICE
2	GARLIC CLOVES, MINCED
2 TABLESPOONS	SWEET GREEN PEPPERS, SLICED
1 TEASPOON	HONEY
1/2 TEASPOON	BRAGG'S AMINOES
3/4 TEASPOON	DILL SEED, GROUND
1 1/2 CUPS	CARROTS, SLICED
1 1/2 CUPS	GREEN SNAP BEANS, SNIPPED AND CUT
1 CUP	CHOPPED ONIONS
4	ROMAINE LETTUCE LEAVES

Place washed head of cauliflower in pan with 1" boiling water, bring to boil without cover and boil 5 minutes. Cover, cook 10 minutes more, turning head. Drain. Combine vinegar, oil, lemon juice, garlic, green pepper, honey, dill seed. Pour over cauliflower. Add cooked carrots, snap beans, and onion rings. Marinate overnight in refrigerator. To serve, place cauliflower on lettuce, surrounded by rest of vegetables. Serves 4.

CARROT-CABBAGE-CELERY-GINGER JUICE

10	CARROTS
1 CUP	GREEN CABBAGE
1 STALK	CELERY
1 SLICE	GINGER ROOT, 1/8" THICK

Wash all produce, remove carrot tops, cut to fit opening of juicer and process. Serves 2.

GREEN SALAD

8	ROMAINE LETTUCE LEAVES
1/2 CUP	BROCCOLI, CHOPPED
2 STALKS	CELERY, DICED
1	SWEET GREEN PEPPER, SLICED
1 CUP	CHINESE CABBAGE, PAK-CHOI OR BOK CHOY,SHREDDED
1/2 CUP	RED CABBAGE, SHREDDED

Assemble all ingredients in salad bowl and toss gently with Dijon Dressing. Serves 4.

DIJON DRESSING

1/2 CUP	WATER
2 TEASPOONS	PAPRIKA
1/4 CUP	WHOLE WHEAT FLOUR
1	GARLIC CLOVE, MINCED
1/2 CUP	LEMON JUICE
1 TABLESPOON	DIJON MUSTARD

Put first 3 ingredients into blender and mix. Transfer mixture to a small saucepan and cook on low for about 10 minutes, stirring occasionally. Return to blender and add rest of ingredients. Blend until smooth. Serves 4.

BAKED BUTTERNUT SQUASH

4 CUPS	BUTTERNUT WINTER SQUASH
1/2 TEASPOON	GROUND CINNAMON
1 TABLESPOON	OLIVE OIL
1/4 CUP	WATER
1 TEASPOON	HONEY
2	GARLIC CLOVES, MINCED
1/2 TEASPOON	JENSEN'S BROTH AND SEASONING

Peel squash, remove seeds and fiber, cut into 1" cubes. Place in oiled casserole dish, sprinkling on cinnamon and adding a little water, oil and honey. Bake covered at 350° F. for 45 minutes. Before serving, add minced garlic and Jensen's Broth to taste. Serves 4.

WHEAT RICE

2 CUPS	BROWN RICE,DRY
1 CUP	BULGUR, DRY
5 CUPS	WATER
1/4 CUP	SUNFLOWER SEED

Place all ingredients in a 4 quart pot. Bring to boil, reduce heat, cover, and simmer for 1 hour. Turn off heat and let sit for 10 minutes. Uncover, fluff with a wooden spoon. Serves 4.

• MENU FOR DAY SIX •

BREAKFAST

JAY'S LEMONADE
KIWI FRUIT SALAD
BANANA-LIME DRESSING

LUNCH

CARROT-CELERY JUICE
VEGETABLE DELIGHT
HUMMUS

DINNER

CARROT-APPLE-RED CABBAGE JUICE
SPRING SALAD
CUCUMBER DRESSING
STEAMED GREEN BEANS PLUS
BAKED POTATOES

NUTRIENTS	
Protein (gm)	31
Total Fat (gm)	26
Complex Carb (gm)	338
Dietary Fiber (gm)	44
Cholesterol (mg)	0
Sodium (mg)	1193
Potassium (mg)	7878
Vitamin A (RE)	23937
Vitamin C (mg)	556
Iron (mg)	23
Calcium (mg)	721
Phosphorus (mg)	1242

TOTAL DAILY CALORIES 1801

13% OF CALORIES ARE FROM FAT

RECIPES

JAY'S LEMONADE

4 APPLES
1 LEMON

Wash produce. Cut to fit opening of juicer. Serves 2.

KIWI FRUIT SALAD

2 PEARS
2 APPLES
2 PEACHES
4 KIWIFRUIT

Wash fruit. Core apple and pear, pit the peach, skin the kiwi. Cube the apple and pear. Slice the peach and kiwi. Combine all fruit in a serving bowl, add Banana-Lime Dressing and serve. Serves 2.

BANANA-LIME DRESSING

2 BANANAS
1 LIME

Blend ingredients with hand blender. Or mash banana, add lime juice, and whip by hand. Serves 2.

CARROT-CELERY JUICE

10 CARROTS
1 STALK CELERY
1 APPLE
1/2 CUP PARSLEY, CHOPPED

Wash, dry and cut vegetables to fit opening of juicer. Serves 2.

VEGETABLE DELIGHT

1 CUP	CAULIFLOWER
2	CARROTS
1 CUP	BROCCOLI

Wash, dry vegetables and cut into finger food size pieces. Use hummus as vegetable dip. Serves 2.

HUMMUS

1/4 CUP	TAHINI SESAME BUTTER
1 TABLESPOON	LEMON JUICE
1 TABLESPOON	BRAGG'S AMINOES
1 TEASPOON	CUMIN SEED, GROUND
1 TEASPOON	ONION POWDER
1 CUP	DRIED GARBANZO BEANS

Soak garbanzos overnight in pure water to cover, or use pre-cooked beans. Replace water, cook beans over medium heat for 2 hours or until tender (lid slightly ajar). Place cooked garbanzo beans in heavy duty blender with enough water to allow the food to process along with the rest of the ingredients. Blend well. May have to do this in two batches in blender. Remove from blender and store in airtight container. Use as vegetable dip. Serves 4.

CARROT-APPLE-RED CABBAGE JUICE

10	CARROTS
1	APPLE
1/2 CUP	RED CABBAGE, COARSELY CUT

Wash, dry and cut vegetables to fit juicer opening. Serves 2.

SPRING SALAD

8	BUTTERHEAD LETTUCE LEAVES, COARSELY CHOPPED (OR TORN)
1 CUP	PEAS, EDIBLE PODS
8 SPEARS	ASPARAGUS SPEARS, COARSELY CHOPPED
1/2 CUP	RADISHES, SLICED

Wash and dry greens and vegetables. Assemble ingredients and arrange on plate. Add cucumber dressing. Serves 2.

CUCUMBER DRESSING

1	CUCUMBER, COARSELY CUT
1/4 CUP	ONIONS, CHOPPED
1	GARLIC CLOVE, MINCED
1 TABLESPOON	LEMON JUICE
2 TABLESPOONS	WHITE WINE VINEGAR
2 TABLESPOONS	HONEY
1 TABLESPOON	TAHINI SESAME BUTTER
1 TABLESPOON	DILL WEED, GROUND
3/4 CUP	SOYMILK

Place all ingredients except soymilk and dill in blender and process briefly. Add soymilk and dill and process briefly again. Store in small airtight container. Serves 4.

STEAMED GREEN BEANS PLUS

2 CUPS	GREEN SNAP BEANS
2	CARROTS, SLICED
1 CUP	BROCCOLI, COARSELY CHOPPED
1/2 CUP	ONIONS, CHOPPED
1/2 CUP	MUSHROOMS, SLICED
1 TABLESPOON	BRAGG'S AMINOES
1/2 TEASPOON	JENSEN'S BROTH AND SEASONING

Steam all vegetables together over medium heat until crisp tender. Before serving, season with Jensen's Broth and Bragg's Aminoes. Serves 4.

BAKED POTATOES

4	POTATOES
4 TABLESPOONS	OLIVE OIL
1 TEASPOON	JENSEN'S BROTH AND SEASONING, OR TO TASTE

Scrub potatoes, prick with fork in several spots, bake at 350° F. for 1 hour or until done. When serving, add Jensen's Broth to taste and 1 tablespoon of olive oil per potato. Serves 4.

• MENU FOR DAY SEVEN •

BREAKFAST

WATERMELON JUICE
FRESH MELON SALAD

LUNCH

CARROT COOLER
CUCUMBER SALAD
TABOULI SALAD

LUNCH SNACK

CHERRIES*

DINNER

CARROT-BOK CHOY JUICE
SPINACH SALAD WITH TOMATO-LEMON DRESSING
BROCCOLI WITH TOMATO SAUCE
ESSENE BREAD (SPROUTED WHOLE GRAIN BREAD)*

**indicates no recipe included*

NUTRIENTS	
Protein (gm)	44
Total Fat (gm)	23
Complex Carb (gm)	351
Dietary Fiber (gm)	43
Cholesterol (gm)	0
Sodium (mg)	1920
Potassium (mg)	8422
Vitamin A (RE)	22483
Vitamin C (mg)	676
Iron (mg)	27
Calcium (mg)	998
Phosphorus (mg)	1586
TOTAL DAILY CALORIES	**1830**

11% OF CALORIES ARE FROM FAT

RECIPES

WATERMELON JUICE

1 WATERMELON

Wash outside of watermelon thoroughly. Slice watermelon in 1" slices. Cut strips of watermelon to fit opening of juicer and process. Serves 2.

FRESH MELON SALAD

1 CANTALOUPE MELON
1 HONEYDEW MELON
4 WATERMELON SLICES

Cut cantaloupe and honeydew in half and remove seeds. Remove seeds from slices of watermelon. Using melon baller, scoop melon balls from fruit and place in serving dish. Toss gently. Garnish with fresh mint leaves.

Serves 3.

CARROT COOLER

10 CARROTS
2 STALKS CELERY
1/2 CUCUMBER
1/2 SWEET GREEN PEPPER

Wash and prepare all vegetables. Remove carrot tops. Prepare vegetables for processing through juicer. Serves 2.

CUCUMBER SALAD

4	CUCUMBERS, SLICED
2 STALKS	CELERY, DICED
1	SWEET GREEN PEPPER, DICED
3 TABLESPOONS	LEMON JUICE
1	GARLIC CLOVE, MINCED
4 TABLESPOONS	OLIVE OIL
1 TABLESPOON	BRAGG'S AMINOES

Assemble all ingredients together in large bowl. Toss gently. Serves 4.

TABOULI SALAD

4 CUPS	WATER
2 CUPS	BULGUR, DRY
2	TOMATOES, CHOPPED
1/4 CUP	CHOPPED ONIONS
1 CUP	PARSLEY, CHOPPED
3 TABLESPOONS	BRAGG'S AMINOES
2 TABLESPOONS	OLIVE OIL
2	GARLIC CLOVES, MINCED
1 TEASPOON	PEPPERMINT
2 TABLESPOONS	LEMON JUICE

Place water in large saucepan over medium heat, bring to boil. Add bulgur, turn off heat, leaving lid on. Bulgur will become soft and absorb all liquid in about 20 minutes. Allow to cool. Transfer to serving bowl. Add rest of ingredients, toss gently. Garnish with fresh parsley or sprig of mint.

Serves 4.

CARROT-BOK CHOY JUICE

10	CARROTS
1/2 CUP	CHINESE CABBAGE, PAK-CHOI OR BOK CHOY
1	APPLE
2 STALKS	CELERY

Wash and prepare produce. Remove carrot tops, cut to fit opening of juicer. Serves 2.

SPINACH SALAD WITH TOMATO-LEMON DRESSING

6 CUPS	SPINACH, CHOPPED
2	TOMATOES, QUARTERED
1 CUP	MUSHROOMS, SLICED
1/2 CUP	LEMON JUICE
1/2 CUP	TOMATO JUICE
1	GARLIC CLOVE, MINCED
1/4 CUP	PARSLEY, CHOPPED
1/2 CUP	CELERY, DICED

Toss spinach, tomato and mushrooms in large bowl. Sprinkle with soy baco-bits if desired. Make dressing by putting all dressing ingredients in blender and process until well mixed. Pour on salad and toss right before serving. Serves 4.

BROCCOLI WITH TOMATO SAUCE

1/4 CUP	CHOPPED ONIONS
2	GARLIC CLOVES, MINCED
2 TABLESPOONS	WATER
1/2 CUP	TOMATOES, CHOPPED
1/2 CUP	WATER
1 TABLESPOON	PARSLEY, CHOPPED
1/4 TEASPOON	TARRAGON
1 TABLESPOONS	TOMATO PASTE
2 POUNDS	BROCCOLI, SPEARS

Steam broccoli until crisp, tender. Saute onions and garlic in water until lightly browned. Add tomato, water, parsley, salt (optional), tarragon, and tomato paste. Stir and cook until hot. Serve over hot broccoli. Serves 4.

STAGE III DESSERTS

RECIPES

FIG AND DATE PIE

10	DRIED FIGS
1 CUP	DATES, PITTED
1 CUP	SEEDLESS RAISINS
1 CUP	UNSWEETENED, DRIED COCONUT
1/2 CUP	SUNFLOWER SEEDS
2 TABLESPOONS	WHEAT GERM
1/4 TEASPOON	CINNAMON
2 TABLESPOONS	SAFFLOWER OIL
3 TABLESPOONS	WATER
1 TABLESPOON	HONEY
2	NECTARINES

Soak dried fruit in pure water to cover for 12 hours. Blend, adding enough water only to blend. Keep thick. Pour into pie crust and chill to set before serving. Can thicken with 2 teaspoons of agar-agar that has been soaked in small amount of water and then boiled. This will help thicken mixture. Top with sliced peaches or nectarines. For crust: mix next 4 ingredients, add oil, water, and honey, mix well. Press into pie pan, building up edges. May be eaten as is or baked 12 minutes at 325° F. before adding filling. Allow to cool before adding filling. For a strict Stage III Diet, use sliced bananas for the crust instead of the given recipe. Serves 8.

BANANA POPS

6 LARGE	BANANAS, PEELED
1/2 CUP	DATES, PITTED, SOAKED IN 1/4 CUP WATER FOR 1 HOUR
1/2 CUP	ALMONDS, COARSELY GROUND
1/4 CUP	COCONUT, SHREDDED

Cut bananas in half. Push ice cream stick into cut end of each half. Puree dates in soak water until smooth. Dip each banana in date puree, roll in almonds, sprinkle with coconut. Place on tray covered with wax paper and freeze at least 5 hours. May be kept up to one week in refrigerator.

Serves 12.

APPLE CRUMB PIE

1 CUP	ALMONDS, SOAKED 5 HOURS IN 2 CUPS WATER
1/4 CUP	DATES, PITTED, SOAKED 1 HOUR IN 1/8 CUP WATER
1/2 TEASPOON	CINNAMON
1/4 CUP	COCONUT, SHREDDED
7	APPLES, MEDIUM-SIZED
3/4 CUP	DATES, SOAKED 1 HOUR IN 1/2 CUP WATER
1 TEASPOON	LEMON PEEL, GRATED
1 TEASPOON	CINNAMON
1/8 TEASPOON	CLOVES
3/4 CUP	ALMONDS, GROUND
1/4 CUP	SEEDLESS RAISINS
1/4 CUP	COCONUT, SHREDDED
1 TABLESPOON	LEMON JUICE

Drain almonds and dates, discard water. Grind almonds, dates, and cinnamon together in food processor until sticky and coarse. Mix in coconut. Press into 9" pie plate. Make fluted edge. For filling: Coarsely grate 4 apples. Cut 2 more into bite-size pieces. Drain dates and puree with lemon peel, cinnamon, clove. Mix apples, date puree, 1/2 cup ground almonds, and currants. Fold into pie shell, pat down slightly. Mix remaining ground almonds with coconut and sprinkle over top of pie. Cut remaining apple into thick wedges, sprinkle with lemon juice, and arrange in circle in center of pie. Refrigerate and serve as soon as possible. Serves 10.

FRESH BLUEBERRY-BANANA PIE

2	BANANAS
1 1/4 CUPS	ALMONDS, GROUND
1/4 TEASPOON	PURE VANILLA EXTRACT
4 CUPS	BLUEBERRIES
3/4 CUP	DATES, PITTED, SOAKED 1 HR. IN 1/4 CUP WATER
2 TEASPOONS	FLAX SEEDS, GROUND
2	BANANAS, LARGE, PEELED

Crust: Mash bananas until creamy. Mix in ground almonds and vanilla. Smooth into bottom of pie pan. Filling: Blend 1 cup blueberries with dates, soak water, flax seed (or psyllium, optional), and bananas until creamy. Stir in remaining blueberries. Pour filling into crust. Refrigerate until ready to serve. Serves 10.

DATE-NUT CANDY

1 CUP	DATES, PITTED, SOAKED 2 HOURS IN 1/2 CUP WATER
2 CUPS	PINE NUTS
1/8 TEASPOON	PURE VANILLA EXTRACT
1 1/3 CUPS	COCONUT, GROUND

Drain dates. Grind dates, pine nuts, and vanilla in food processor until smooth, adding a little soak water if needed. Blend in 1 cup of ground coconut. Refrigerate 4 hours or overnight. Form dough into small balls, roll in remaining coconut, shape into cubes. Refrigerate until ready to serve. Serves 12.

CHAPTER 12

Intuitive Eating as a Way of Life

THE nature of life is that it is literally "all one piece." You make a change in one area and, like pushing over the first domino in a line, you start a chain reaction. While the subject of this book has been food, nutrition, and habits of eating, it is impossible to alter something in this arena without affecting many other aspects of your life.

Think about it. Food is necessary to support your life. As an infant you were totally dependent on others to supply that need. Consequently, feeding, or the lack of it, became emeshed with your primal sense of well-being. Your relationship to food today is still being influenced by those initial experiences. Even though you may not lack resources to support your life, food and eating are still intimately connected to your sense of security in the world, and to your self-esteem.

I believe that as you take responsibility for the quality of your food and your eating habits, and start giving attention to the innate wisdom of your body, you will be taking a huge leap in personal growth. Instead of being a victim of the TV, the food advertising companies, or even your childhood eating patterns, you will instead be taking a stand for health, for energy, and for longevity. It's that simple, and that profound. *Intuitive Eating* is a way of life.

EVERYTHING CHANGES

Let's take a look at some of the ways in which *Intuitive Eating* will affect you.

First, it will make a difference financially — certainly a plus for those who need to watch their budgets. The use of fresh fruits and vegetables, whole grains, nuts and seeds, etc., even if you purchase the highest quality, and sometimes most expensive organic varieties, is much less costly than a diet of processed (and packaged) foods, meats, and dairy products.

Following the dietary guildelines suggested in the three transitional stages, moreover, will soon affect your overall health. With less common ailments, allergies, digestive problems, etc., there will be little need for over-the-counter drugs, less need for visits to your doctor, and less time lost from necessary occupations and vacations. All plusses where your finances are concerned.

Then there is the area of personal energy conservation. As I have mentioned before, I experience vibrant health on minimal sleep. Just think of all the things you would like to do that you now say you have no time or energy to accomplish. Just think of having the luxury to take time daily to nurture yourself, read for enjoyment, play with your kids, or whatever, and still have energy to spare.

There is no doubt in my mind that your eating habits are affecting your stress level — either for good or ill. By becoming an intuitive eater you will eat in a way that optimizes digestion and provides minimal stress to your system. Then you will be eating for energy — the energy that supports your life. You will have available reserves of energy that you can call on when needed for handling a health crisis, or for getting you through other hard times.

Intuitive Eating is a conscious process which can transform ordinary *feeding* into a type of *communion* — both with yourself and others. Food can then be recognized as sacred, as your participation in the chain of existance, and your way of nourishing the body which many Scriptures refer to as a temple of God. It is not uncommon to find that by changing your food and eating habits you will be changing the "vibe" around your dinner table, in your kitchen, and throughout your entire house. Suddenly, your table and kitchen become places for healing and nourishment of body and soul.

Your social life may also change as you start eating differently. If socializing was constellated around drinking alcohol, or coffee, or eating lots of fast food, or processed foods, you may find that you will start hanging out with different friends, or start becoming more creative in the types of activities you plan. Instead of meeting in a cafe, or a bar, or at a hamburger stand, you may meet for a walk or a picnic in the park. Those friends who can't make the adjustment may simply move on. Those friends who support you in your lifestyle change will encourage it, and may even be inspired to do some re-evaluating of their own.

THE DOWNSIDE OF UP

Changes can be threatening — and not only for yourself. Realize that as you alter your relationship to food you will be challenging some deeply-ingrained programming in other members of your family, and even among more casual acquaintances. It's a bit like removing one block from a child's block tower — depending upon where the block was, it can topple the whole structure.

Even though we suggest dietary changes in a slow, graduated manner, they can still be disruptive for some people, and may trigger old memories, fears, and insecurities. Since many of us have used food for years to dull our senses, to fill up the emotional or spiritual emptiness, or to comfort ourselves, changing our eating habits may be accompanied, at least in the initial stages, by some emotional pain. Like any symptoms, consider these emotional states as part of the Healing Crisis (see Chapter 7) and handle them accordingly. Remember that often things need to get worse just before they take a turn for the better.

Emotional pain and self-questioning can be dealt with by getting professional help — i.e. psychological counseling, or consultation with your health professional. Don't try to pretend you are strong when you're not feeling that way. You are a human being, and humans are allowed to feel pain.

Some people keep a journal in which they write about their own process and literally guide themselves through the transition. In every case, a support system of good friends, especially those who have made similar life changes, can be invaluable. Talk about the strong and strange emotions you may be having. Talk about your questions, your fears, and about your goals and how good you are beginning to feel too. It is just important to remember not to be shocked by what "comes up" as you engage this process. It's normal to feel challenged, or even threatened.

INTUITION FOR EVERYONE

All people can become more intuitive, particularly in regards to knowing what they know and need for health and nutrition.

Becoming an intuitive eater means that your awareness of body feedback will be heightened in so many ways. You will actually start to "read" the effects of your food before you actually eat it, and immediately after as well. Your sensitivities to the workings of your organs — the proper functioning of your digestive system, your eliminative system, etc. — will be intensified. You will be much more attuned to your energy level, knowing which foods make you feel light and strong, or which foods weigh you down. Some people even report that the liver will "talk" to them about what foods to eat, or not eat, and when. One woman I know experiences a slight pain in the area of her liver when she even thinks about drinking coffee or beer. As Doctor Scott said, a generalized sensitivity and a heightened immune system are the prices you pay for this degree of health.

Being able to test your urinary pH and analyze the efficiency of your digestion by examining your bowel movements, will be a beginning step in growing intuition. Soon, you will use even more subtle ways to "put two and two together" about what your body is wanting and needing. You will be a full-fledged intuitive eater when you naturally crave the things you need.

As your food serves to cleanse your whole system you will become more attuned to the all influences in your environment. It is possible that you may find yourself naturally picking up other people's thoughts, or unexpressed emotions more readily. You might even see "auras" around others. You may become more psychic, in general. While this is certainly not one of the goals of this program, I want you to be ready for it. The human being has untapped potential that will start being available to you as you eat differently.

Greater self-awareness and intuition means that you will have a transformed relationship to health and illness, and a deepened appreciation of the miracle of your body. Instead of asking "out there" for drugs or diagnoses, your first line of approach will be to check "in here" to see what is going on. This enhanced self-appreciation will give you a better sense of who you are as a person, and help you to clarify what your beliefs are. Liking yourself, and feeling in tune with your body, will transform all your relationships. It's that simple.

THE GLOBAL PLAN

Once you are well established as an intuitive eater you will be eating in harmony with the universe. You will be eating low on the food-chain and hence not supporting the wastefulness and greed that characterize the relationship to food that is present in most industrialized countries. You will be making a stand for the fact that there is enough food — real food — to feed the planet, if people would only reexamine the facts of the case, especially with regard to the global implications of meat-eating in rich countries.

By living your practice of *Intuitive Eating,* you will be making a stand for the health of the whole planet, because whatever happens in the microdimension — your body — will have its effect upon the macrodimension — the body of humans — as well. It all starts with you.

PART 4

APPENDICES

APPENDIX A

U.S. RECOMMENDED DAILY ALLOWANCES (U.S. RDA)

Vitamins Minerals, and Protein	Unit of Measurement	Infants	Adults and Children 4 or More Years of Age	Children Under 4 Years of Age	Pregnant or Lactating Women
Fat-Soluble Vitamins					
Vitamin A	IU	1,500.0	5,000.0	2,500.00	8,000.0
Vitamin D	IU	400.0	400.0	400.00	400.0
Vitamin E	IU	5.0	30.0	10.00	30.0
Water-Soluble Vitamins					
Vitamin C	Mg	35.0	60.0	40.00	60.0
Folic Acid	Mg	0.1	0.4	0.20	0.8
Thiamine	Mg	0.5	1.5	0.70	1.7
Riboflavin	Mg	0.6	0.7	0.80	2.0
Niacin	Mg	8.0	20.0	9.00	20.0
Vitamin B_6	Mg	0.4	2.0	0.70	2.5
Vitamin B_{12}	Mcg	2.0	6.0	3.00	8.0
Biotin	Mg	0.5	0.3	0.15	0.3
Pantothenic Acid	Mg	3.0	10.0	5.00	10.0
Major Minerals					
Calcium	G	0.6	1.0	0.80	1.3
Phosphorus	G	0.5	1.0	0.80	1.3
Trace Minerals					
Iodine	Mcg	45.0	150.0	70.00	150.0
Iron	Mg	15.0	18.0	10.00	18.0
Magnesium	Mg	70.0	400.0	200.00	450.0
Copper	Mg	0.6	2.0	1.00	2.0
Zinc	Mg	5.0	15.0	8.00	15.0
Macronutrients					
Protein	G	18.0	45.0	20.00	

IU = International Units
Mg = Milligram
Mcg = Microgram
G = Gram

Source: FDA, 1981.

APPENDIX B

NUTRITIVE VALUES OF FOOD
(per 100 grams)

FOOD	WEIGHT OF COMMON PORTION	
	Common Portion	Amount in Grams
GRAINS AND FLOUR		
amaranth	1/2 cup	98
arrowroot	1/3 cup	43
barley, pearled, cooked	1/2 cup	79
buckwheat groats, roasted, cooked	1/2 cup	99
buckwheat flour, whole groat	1/2 cup	60
bulgur, cooked	1/2 cup	91
cornmeal, whole-grain	1/4 cup	30
couscous, cooked	1/2 cup	90
millet, cooked	1/2 cup	120
oats, rolled cooked	1 cup	234
quinoa	1/2 cup	85
rice, brown, long-grain, cooked	1/2 cup	98
rice flour, brown	1/2 cup	79
rye flour, dark	1/2 cup	64
triticale flour, whole grain	1/2 cup	65
wheat flour, whole grain	1/2 cup	60
wheat, sprouted	1/3 cup	36
wild rice, cooked	1/2 cup	82
LEGUMES		
adzuki beans, cooked, boiled	1/2 cup	115
black beans, cooked, boiled	1/2 cup	86
kidney beans, cooked, boiled	1/2 cup	88
navy beans, cooked, boiled	1/2 cup	91

NA = DATA NOT AVAILABLE

NUTRITIVE VALUES OF FOOD

(per 100 grams)

	Calories (kcal)	Protein (gm)	Fat (gm)	Carbohydrates (gm)	Fiber (gm)	Cholesterol (mg)
	374	14.45	6.51	66.17	3.77	
	357	0.30	0.10	88.15		
	123	2.26	0.44	28.22	0.23	
	92	3.38	0.62	19.94	0.52	
	335	12.62	3.10	70.59		
	83	3.08	0.24	18.58	0.35	
	362	8.12	3.59	76.89	1.84	
	112	3.79	0.16	23.22	0.14	
	119	3.51	1.00	23.67	0.36	
	62	2.6	1.0	10.80	0.2	
	374	13.10	5.8	68.90		
	111	2.58	0.90	22.96	0.34	
	363	7.23	2.78	76.48	1.29	
	324	14.03	2.69	68.74		
	338	13.18	1.81	73.14	1.50	
	339	13.70	1.87	72.57	2.10	
	198	7.49	1.27	42.53		
	101	3.99	0.34	21.34	0.33	
	128	7.52	0.10	24.77	2.02	
	132	8.86	0.54	23.71	2.03	
	127	8.67	0.50	22.81	2.81	
	142	8.70	0.57	26.31	3.14	

NUTRITIVE VALUES OF FOOD (per 100 grams)

FOOD	Common Portion	Amt. Grams
pinto beans, cooked, boiled	1/2 cup	85
white beans, cooked, boiled	1/2 cup	90
chick peas, cooked, boiled	1/2 cup	82
lentils, cooked, boiled	1/2 cup	99
lima beans, cooked, boiled	1/2 cup	94
mung beans, cooked, boiled	1/2 cup	101
split peas, cooked, boiled	1/2 cup	98
peanuts, all types, raw	1 oz	28
soybeans, cooked, boiled	1/2 cup	86
SOY PRODUCTS		
miso	1/2 c	138
tempeh	1/2 cup	83
soymilk	1/2 cup	120
tamari soy sauce	1 teaspoon	18
tofu, raw, firm	1/4 block	81
NUTS AND SEEDS		
almonds, dried, unblanched	1 oz	28.4
brazil nuts, dried, unblanched	1 oz	28.4
cashew nuts, dry, roasted	1 oz	28.4
filberts or hazelnuts, dried, unblanched	1 oz	28.4
flaxseed	1 oz	28
pecans, dried	1 oz	28.4
pinenuts, dried	1 oz	28.4
pistachio nuts, dried	1 oz	28.4
walnuts, dried	1 oz	28.4
pumpkin & squash seeds, dried	1 oz	28.4
sesame seeds, whole, dried	1 Tbsp.	9
sunflower seed kernels, dried	1 oz	28.4

NUTRITIVE VALUES OF FOOD (per 100 grams)

Calories (kcal)	Protein (gm) (gm)	Fat (gm)	Carbohydrates (gm)	Fiber (gm)	Cholesterol (mg)
137	8.21	0.52	25.65	3.02	
139	9.73	0.35	25.10	2.49	
164	8.86	2.59	27.41	2.50	
116	9.02	0.38	20.14	2.76	
115	7.80	0.38	20.89	3.09	
105	7.02	0.38	19.14	0.46	
118	8.34	0.39	21.11	1.97	
567	25.80	49.24	16.14	4.85	
173	16.64	8.97	9.92	2.03	
206	11.81	6.07	27.96	2.47	
199	18.95	7.68	17.03	2.99	
33	2.75	1.91	1.81		
60	10.51	0.10	5.57		
145	15.78	8.72	4.28	0.15	
589	19.95	52.21	20.40	2.71	
656	14.34	66.22	12.80	2.29	
574	15.31	46.35	32.69	0.70	
632	13.04	62.64	15.30	3.80	
498	18.00	34.08	37.20	8.80	
667	7.75	67.64	18.24	1.60	
515	24.00	50.70	14.22	0.80	
577	20.58	48.39	24.81	1.88	
607	24.35	56.58	12.10	6.46	
541	24.54	45.85	17.81	2.22	
573	17.73	49.67	23.45	4.60	
570	22.78	49.57	18.76	4.16	

NUTRITIVE VALUES OF FOOD (per 100 grams)

FOOD	Common Portion	Amt. Grams	
FRUITS			
apples, raw with skin	1 fruit	138	
apricots, raw	3 fruits	106	
avocadoes, raw	1 fruit	201	
bananas	1 fruit	114	
backberries, raw	1/2 cup	72	
blueberries, raw	1 cup	145	
carambola, raw	1 fruit	127	
cherries, sweet, raw	10 fruit	68	
cranberries, raw	1 cup	95	
dates, domestic, natural dry	10 fruit	83	
figs, raw	1 medium	50	
figs, dried, uncooked	10 fruit	187	
grapefruit, raw, pink, red, white, all sizes	1/2 fruit	120	
grapes (American type) raw	10 fruit	24	
guavas, raw	1 fruit	90	
kiwi fruit, raw	1 fruit	76	
lemons, raw	1 fruit	58	
limes, raw	1 fruit	67	
mangoes	1 fruit	207	
melons, cantaloupe, raw	1/2 fruit	267	
casaba, raw	1/10 fruit	164	
honeydew, raw	1/10 fruit	129	
nectarines, raw	1 fruit	136	
oranges, raw, all varieties	1 fruit	131	
papayas, raw	1 fruit	304	
peaches, raw	1 fruit	87	
pears, raw	1 fruit	166	
persimmons, raw	1 fruit	168	
pineapple, raw	1 slice	84	
plums, raw	1 fruit	66	
pomegranates	1 fruit	154	

NUTRITIVE VALUES OF FOOD (per 100 grams)

Calories (kcal)	Protein (gm) (gm)	Fat (gm)	Carbohydrates (gm)	Fiber (gm)	Cholesterol (mg)
59	0.19	0.36	15.25	0.77	
48	1.40	0.39	11.12	0.60	
161	1.98	15.32	7.39	2.11	
92	1.03	0.48	23.43	0.50	
52	0.72	0.39	12.76	4.10	
56	0.67	0.38	14.13	1.30	
33	0.54	0.35	7.83	0.92	
72	1.20	0.96	16.55	0.40	
49	0.39	0.20	12.68	1.20	
275	1.97	0.45	73.51	2.20	
74	0.75	0.30	19.18	1.20	
255	3.05	1.17	65.35	4.80	
32	0.63	0.10	8.08	0.20	
63	0.63	0.35	17.15	0.76	
51	0.82	0.60	11.88	5.60	
61	0.99	0.44	14.88	1.10	
29	1.10	0.30	9.32	0.40	
30	0.70	0.20	10.54	0.50	
65	0.51	0.27	17.00	0.84	
35	0.88	0.28	8.36	0.36	
26	0.90	0.10	6.20	0.50	
35	0.46	0.10	9.18	0.60	
49	0.94	0.46	11.78	0.40	
47	0.94	0.12	11.75	0.43	
39	0.61	0.14	9.81	0.77	
43	0.70	0.09	11.10	0.64	
59	0.39	0.40	15.11	1.40	
70	0.58	0.19	18.59	1.48	
49	0.39	0.43	12.39	0.54	
55	0.79	0.62	13.01	0.60	
68	0.95	0.30	17.17	0.20	

NUTRITIVE VALUES OF FOOD (per 100 grams)

FOOD	Common Portion	Amt. Grams
raisins, seedless	1 cup not packed	145
raspberries, raw	1 cup	123
strawberries, raw	1 cup	149
tangarines, raw	1 fruit	84
watermelon	1/16 fruit	482
VEGETABLES AND SPROUTS		
alfalfa seeds, sprouted, raw	1 cup	33
artichokes, raw	1 cup	128
asparagus, raw	1/2 cup	67
beans, lima, cooked, boiled, drained	1/2 cup	85
mung beans, sprouted, raw	1/2 cup	52
beans, snap, cooked	1/2 cup	62
beets, raw	1/2 cup	68
beets, cooked	1/2 cup	85
beet greens, raw	1/2 cup	19
beet greens, cooked	1/2 cup	72
broad beans, cooked	1/2 cup	NA
broccoli, raw	1/2 cup	44
brussel sprouts, raw	1 sprout	19
brussel sprouts, cooked	1 sprout	21
cabbage, raw	1/2 cup	35
cabbage, cooked	1/2 cup	75
cabbage, red, raw	1/2 cup	35
carrots, raw	1/2 cup	55
carrots, cooked	1/2 cup	78
cauliflower,raw	1/2 cup	50
cauliflower, cooked	1/2 cup	62
celery, raw	1 stalk	40
swiss chard, raw	1/2 cup	18
collards, raw	1/2 cup	93

NUTRITIVE VALUES OF FOOD (per 100 grams)

Calories (kcal)	Protein (gm) (gm)	Fat (gm)	Carbohydrates (gm)	Fiber (gm)	Cholesterol (mg)
302	3.39	0.46	79.52	1.43	
49	0.91	0.55	11.57	3.00	
30	0.61	0.37	7.02	0.53	
44	0.63	0.19	11.19	0.33	
32	0.62	0.43	7.18	0.30	
29	3.99	0.69	3.78	1.64	
51	2.66	0.20	11.94	1.06	
22	3.06	0.22	3.68	0.83	
123	6.81	0.32	23.64	2.09	
30	3.04	0.18	5.93	0.81	
35	1.89	0.28	7.89	1.43	
44	1.48	0.14	10.00	0.80	
31	1.06	0.05	6.69	0.85	
19	1.82	0.06	3.97	1.30	
27	2.57	0.20	5.46	1.05	
56	4.80	0.50	10.10	1.90	
28	2.98	0.35	5.24	1.11	
43	3.38	0.30	8.96	1.51	
39	2.55	0.51	8.67	1.37	
24	1.21	0.18	5.37	0.80	
21	0.96	0.25	4.77	0.60	
27	1.39	0.26	6.12	1.00	
43	1.03	0.19	10.14	1.04	
45	1.09	0.18	10.48	1.47	
24	1.99	0.18	4.92	0.85	
24	1.87	0.17	4.62	0.82	
16	0.66	0.12	3.63	0.69	
19	1.80	0.20	3.74	0.80	
19	1.57	0.22	3.76	0.57	

NUTRITIVE VALUES OF FOOD (per 100 grams)

FOOD	Common Portion	Amt. Grams
sweet corn, raw	1/2 cup	77
sweet corn, cooked	1/2 cup	82
cucumber, raw	1/2 cup	52
dandelion greens, raw	1/2 cup	28
dandelion greens, cooked	1/2 cup	52
eggplant, cooked	1/2 cup	48
endive, raw	1/2 cup	25
garlic, raw	1 clove	3
ginger root, raw	5 slices	11
kale, raw	1/2 cup	34
kale, cooked	1/2 cup	65
kohlrabi, raw	1/2 cup	70
leeks, raw	1/4 cup	26
lentils, sprouted, raw	1/2 cup	38
lettuce, romaine	1/2 cup	28
mushrooms, raw	1/2 cup	35
mustard greens, raw	1/2 cup	28
okra, cooked	1/2 cup	80
onions, raw	1 tablespoon	10
parsley, raw	10 sprigs	10
parsnips, raw	1/2 cup	67
peas, edible - podded, raw	1/2 cup	72
peas, green, raw	1/2 cup	78
peas, mature, sprouted, raw	1/2 cup	60
peppers, sweet, raw	1 pepper	74
potato, baked, flesh & skin	1 potato	202
pumpkin, cooked	1/2 cup	122
radishes, raw	10 radishes	45
radish, seeds, sprouted, raw	1/2 cup	19
rutabagas, cooked	1/2 cup	85
soybeans, sprouted, raw	1/2 cup	35

NUTRITIVE VALUES OF FOOD (per 100 grams)

Calories (kcal)	Protein (gm) (gm)	Fat (gm)	Carbohydrates (gm)	Fiber (gm)	Cholesterol (mg)
86	3.22	1.18	19.02	0.70	
108	3.32	1.28	25.11	0.60	
13	0.54	0.13	2.91	0.60	
45	2.70	0.70	9.20	1.60	
33	2.00	0.60	6.40	1.30	
28	0.83	0.23	6.64	0.97	
17	1.25	0.20	3.35	0.90	
149	6.36	0.50	33.07	1.50	
69	1.74	0.73	15.09	1.03	
50	3.30	0.70	10.01	1.50	
32	1.90	0.40	5.63	0.80	
27	1.70	0.10	6.20	1.00	
61	1.50	0.30	14.15	1.51	
106	8.96	0.55	22.14	3.05	
16	1.62	0.20	2.37	0.70	
25	2.09	0.42	4.65	0.75	
26	2.70	0.20	4.90	1.10	
32	1.87	0.17	7.21	0.90	
34	1.18	0.26	7.32	0.44	
33	2.20	0.30	6.91	1.20	
75	1.20	0.30	17.99	2.00	
42	2.80	0.20	7.56	2.50	
81	5.41	0.40	14.46	2.21	
128	8.80	0.68	28.26	2.78	
25	0.85	0.45	5.31	1.20	
109	2.30	0.10	25.23	0.66	
20	0.72	0.07	4.89	0.83	
17	0.60	0.54	3.59	0.54	
41	3.81	2.53	3.06	-	
34	1.10	0.19	7.74	1.04	
128	13.09	6.70	11.17	2.30	

NUTRITIVE VALUES OF FOOD (per 100 grams)

FOOD	Common Portion	Amt. Grams
soybeans, green, cooked	1/2 cup	90
spinach, raw	1/2 cup	28
summer squash, raw, all varieties	1/2 cup	65
summer squash, cooked	1/2 cup	90
winter squash, all varieties, baked	1/2 cup	102
sweet potato, baked in skin	1 potato	114
tomatoes, red, ripe, raw	1 tomato	123
turnips, raw	1/2 cup	65
turnip greens, raw	1/2 cup	28
watercress, raw	1/2 cup	17
yams, baked	1/2 cup	75
DAIRY PRODUCTS		
cheese, cheddar	1 oz	28
cottage cheese, 1% fat	4 oz	113
cheese, feta	1 oz	28
cottage cheese, dry curd	4 oz	113
cheese, monterey	1 oz	28
cheese, mozzerella, part skin	1 oz	28
cheese, parmesan, grated	1 oz	28
cheese, ricotta (part skim)	1/2 cup	124
cheese, swiss	1 oz	28
cheese, American	1 oz	28
whole milk	1 cup	244
milk, low fat 2%	1 cup	244
skim milk	1 cup	245
buttermilk	1 cup	245
yogurt, plain, low fat	1 8 oz container	227
egg, chicken, whole, hard cooked	1 white	50

NUTRITIVE VALUES OF FOOD (per 100 grams)

Calories (kcal)	Protein (gm) (gm)	Fat (gm)	Carbohydrates (gm)	Fiber (gm)	Cholesterol (mg)
141	12.35	6.40	11.05	1.85	
22	2.86	0.35	3.50	0.89	
20	1.18	0.21	4.35	0.60	
20	0.91	0.31	4.31	0.60	
39	0.89	0.63	8.75	0.71	
103	1.72	0.11	24.27	0.80	
19	0.89	0.21	4.34	0.47	
27	0.90	0.10	6.23	0.90	
27	1.50	0.30	5.73	0.80	
11	2.30	0.10	1.29	0.70	
118	1.53	0.17	27.89	-	
403	24.90	33.14	1.28	0	105
72	12.39	1.02	2.72	0	4
264	14.21	21.28	4.0	0	89
85	17.27	0.42	1.85	0	7
373	24.48	30.28	0.68	0	-
254	24.26	15.92	2.77	0	58
456	41.56	30.02	3.74	0	79
138	11.39	7.91	5.14	0	31
376	28.43	27.45	3.38	0	92
375	22.15	31.25	1.60	0	94
61	3.29	3.34	4.66	0	14
50	3.33	1.92	4.80	0	8
35	3.41	0.18	4.85	0	2
40	3.31	0.88	4.79	0	4
61	3.47	3.25	4.66	0	13
158	12.14	11.115	1.20	0	548

NUTRITIVE VALUES OF FOOD (per 100 grams)

FOOD	Common Portion	Amt. Grams
FISH		
bass, fresh water	1 fillet	79
cod, cooked	1 fillet	180
haddock	1 fillet	150
halibut	1 fillet	159
herring, cooked	1 fillet	143
mackerel, cooked	1 fillet	88
ocean perch	1 fillet	50
salmon, pink, canned	3 oz	85
trout, rainbow, cooked	1 fillet	62
tuna, canned in water	3 oz	85
POULTRY		
chicken, broilers or fryers, fresh only, roasted	1 cup	140
chicken, dark, with skin, roasted	1 cup	140
chicken, light without skin, roasted	1 cup	140
turkey, fryer-roasters, fresh only, roasted	1 cup	140
turkey, light, without skin, roasted	1 cup	140
turkey, dark without skin, roasted	1 cup	140

SOURCES: Composition of Food - by Nutrition Minotoring Division, USDA Human Nutrition Information Service:

- *Cereal Grains and Pasta Agriculture Handbook 8-20 revised, Oct. 1989*
- *Dairy and Egg Products Agriculture Handbook 8-1 Nov. 1976*
- *Finfish and Shellfish Products Sept. 1987*
- *Fruits and Fruit Juices Agriculture Handbook 8-9 revised, Aug. 1982*
- *Legumes and Legume Products Agriculture Handbook 8-16 revised, Dec. 1986*
- *Nut and Seed Products Agriculture Handbook 8-12 revised, Sept. 1984*
- *Poultry Products Agriculture Handbook 8-5 Aug. 1979*
- *Vegetable and Vegetable Products Agriculture Handbook 8-11 revised, Aug. 1984*

NUTRITIVE VALUES OF FOOD (per 100 grams)

Calories (kcal)	Protein (gm) (gm)	Fat (gm)	Carbohydrates (gm)	Fiber (gm)	Cholesterol (mg)
114	18.86	3.69	0.00	0.00	68
105	22.83	0.86	0.00	0.00	55
112	24.24	0.93	0.00	0.00	74
140	26.69	2.94	0.00	0.00	41
203	23.03	11.59	0.00	0.00	77
262	23.85	17.81	0.00	0.00	75
121	23.88	2.09	0.00	0.00	54
139	19.78	6.05	0.00	0.00	-
151	26.34	4.31	0.00	0.00	73
131	29.58	0.50	0.00	0.00	-
190	28.93	7.41	0.00	0.00	89
205	27.37	9.73	0.00	0.00	93
173	30.91	4.51	0.00	0.00	85
150	29.56	2.63	0.00	0.00	98
140	30.19	1.18	0.00	0.00	86
162	28.84	4.31	0.00	0.00	112

APPENDIX C

NUTRITIVE VALUES OF FOOD - MINERALS

(per 100 grams)

FOOD	WEIGHT OF COMMON PORTION		Ca (mg)
	Common Portion	Weight (in grams)	
GRAINS AND FLOUR:			
amaranth	1/2 c	98	153
arrowroot	1/2 c	43	40
barley, pearled, cooked	1/2 c	79	11
buckwheat groats, roasted, cooked	1/2 c	99	7
buckwheat flour, whole groat	1/2 c	60	41
bulgur, cooked	1/2 c	91	10
cornmeal, wholegrain	1/4 c	30	6
couscous, cooked	1/2 c	90	8
millet, cooked	1/2 c	120	3
oats, rolled or oatmeal, cooked	1 c	234	8
quinoa	1/2 c	85	60
rice, brown, long-grain, cooked	1/2 c	98	10
rice flour, brown	1/2 c	79	11
rye flour, dark	1/2 c	64	56
triticale flour, whole grain	1/2 c	65	35
wheat flour, whole grain	1/2 c	60	34
wheat, sprouted	1/3 c	36	28
wild rice, cooked	1/2 c	82	3
LEGUMES			
adzuki beans, cooked, boiled	1/2 c	115	28
black beans, cooked, boiled	1/2 c	86	27
kidney beans, cooked, boiled	1/2 c	88	28

Ca - calcium **P** - phosphorus **Mg** - magnesium **K** - potassium **Na** - sodium

NA = DATA NOT AVAILABLE

NUTRITIVE VALUES OF FOOD - MINERALS

(per 100 grams)

MINERALS							
P (mg)	Mg (mg)	K (mg)	Na (mg)	Fe (mg)	Cu (mg)	Mn (mg)	Zn (mg)
455	266	366	21	7.59	0.777	2.260	3.18
5	3	11	2	0.33	0.040	0.470	0.07
54	22	93	3	1.33	0.105	0.259	0.82
70	51	88	4	0.80	0.146	0.403	0.61
337	251	577		4.06	0.515	2.030	3.12
40	32	68	5	0.96	0.075	0.609	0.57
241	127	287	35	3.45	0.193	0.498	1.82
22	8	58	5	0.38	0.041	0.084	0.26
100	44	62	2	0.63	0.161	0.272	0.91
76	24	56	1	0.68	0.055	0.585	0.49
410	210	740		9.25	0.820		3.30
83	43	43	5	0.42	0.100	0.905	0.63
337	112	289	8	1.98	0.230	4.013	2.45
632	248	730	1	6.45	0.750	5.620	
321	153	466	2	2.59	0.559	4.185	2.66
346	138	405	5	3.88	0.382	3.799	2.93
200	82	169	16	2.14	0.261	1.858	1.65
82	32	101	3	0.60	0.121	0.282	1.34
168	52	532	8	2.00	0.298	0.573	1.77
140	70	355	1	2.10	0.209	0.444	1.12
142	45	403	2	2.94	1.07	0.477	1.07

Fe - iron **Cu** - copper **Mn** - manganese **Zn** - zinc **mg** - milligrams

NUTRITIVE VALUES OF FOOD - MINERALS (PER 100 GRAMS)

FOOD	Common Portion	Weight (in grams)	Ca (mg)
navy beans, cooked, boiled	1/2 c	91	70
pinto beans, cooked, boiled	1/2 c	85	48
white beans, cooked, boiled	1/2 c	90	90
chickpeas, cooked, boiled	1/2 c	82	49
lentils, cooked, boiled	1/2 c	99	19
lima beans, cooked, boiled	1/2 c	94	17
mungbeans, cooked, boiled	1/2 c	101	27
split peas, cooked, boiled	1/2 c	98	14
peanuts, all types, raw	1 oz.	28	92
soybeans, cooked, boiled	1/2 c	86	102
SOY PRODUCTS			
miso	1/2 c	138	66
tamari	1 tsp	18	20
tempeh	1/2 c	83	93
soymilk	1/2 c	120	4
tofu, raw, firm	1/4 block	81	205
NUTS AND SEEDS			
almonds, dried, unblanched	1 oz.	28.4	266
brazil nuts, dried, unblanched	1 oz.	28.4	176
cashew nuts, dry, roasted	1 oz.	28.4	45
filbert nuts or hazelnuts, dried, unblanched	1 oz.	28.4	188
flax seed	1 oz.	18	271
pecans, dried	1 oz.	28.4	36
pinenuts, dried, pignolia	1 oz.	28.4	26
pistachio nuts, dried	1 oz.	28.4	135
walnuts, dried	1 oz.	28.4	58
pumpkin/squash seeds, dried	1 oz.	28.4	43
sesame seeds, whole, dried	1 Tbsp.	9	975
sunflower seed kernels, dried	1 oz.	28.4	116

NUTRITIVE VALUES OF FOOD - MINERALS (PER 100 GRAMS)

	P (mg)	Mg (mg)	K (mg)	Na (mg)	Fe (mg)	Cu (mg)	Mn (mg)	Zn (mg)
	157	59	368	1	2.48	0.295	0.556	1.06
	160	55	468	2	2.61	0.257	0.556	1.08
	113	63	561	6	3.70	0.287	0.636	1.38
	168	48	291	7	2.89	0.352	1.030	1.53
	180	36	369	2	3.33	0.251	0.494	1.27
	111	43	508	2	2.39	0.235	0.516	0.95
	99	48	266	2	1.40	0.156	0.298	0.84
	99	36	362	2	1.29	0.181	0.396	1.00
	376	168	705	18	4.58	1.144	1.934	3.27
	245	86	515	1	5.14	0.407	0.824	1.15
	153	42	164	3,647	2.74	0.437	0.859	3.32
	130	40	212	5,586	2.38	-	-	0.43
	206	70	367	6	2.26	0.670	1.430	1.81
	49	19	141	12	0.58	0.120	0.170	12
	190	94	237	14	10.47	0.378	1.181	1.57
	520	296	732	11	3.66	0.942	2.273	2.92
	600	225	600	2	3.40	1.770	0.774	4.59
	490	260	565	16	6.00	2.220	-	5.60
	312	285	445	3	3.27	1.509	2.016	2.40
	462	-	-	30	43.80	-	-	-
	291	128	392	1	2.13	1.182	4.506	5.47
	508	-	599	4	9.20	1.026	-	4.25
	503	158	1,093	6	6.78	1.189	0.327	1.34
	464	202	524	1	3.07	1.020	4.271	3.42
	1,174	535	807	18	14.97	1.387	-	7.46
	629	351	468	11	14.55	4.082	2.460	7.75
	705	354	689	3	6.77	1.752	2.020	5.06

NUTRITIVE VALUES OF FOOD - MINERALS (PER 100 GRAMS)

FOOD	Common Portion	Weight (in grams)	Ca (mg)
FRUITS			
apples, raw with skin	1 fruit	138	7
apricots, raw	3 fruits	106	14
avocadoes, all types, raw	1 fruit	201	11
bananas, raw	1 fruit	114	6
blackberries, raw	1/2 c	72	32
blueberries, raw	1 c	145	6
carambola, raw	1 fruit	127	4
cherries, raw, sweet	10 fruit	68	15
cranberries, raw	1 c	95	7
dates, domestic, natural dry	10 fruit	83	32
figs, raw	1 med.	50	35
figs, dried, uncooked	10 fruit	187	144
grapefruit, red, white, pink, all sizes	1/2 fruit	120	12
grapes (American type) raw	10 fruit	24	14
guavas, raw, commercial	1 fruit	90	20
kiwi fruit, raw	1 fruit	76	26
lemons, raw, w/o peel	1 fruit	58	26
limes, raw	1 fruit	67	33
mangos, raw	1 fruit	207	10
melons, cantaloupe	1/2 fruit	267	11
casaba	1/10 fruit	164	5
honeydew, raw	1/10 fruit	129	6
nectarines, raw	1 fruit	136	5
oranges, raw, all varieties	1 fruit	131	40
papayas, raw	1 fruit	304	24
peaches, raw	1 fruit	87	5
pears, raw	1 fruit	166	11
persimmons, raw	1 fruit	168	8
pineapple, raw	1 slice	84	7
plums, raw	1 fruit	66	4
pomegranates, raw	1 fruit	154	3

NUTRITIVE VALUES OF FOOD - MINERALS (PER 100 GRAMS)

	P (mg)	Mg (mg)	K (mg)	Na (mg)	Fe (mg)	Cu (mg)	Mn (mg)	Zn (mg)
	7	5	115	0	0.18	0.041	0.045	0.04
	19	8	296	1	0.54	0.089	0.079	0.26
	41	39	599	10	1.02	0.262	0.226	0.42
	20	29	396	1	0.31	0.104	0.152	0.16
	21	20	196	0	0.57	0.140	1.291	0.27
	10	5	89	6	0.17	0.061	0.282	0.11
	16	9	163	2	0.26	0.120	0.082	0.11
	19	11	224	0	0.39	0.095	0.092	0.06
	9	5	71	1	0.20	0.058	0.157	0.13
	40	35	652	3	1.15	0.288	0.298	0.29
	14	17	232	1	0.37	0.070	0.128	0.15
	68	59	712	11	2.23	0.313	0.388	0.51
	8	8	139	0	0.09	0.047	0.012	0.07
	10	5	191	2	0.29	0.040	0.718	0.04
	25	10	284	3	0.31	0.103	0.144	0.23
	40	30	332	5	0.41	-	-	-
	16	-	138	2	0.60	0.037	-	0.06
	18	-	102	2	0.60	0.11	0.065	0.11
	11	9	156	2	0.13	0.110	0.027	0.04
	17	11	309	9	0.21	0.042	0.047	0.16
	7	8	210	-	0.40	-	-	-
	10	7	271	10	0.07	0.041	0.018	-
	16	8	212	0	0.15	0.073	0.044	0.09
	14	10	181	0	0.10	0.045	0.025	0.07
	5	10	257	3	0.10	0.016	0.11	0.07
	12	7	197	0	0.11	0.068	0.047	0.14
	11	6	125	0	0.25	0.113	0.076	0.12
	17	9	161	1	0.15	0.113	0.355	0.11
	7	14	113	1	0.37	0.110	1.649	0.08
	10	7	172	0	0.10	0.043	0.049	0.10
	8	-	259	3	0.30	-	-	-

NUTRITIVE VALUES OF FOOD - MINERALS (PER 100 GRAMS)

FOOD	Common Portion	Weight (in grams)	Ca (mg)
raisins, seedless	1 c not packed	145	53
raspberries, raw	1 c	123	22
strawberries	1 c	149	14
tangerines	1 c	84	14
watermelon	1/16 fruit	482	8
VEGETABLES AND SPROUTS:			
alfalfa seeds, sprouted, raw	1 c	33	32
artichokes, raw	1 artichoke	128	48
asparagus, raw	1/2 c	67	22
beans, lima, cooked, boiled, drained	1/2 c	85	32
mung beans, sprouted, raw	1/2 c	52	13
beans, snap, cooked	1/2 c	62	46
beets, raw	1/2 c	68	16
beets, cooked	1/2 c	85	11
beet greens, raw	1/2 c	19	119
beet greens, cooked	1/2 c	72	114
broad beans, cooked	1/2 c	NA	18
broccoli, raw	1/2 c	44	44
brussel sprouts, raw	1 sprout	19	42
brussel sprouts, cooked	1 sprout	21	36
cabbage, raw	1/2 c	35	47
cabbage, cooked	1/2 c	75	33
cabbage, red, raw	1/2 c	35	51
carrots, raw	1/2 c	55	27
carrots, cooked	1/2 c	78	31
cauliflower,raw	1/2 c	50	29
cauliflower, cooked	1/2 c	62	27
celery, raw	1 stalk	40	36
swiss chard, raw	1/2 c	18	51
collards, raw	1/2 c	93	117
sweet corn, raw	1/2 c	77	2

NUTRITIVE VALUES OF FOOD - MINERALS (PER 100 GRAMS)

	P (mg)	Mg (mg)	K (mg)	Na (mg)	Fe (mg)	Cu (mg)	Mn (mg)	Zn (mg)
	115	35	746	12	1.79	0.363	0.308	0.32
	12	18	152	0	0.57	0.074	1.013	0.46
	19	10	166	1	0.38	0.049	0.290	0.13
	10	12	157	1	0.10	0.028	0.032	-
	9	11	116	2	0.17	0.032	0.037	0.07
	70	27	79	6	0.96	0.157	0.188	0.92
	77	47	339	80	1.64	0.074	0.333	0.44
	52	18	302	2	0.68	0.153	0.214	0.70
	130	74	570	17	2.45	0.305	1.252	0.79
	54	21	149	6	0.91	0.164	0.188	0.41
	39	25	299	3	1.28	0.103	0.294	0.36
	48	21	324	72	0.91	0.083	0.352	0.37
	31	37	312	49	0.62	0.057	0.240	0.25
	40	72	547	201	3.3	0.38	0.191	0.38
	41	68	909	241	1.9	0.251	-	0.50
	73	31	193	41	1.50	-		
	66	25	325	27	0.88	0.045	0.229	0.40
	69	23	389	25	1.40	0.070	0.337	0.42
	56	20	317	21	1.20	0.083	0.227	0.33
	23	15	246	18	0.56	0.023	0.159	0.18
	25	15	205	19	0.39	0.028	0.129	0.16
	42	15	206	11	0.49	0.097	0.180	0.21
	44	15	323	35	0.50	0.047	0.142	0.20
	30	13	227	66	0.62	0.134	0.752	0.30
	46	14	355	15	0.58	0.032	0.203	0.18
	35	11	323	6	0.42	0.091	0.178	0.24
	26	12	284	88	0.48	0.035	0.136	0.17
	46	81	379	213	1.80	-	-	-
	16	17	148	28	0.62	0.260	0.369	0.96
	89	37	270	15.2	0.52	0.054	0.161	0.45

NUTRITIVE VALUES OF FOOD - MINERALS (PER 100 GRAMS)

FOOD	Common Portion	Weight (in grams)	Ca (mg)
sweet corn, cooked	1/2 c	82	2
cucumber, raw	1/2 c	52	14
dandelion greens, raw	1/2 c	28	187
dandelion greens, cooked	1/2 c	52	140
eggplant, cooked	1/2 c	48	6
endive, raw	1/2 c	25	52
garlic, raw	1 clove	3	181
ginger root, raw	5 slices	11	18
kale, raw	1/2 c	34	135
kale, cooked	1/2 c	65	72
kohlrabi, raw	1/2 c	70	24
leeks, raw	1/4 c	26	59
lentils, sprouted, raw	1/2 c	38	25
lettuce, romaine	1/2 c	28	36
mushrooms, raw	1/2 c	35	5
mustard greens, raw	1/2 c	28	103
okra, cooked	1/2 c	80	63
onions, raw	1 tablespoon	10	25
parsley, raw	10 sprigs	10	130
parsnips, raw	1/2 c	67	36
peas, edible - podded, raw	1/2 c	72	43
peas, green, raw	1/2 c	78	25
peas, mature, sprouted, raw	1/2 c	60	36
peppers, sweet, raw	1 pepper	74	6
potato, baked, flesh & skin	1 potato	202	10
pumpkin, cooked	1/2 c	122	15
radishes, raw	10 radishes	45	21
radish, seeds, sprouted, raw	1/2 c	19	51
rutabagas, cooked	1/2 c	85	42
soybeans, sprouted, raw	1/2 c	35	67
soybeans, green, cooked	1/2 c	90	145
spinach, raw	1/2 c	28	99

NUTRITIVE VALUES OF FOOD - MINERALS (PER 100 GRAMS)

P (mg)	Mg (mg)	K (mg)	Na (mg)	Fe (mg)	Cu (mg)	Mn (mg)	Zn (mg)
103	32	249	17	0.61	0.053	0.194	0.48
17	11	149	2	0.28	0.040	0.061	0.23
66	36	397	76	3.10	-	-	-
42	-	232	44	1.80	-	-	-
22	13	248	3	0.35	0.108	0.136	0.15
28	15	314	22	0.83	0.099	0.420	0.79
153	25	401	17	1.70	-	-	-
27	43	415	13	0.50	-	-	-
56	34	447	43	1.70	0.290	0.774	0.44
28	18	228	23	0.90	0.156	0.416	0.24
46	19	350	20	0.40	-	-	-
35	28	180	20	2.10	-	-	-
173	37	322	11	3.21	0.352	0.506	1.51
45	6	290	8	1.10	-	-	-
104	10	370	4	1.24	0.492	0.112	0.73
43	32	354	25	1.46	-	-	-
56	57	322	5	0.45	0.086	0.911	0.55
29	10	155	2	0.37	0.040	0.133	0.18
41	44	536	39	6.2	0.055	0.160	0.73
71	29	375	10	0.59	0.120	0.560	0.59
53	24	200	4	2.08	-	-	-
108	33	244	5	1.47	0.176	0.410	1.24
165	56	38	120	2.26	0.272	0.438	1.05
22	14	195	3	1.27	0.103	0.140	0.18
57	27	418	8	1.36	0.305	0.229	0.32
30	9	230	1	0.57	-	-	-
18	9	232	24	0.29	0.040	0.70	0.30
113	44	86	6	0.86	0.120	0.260	0.56
49	21	287	18	0.47	0.036	0.153	0.30
164	72	484	14	2.10	0.427	0.702	1.17
158	-	-	-	2.50	-	-	-
49	79	558	79	2.71	0.130	0.897	0.53

NUTRITIVE VALUES OF FOOD - MINERALS (PER 100 GRAMS)

FOOD	Common Portion	Weight (in grams)	Ca (mg)
summer squash, raw, all varieties	1/2 c	65	20
summer squash, cooked	1/2 c	90	27
winter squash, all varieties, baked	1/2 c	102	14
sweet potato, baked in skin	1 potato	114	28
tomatoes, red, ripe, raw	1 tomato	123	7
turnips, raw	1/2 c	65	30
turnip greens, raw	1/2 c	28	190
watercress, raw	1/2 c	17	120
yams, baked	1/2 c	75	17
DAIRY PRODUCTS			
cheese, cheddar	1 oz	28	721
cottage cheese, 1% fat	4 oz	113	61
cheese, feta	1 oz	28	492
cottage cheese, dry curd	4 oz	113	32
cheese, monterey	1 oz	28	746
cheese, mozzerella, part skin	1 oz	28	646
cheese, parmesan, grated	1 oz	28	1,376
cheese, ricotta (part skim)	1/2 c	124	272
cheese, swiss	1 oz	28	961
cheese, American	1 oz	28	616
whole milk	1 c	244	119
milk, low fat 2%	1 c	244	122
skim milk	1 c	245	123
buttermilk	1 c	245	116
yogurt, plain, low fat	1 8 oz container	227	121
egg, chicken, whole, hard cooked	1 white	50	56
FISH			
bass, fresh water	1 fillet	79	80
cod, cooked	1 fillet	180	14
haddock	1 fillet	150	42

NUTRITIVE VALUES OF FOOD - MINERALS (PER 100 GRAMS)

P (mg)	Mg (mg)	K (mg)	Na (mg)	Fe (mg)	Cu (mg)	Mn (mg)	Zn (mg)
35	23	195	2	0.46	0.076	0.157	0.25
39	24	192	1	0.36	0.103	0.213	0.39
20	8	437	1	0.33	0.095	0.211	0.26
55	20	348	10	0.45	0.208	0.560	0.29
23	11	207	8	0.48	0.077	0.122	0.11
27	11	191	67	0.30	-	-	-
42	31	296	40	1.10	0.350	0.466	0.19
60	21	330	41	0.20	-	-	-
55	21	816	9	0.54	0.24	0.178	9
512	28	98	620	0.68	-	-	3.11
134	5	86	406	0.14	-	-	0.38
337	19	62	1,116	0.65	-	-	2.88
104	4	32	13	0.23	-	-	0.47
444	27	81	536	0.72	-	-	3.00
463	23	84	466	0.22	-	-	2.76
807	51	107	1,862	0.95	-	-	3.19
183	15	125	125	0.44	-	-	1.34
605	36	111	260	0.17	-	-	3.90
745	22	162	1,430	0.39	-	-	2.99
93	13	152	49	0.05	-	-	0.38
95	14	154	50	0.05	-	-	0.39
101	11	166	52	0.04	-	-	0.40
89	11	151	105	0.05	-	-	0.42
95	12	155	46	0.05	-	-	0.59
180	12	130	138	2.09	-	-	1.44
200	30	356	70	1.49	0.093	0.889	0.65
138	42	244	78	0.49	0.036	-	0.58
241	50	399	87	1.35	0.033	-	0.48

NUTRITIVE VALUES OF FOOD - MINERALS (PER 100 GRAMS)

FOOD	Common Portion	Weight (in grams)	Ca (mg)
halibut	1 fillet	159	60
herring, cooked	1 fillet	143	74
mackerel, cooked	1 fillet	88	15
ocean perch	1 fillet	50	137
salmon, pink, canned	3 oz	85	213
trout, rainbow, cooked	1 fillet	62	86
tuna, canned in water	3 oz	85	12
POULTRY			
chicken, broilers or fryers, fresh only, roasted	1 c	140	15
chicken, dark, with skin, roasted	1 c	140	15
chicken, light, without skin, roasted	1 c	140	15
turkey, fryer, roasters, flesh only roasted	1 c	140	20
turkey, light, without skin, roasted	1 c	140	15
turkey, dark without skin, roasted	1 c	140	26

NUTRITIVE VALUES OF FOOD - MINERALS (PER 100 GRAMS)

P (mg)	Mg (mg)	K (mg)	Na (mg)	Fe (mg)	Cu (mg)	Mn (mg)	Zn (mg)
285	107	576	69	1.07	0.035	-	0.53
303	41	419	115	1.41	0.118	-	-
278	97	401	83	1.57	0.094	-	0.94
277	39	350	96	1.18	0.033	-	0.61
329	34	326	554	0.84	0.102	-	0.92
321	39	634	34	2.44	0.141	-	1.39
186	29	314	356	3.20	0.011	-	0.44
195	25	243	86	1.21	0.067	0.019	2.10
179	23	240	93	1.33	0.080	0.021	2.80
216	27	247	77	1.06	0.050	0.017	1.23
207	26	263	67	1.96	0.150	0.025	3.04
216	28	277	56	1.57	0.086	0.025	2.08
196	24	246	79	2.41	0.223	0.025	4.13

CHART C-2

GOOD SOURCES OF SELENIUM*

FOOD	Portion	amount in micrograms
whole wheat bread	1 slice	15.5
whole wheat flour	1 cup	77.4
wheat bran	1 cup	35.9
brown rice	1 cup	77.2
apple	1	0.7
avocado	1	1.5
orange	1	2.5
peach	1	0.46
pear	1	1.2
pineapple	1 cup	0.93
almonds	1 cup	2.8
brazil nuts	1 cup	144
hazelnuts	1 cup	2.7
pecans	1 cup	3.24
cabbage, common	1 cup	1.54
carrots	1 cup	3.3
cauliflower	1 cup	0.7
corn	1 cup	0.495
green beans	1 cup	0.66
mushrooms	1 cup	8.54
onions, mature	1 cup	2.55
peppers, green	1 cup	0.48
radish	10 med.	2.1

SOURCE: Nutrition Almanac (2nd Edition). Nutrition Search, Inc.: John D. Kirschmann, Director; Lavon J. Dunne, co-author. NY: McGraw Hill Book Company, 1984.

CHART C-3

CHROMIUM CONTENT OF FOODS

FOOD	Concentration mcg/100 gram	portion size size	amount of portion (gram)	amount of Chromium mcg/portion
apple	24	1 medium	150	36
asparagus	11	1 cup	100	11
baked beans	24	1 cup	100	24
banana	11	1 medium	150	16
barley	17	1/4 cup	50	8.5
beets	5	1 cup	140	7
blueberries	5	1 cup	140	7
broccoli	19	1 head	180	34
brown rice	9	1/4 cup	50	4.5
brussel sprouts	14	4 small	140	20
buckwheat	38	1/3 cup	33	13
cabbage	15	1 cup	90	13
carrots	8	1 medium	80	6.4
cauliflower	3	1 cup	100	3
celery	18	1 cup	120	21
chard	6	1 cup raw	115	8
chickpeas	10	1/4 cup	50	5
corn	37	1 ear	140	52
cornmeal	11	1 cup	100	11
cracked wheat (dry)	60	1/3 cup	50	30
cucumber	17	1 small	180	30
dates	19	5	40	7.6
eggplant	2	1 cup	200	4
figs	25	1	40	10
garbanzo beans	10	1/2 cup raw	100	10
green beans	4	1 cup	100	4
green pepper	19	1 cup	100	19
kale	4	1/4 lb.	115	4.6
leeks	8	3 to 4	100	8

mcg = micrograms

CHROMIUM CONTENT OF FOODS				
FOOD	Concentration mcg/100 gram	portion size size	amount of portion	amount of Chromium mcg/portion
lentils	11	1/2 cup	100	11
lettuce, romaine	20	2 cups	90	15
lima beans	10	1/2 cup	100	10
melon	13	1/4	100	13
millet	8	1/4 cup raw	25	2
mushrooms	47	1 cup raw	70	33
onions	19	1 cup chopped	160	30
orange	5	1 medium	180	9
parsnips	13	1 cup	100	13
peach	8	1 medium	100	8
peanuts	90	1 Tablespoon	9	8
pear	44	1 small	75	33
peas	38	1 cup	100	38
pinto beans	17	1/2 cup, cooked	100	17
plum	10	2 medium	100	10
popcorn	9	3 cups	42	3.8
potato	21	1 medium	250	42
prunes	100	5	50	25
red pepper (sweet)	10	1 cup	100	10
rolled oats	9	1 cup	80	7.2
rye bread	30	2 slices	50	15
spinach	20	1 cup (raw)	55	11
split peas	18	1/2 cup (raw)	100	18
squash (winter)	18	3/4 cup	100	18
strawberries	3	1 cup	150	4.5
sunflower seeds	34	1 Tablespoon	18	3
sweet potato/yams	20	1 medium	180	36
thyme	1,000	1/4 teaspoon	1.25	12.5
tomato	24	1 medium	100	24
turnip greens	5	1/4 lb.	115	5.6

CHROMIUM CONTENT OF FOODS				
FOOD	Concentration mcg/100 gram	portion size size	amount of portion	amount of Chromium mcg/portion
walnuts	48	1 Tablespoon	8	4
watercress	16	1 cup	120	19
wheat bran	38	1/4 cup	25	9.5
wheat germ	25	1/4 cup	25	6
whole wheat (berries)	29	1 cup cooked	125	36
zucchini	3	1 cup	205	6

Source: excerpted from Fisher, Jeffrey, A. M.D., The Chromium Program, *N.Y.: Harper and Row, 1990.*

APPENDIX D

NUTRITIVE VALUES OF FOOD - VITAMINS
(per 100 grams)

	WEIGHT OF COMMON PORTION			
FOOD	Common Portion	Weight (in grams)	A (mg)	C (mg)
GRAINS AND FLOUR:				
amaranth	1/2 c	98		4.2
arrowroot	1/2 c	43		
barley, pearled, cooked	1/2 c	79		
buckwheat groats, roasted, cooked	1/2 c	99		
buckwheat flour, whole groat	1/2 c	60		
bulgur, cooked	1/2 c	91		
cornmeal, wholegrain	1/4 c	30		
couscous, cooked	1/2 c	90		
millet, cooked	1/2 c	120		
oats, rolled, cooked	1 c	234		
quinoa	1/2 c	85		
rice, brown, long-grain, cooked	1/2 c	98		
rice flour, brown	1/2 c	79		
rye flour, dark	1/2 c	64		
triticale flour, whole grain	1/2 c	65		
wheat flour, whole grain	1/2 c	60		
wheat, sprouted	1/3 c	36		
wild rice, cooked	1/2 c	82		
LEGUMES				
adzuki beans, cooked, boiled	1/2 c	115		
black beans, cooked, boiled	1/2 c	86		
kidney beans, cooked, boiled	1/2 c	88		1.2

I.U. - international units **mg** - milligram **mcg** - microgram **RE** - retinol equivalents

NA = DATA NOT AVAILABLE

NUTRITIVE VALUES OF FOOD - VITAMINS

(per 100 grams)

	MINERALS						
	Thiamine (mg)	Riboflavin (mg)	Niacin (mg)	B-6 (mg)	Folacin (mg)	B-12 (mg)	Pantothenic (mg)
	0.080	0.208	1.286	0.223	49	-	1.047
	0.001	0.000	0.000	0.005	7		0.130
	0.083	0.062	2.063	0.115	16	-	0.135
	0.040	0.039	0.940	0.077	14		0.359
	0.417	0.190	6.150	0.582	54		0.440
	0.057	0.028	1.000	0.083	18		0.344
	0.385	0.201	3.632	0.304			0.425
	0.063	0.027	0.983	0.051	15		0.371
	0.106	0.082	1.330	0.108			0.171
	0.11	0.02	0.13	0.020	4		0.200
	0.198	0.396	2.930				
	0.096	0.025	1.528	0.145	4		0.285
	0.443	0.080	6.340	0.736	16		1.591
	0.316	0.251	4.270	0.443	60		1.456
	0.378	0.132	2.860	0.403	74		2.167
	0.447	0.215	6.365	0.341	44		1.008
	0.225	0.155	3.087	0.265			0.947
	0.052	0.087	1.287	0.135	26		0.154
	0.115	0.064	0.717				
	0.244	0.059	0.505	0.069	148.8		0.242
	0.160	0.058	0.578	0.120	129.6		0.220

NUTRITIVE VALUES OF FOOD - VITAMINS (PER 100 GRAMS)

FOOD	Common Portion	Weight (in grams)	A (mg)	C (mg)
navy beans, cooked, boiled	1/2 c	91		0.9
pinto beans, cooked, boiled	1/2 c	85		2.1
white beans, cooked, boiled	1/2 c	90		
chickpeas, cooked, boiled	1/2 c	82		1.3
lentils, cooked, boiled	1/2 c	99		1.5
lima beans, cooked, boiled	1/2 c	94		
mungbeans, cooked, boiled	1/2 c	101		1.0
split peas, cooked, boiled	1/2 c	98		0.4
peanuts, all types, raw	1 oz.	28		
soybeans, cooked, boiled	1/2 c	86		1.7
SOY PRODUCTS				
miso	1/2 c	138		
tamari	1 t	18		
tempeh	1/2 c	83		
soymilk	1/2 c	120		
tofu	1/4 block	81		0.2
NUTS AND SEEDS				
almonds, dried, unblanched	1 oz.	28.4		0.6
brazil nuts, dried, unblanched	1 oz.	28.4		0.7
cashew nuts, dry, roasted	1 oz.	28.4		
filbert nuts or hazelnuts, dried, unblanched	1 oz.	28.4		1.0
flax seed	1 oz.			
pecans, dried	1 oz.	28.4		2.0
pinenuts, dried, pignolia	1 oz.	28.4		
pistachio nuts, dried	1 oz.	28.4		
walnuts, dried	1 oz.	28.4		
pumpkin/squash seeds, dried	1 oz.	28.4		
sesame seeds, whole, dried	1 Tbsp.	9		
sunflower seed kernals, dried	1 oz.	28.4		

NUTRITIVE VALUES OF FOOD - VITAMINS (PER 100 GRAMS)

	Thiamine (mg)	Riboflavin (mg)	Niacin (mg)	B-6 (mg)	Folacin (mg)	B-12 (mg)	Pantothenic (mg)
	0.202	0.061	0.531	0.164	139.9		0.255
	0.186	0.091	0.400	0.155	172.0		0.285
	0.118	0.046	0.140	0.093	80.7		0.229
	0.116	0.063	0.526	0.139	172.0		0.286
	0.169	0.073	1.060	0.178	180.8		0.638
	0.161	0.055	0.421	0.161	83.1		0.422
	0.164	0.061	0.577	0.067	158.8		0.410
	0.190	0.056	0.890	0.048	64.9		0.595
	0.640	0.135	12.066	0.348	239.8		1.767
	0.155	0.285	0.399	0.234	53.8		0.179
	0.097	0.250	0.860	0.215	33.0		0.258
	0.059	0.152	3.951	0.200	18.2		0.376
	0.131	0.111	4.630	0.299	52.0		0.355
	0.161	0.70	0.147	0.041	1.5		0.048
	0.158	0.102	0.381	0.092	29.3		0.133
	0.211	0.779	3.361	0.113	58.7		0.471
	1.000	0.122	1.622	0.251	4.0		0.236
	0.200	0.200	1.400	0.256	69.2		1.217
	0.500	0.110	1.135	0.612	71.8		1.148
	0.17	0.16	1.40				
	0.848	0.128	0.887	0.188	39.2		1.707
	0.810	0.190	3.570	-	-		-
	0.820	0.174	1.080	-	58.0		-
	0.217	0.109	0.690	-	-		-
	0.210	0.320	1.745	-	-		-
	0.791	0.247	4.515	0.790	96.7		0.050
	2.290	0.250	4.500				

NUTRITIVE VALUES OF FOOD - VITAMINS (PER 100 GRAMS)

FOOD	Common Portion	Weight (in grams)	A (mg)	C (mg)
FRUITS				
apples, raw with skin	1 fruit	138	44	5.7
apricots, raw	3 fruits	106	2,612	10.0
avocadoes, raw	1 fruit	201	612	7.9
bananas, raw	1 fruit	114	81	9.1
blackberries, raw	1/2 c	72	165	21.0
blueberries, raw	1 c	145	100	13.0
carambola, raw	1 fruit	127	493	21.2
cherries, raw, sweet	10 fruit	68	214	7.0
cranberries, raw	1 c	95	46	13.5
dates, domestic, natural dry	10 fruit	83	50	0.0
figs, raw	1 med.	50	142	2.0
figs, dried, uncooked	10 fruit	187	133	0.8
grapefruit, red, white, pink, all sizes	1/2 fruit	120	124	34.4
grapes (American type) raw	10 fruit	24	100	4.0
guavas, raw	1 fruit	90	792	183.5
kiwi fruit, raw	1 fruit	76	175	98.0
lemons, raw	1 fruit	58	29	53.0
limes, raw	1 fruit	67	10	29.1
mangos, raw	1 fruit	207	3,894	27.7
melons, cantaloupe	1/2 fruit	267	3,224	42.2
casaba	1/10 fruit	164	30	16.0
honeydew, raw	1/10 fruit	129	40	24.8
nectarines, raw	1 fruit	136	736	5.4
oranges, raw, all varieties	1 fruit	131	205	53.2
papayas, raw	1 fruit	304	2,014	61.8
peaches, raw	1 fruit	87	535	6.6
pears, raw	1 fruit	166	20	4.0
persimmons, raw	1 fruit	168	2,167	7.5
pineapple, raw	1 slice	84	23	15.4
plums, raw	1 fruit	66	323	9.5
pomegranates, raw	1 fruit	154	-	6.1

NUTRITIVE VALUES OF FOOD - VITAMINS (PER 100 GRAMS)

	Thiamine (mg)	Riboflavin (mg)	Niacin (mg)	B-6 (mg)	Folacin (mg)	B-12 (mg)	Pantothenic (mg)
	0.017	0.014	0.077	0.048	2.8		0.061
	0.030	0.040	0.600	0.054	8.6		0.240
	0.108	0.122	0.921	0.280	61.9		0.971
	0.045	0.100	0.540	0.578	19.1		0.260
	0.030	0.040	0.400	0.058	-		0.240
	0.048	0.050	0.359	0.036	6.4		0.093
	0.028	0.027	0.411	-	-		-
	0.050	0.060	0.400	0.036	4.2		0.127
	0.030	0.020	0.100	0.065	1.7		0.219
	0.090	0.100	2.200	0.192	12.6		0.780
	0.060	0.050	0.400	0.113			0.300
	0.071	0.088	0.694	0.224	7.5		0.435
	0.036	0.020	0.250	0.042	10.2		0.283
	0.092	0.057	0.300	0.110	3.9		0.024
	0.050	0.050	1.200	0.143			0.150
	0.020	0.050	0.500				
	0.040	0.020	0.100	0.080	10.6		0.080
	0.030	0.020	0.200	-	8.2		0.217
	0.058	0.057	0.584	0.134			0.160
	0.036	0.021	0.574	0.115	17.0		0.128
	0.060	0.020	0.400				
	0.077	0.018	0.600	0.059	-		0.207
	0.017	0.041	0.990	0.025	3.7		0.158
	0.087	0.040	0.282	0.060	30.3		0.250
	0.027	0.032	0.338	0.019	-		0.218
	0.017	0.041	0.990	0.018	0.170		-
	0.020	0.040	0.100	0.018	7.3		0.070
	0.030	0.020	0.100		7.5		
	0.092	0.036	0.420	0.087	10.6		0.160
	0.043	0.096	0.500	0.081	2.2		0.182
	0.030	0.030	0.300	0.105	-		0.596

NUTRITIVE VALUES OF FOOD - VITAMINS (PER 100 GRAMS)

FOOD	Common Portion	Weight (in grams)	A (mg)	C (mg)
raisins, seedless	1 c not packed	145	44	3.2
raspberries, raw	1 c	123	130	25.0
strawberries	1 c	149	27	56.7
tangerines	1 c	84	920	30.8
watermelon	1/16 fruit	482	366	9.6
VEGETABLES AND SPROUTS:				
alfalfa seeds, sprouted, raw	1 c	33	155	8.2
artichokes, raw	1 artichoke	128	185	10.8
asparagus, raw	1/2 c	67	897	33.0
beans, lima, cooked, boiled, drained	1/2 c	85	370	10.1
mung beans, sprouted, raw	1/2 c	52	21	13.2
beans, snap, cooked	1/2 c	62	666	9.7
beets, raw	1/2 c	68	20	11.0
beets, cooked	1/2 c	85	13	5.5
beet greens, raw	1/2 c	19	6,100	30.0
beet greens, cooked	1/2 c	72	5,100	24.9
broad beans, cooked	1/2 c		270	19.8
broccoli, raw	1/2 c	44	1,542	93.2
brussel sprouts, raw	1 sprout	19	883	85.0
brussel sprouts, cooked	1 sprout	21	719	62.0
cabbage, raw	1/2 c	35	126	47.3
cabbage, cooked	1/2 c	75	86	24.3
cabbage, red, raw	1/2 c	35	40	57.0
carrots, raw	1/2 c	55	28,129	9.3
carrots, cooked	1/2 c	78	24,554	2.3
cauliflower,raw	1/2 c	50	16	71.5
cauliflower, cooked	1/2 c	62	14	55.4
celery, raw	1 stalk	40	127	6.3
swiss chard, raw	1/2 c	18	3,300	30.0
collards, raw	1/2 c	93	3,300	23.3
sweet corn, raw	1/2 c cut	77	281	6.8

NUTRITIVE VALUES OF FOOD - VITAMINS (PER 100 GRAMS)

	Thiamine (mg)	Riboflavin (mg)	Niacin (mg)	B-6 (mg)	Folacin (mg)	B-12 (mg)	Pantothenic (mg)
	0.008	0.191	1.142	0.323	3.3		0.140
	0.030	0.090	0.900	0.057	-		0.57
	0.020	0.066	0.230	0.059	17.7		0.340
	0.105	0.022	0.160	0.067	20.4		0.200
	0.080	0.020	0.200	0.144	2.2		0.212
	0.076	0.126	0.481	0.034	36.0		0.563
	0.078	0.060	0.760	0.112	73.6		0.257
	0.114	0.124	1.138	0.153	119.4		0.174
	0.140	0.096	1.040	0.193	-		0.257
	0.084	0.124	0.749	0.088	60.8		0.380
	0.074	0.097	0.614	0.056	33.3		0.074
	0.050	0.020	0.400	0.046	92.6		0.150
	0.031	0.014	0.273	0.031	53.2		0.097
	0.100	0.220	0.400	0.106	-		0.250
	0.117	0.289	0.499	0.132	-		0.329
		0.128	0.090	1.200	-	-	-
	0.065	0.119	0.638	0.159	71.0		0.535
	0.139	0.090	0.745	0.219	61.1		0.309
	0.107	0.080	0.607	0.178	60.0		0.252
	0.050	0.030	0.300	0.095	56.7		0.140
	0.057	0.055	0.230	0.064	20.3		0.063
	0.050	0.030	0.300	0.210	20.7		0.324
	0.097	0.059	0.928	0.147	14.0		0.197
	0.034	0.056	0.506	0.246	13.9		0.304
	0.076	0.057	0.633	0.231	66.1		0.141
	0.063	0.052	0.552	0.202	51.2		0.122
	0.030	0.030	0.300	0.030	8.9		0.169
	0.040	0.090	0.400	-			0.172
	0.029	0.064	0.374	0.067	11.5		0.064
	0.200	0.060	1.700	0.055	45.8		0.760

NUTRITIVE VALUES OF FOOD - VITAMINS (PER 100 GRAMS)

FOOD	Common Portion	Weight (in grams)	A (mg)	C (mg)
sweet corn, cooked	1/2 c cut	82	217	6.2
cucumber, raw	1/2 c	52	45	4.7
dandelion greens, raw	1/2 c	28	14,000	35.0
dandelion greens, cooked	1/2 c	52	11,700	18.0
eggplant, cooked	1/2 c	48	64	1.3
endive, raw	1/2 c	25	2050	6.5
garlic, raw	1 clove	3	0	31.2
ginger root, raw	5 slices	11	0	5.0
kale, raw	1/2 c	34	8,900	120.0
kale, cooked	1/2 c	65	7,400	41.0
kohlrabi, raw	1/2 c	70	36	62.0
leeks, raw	1/4 c	26	95	12.0
lentils, sprouted, raw	1/2 c	38	45	16.5
lettuce, romaine	1/2 c	28	2,600	24.0
mushrooms, raw	1/2 c	35	0	3.5
mustard greens, raw	1/2 c	28	5.300	70.0
okra, cooked	1/2 c	80	575	16.3
onions, raw	1 tablespoon	10	0	8.4
parsley, raw	10 sprigs	10	5,200	90.0
parsnips, raw	1/2 c	67	0	17.0
peas, edible - podded, raw	1/2 c	72	145	60.0
peas, green, raw	1/2 c	78	640	40.0
peas, mature, sprouted, raw	1/2 c	60	166	10.4
peppers, sweet, raw	1 pepper	74	530	128.0
potato, baked, flesh & skin	1 potato	202	-	12.9
pumpkin, cooked	1/2 c	122	1,082	4.7
radishes, raw	10 radishes	45	8	22.8
radish, seeds, sprouted, raw	1/2 c	19	391	28.9
rutabagas, cooked	1/2 c	85	0	21.9
soybeans, sprouted, raw	1/2 c	35	11	15.3
soybeans, green, cooked	1/2 c	90	156	17.0
spinach, raw	1/2 c	28	6,715	28.1

NUTRITIVE VALUES OF FOOD - VITAMINS (PER 100 GRAMS)

Thiamine (mg)	Riboflavin (mg)	Niacin (mg)	B-6 (mg)	Folacin (mg)	B-12 (mg)	Pantothenic (mg)
0.215	0.072	1.614	0.060	46.4		0.878
0.030	0.020	0.300	0.052	13.9		0.250
0.190	0.260	-	-	-		-
0.130	0.175	-	-	-		-
0.076	0.020	0.600	0.086	14.4		0.075
0.080	0.075	0.400	0.020	142.0		0.900
0.200	0.110	0.700	-	3.1		-
0.023	0.029	0.700	0.160	-		0.203
0.110	0.130	1.000	0.271	29.3		0.049
0.053	0.070	0.500	0.138	13.3		0.049
0.050	0.020	0.400	0.150	-		0.165
0.060	0.030	0.400	-	64.1		-
0.228	0.128	1.128	0.190	99.9		0.578
0.100	0.100	0.500	-	135.7		-
0.102	0.449	4.116	0.097	21.1		2.200
0.080	0.110	0.800	-	-		0.210
0.132	0.055	0.871	0.187	45.7		0.213
0.060	0.010	0.100	0.157	19.9		0.132
0.080	0.110	0.700	0.164	183.1		0.300
0.090	0.050	0.700	0.090	66.8		0.600
0.150	0.080	0.600	0.160	-		0.750
0.265	0.132	2.090	0.169	65.2		0.104
0.225	0.155	3.088	0.265	144.0		1.029
0.085	0.050	0.550	0.164	16.9		0.036
0.107	0.033	1.645	0.347	11.0		0.555
0.031	0.078	0.413	-	-		-
0.005	0.045	0.300	0.071	27.0		0.088
0.102	0.103	2.853	0.285	94.7		0.733
0.072	0.036	0.630	0.090	15.5		0.137
0.340	0.118	1.148	0.176	171.8		0.929
0.260	0.155	1.250	-	-		-
0.078	0.189	0.724	0.195	194.4		0.065

NUTRITIVE VALUES OF FOOD - VITAMINS (PER 100 GRAMS)

FOOD	Common Portion	Weight (in grams)	A (mg)	C (mg)
summer squash, raw, all varieties	1/2 c	65	196	14.8
summer squash, cooked	1/2 c	90	287	5.5
winter squash, all varieties, baked	1/2 c	102	3,557	9.6
sweet potato, baked in skin	1 potato	114	21,822	24.6
tomatoes, red, ripe, raw	1 tomato	123	1,133	17.6
turnips, raw	1/2 c	65	0	21.0
turnip greens, raw	1/2 c	28	7,600	60.0
watercress, raw	1/2 c	17	4,700	43.0
yams, baked	1/2 c	75	0	17.1
DAIRY PRODUCTS				
cheese, cheddar	1 oz	28	1,059	0
cottage cheese, 1% fat	4 oz	113	37	trace
cheese, feta	1 oz	28	-	-
cottage cheese, dry curd	4 oz	113	30	0
cheese, monterey	1 oz	28	950	0
cheese, mozzerella, part skin	1 oz	28	584	0
cheese, parmesan, grated	1 oz	28	701	0
cheese, ricotta (part skim)	1/2 c	124	432	0
cheese, swiss	1 oz	28	845	0
cheese, American	1 oz	28	1,210	0
whole milk	1 c	244	126	0.94
milk, low fat 2%	1 c	244	205	0.95
skim milk	1 c	245	204	0.98
buttermilk	1 c	245	33	0.98
yogurt, plain, low fat	1 8 oz container	227	123	0.53
egg, chicken, whole, hard cooked	1 white	50	520	0
FISH				
bass, fresh water	1 fillet	79	NA	
cod, cooked	1 fillet	180	46	1.0
haddock	1 fillet	150	63	-

NUTRITIVE VALUES OF FOOD - VITAMINS (PER 100 GRAMS)

	Thiamine (mg)	Riboflavin (mg)	Niacin (mg)	B-6 (mg)	Folacin (mg)	B-12 (mg)	Pantothenic (mg)
	0.064	0.037	0.551	0.109	25.6		0.102
	0.044	0.041	0.513	0.065	20.1		0.137
	0.085	0.024	0.701	0.072	28.0		0.350
	0.073	0.127	0.604	0.241	22.6		0.646
	0.060	0.050	0.600	0.048	9.4		0.247
	0.040	0.030	0.400	0.090	14.5		0.200
	0.070	0.100	0.600	0.263	194.4		0.380
	0.090	0.120	0.200	0.129	-		0.310
	0.112	0.032	0.758	0.293	23.0		0.314
	0.027	0.375	0.080	0.074	18	0.827	0.413
	0.021	0.165	0.128	0.068	12	0.633	0.215
	-	-	-	-	-	-	-
	0.025	0.142	0.155	0.082	15	0.825	0.163
	0.390	-	-	-	-	-	-
	0.018	0.303	0.105	0.070	9	0.817	0.079
	0.045	0.386	0.315	0.105	8	-	0.527
	0.021	0.185	0.078	0.020	-	0.291	-
	0.022	0.365	0.092	0.083	6	1.676	0.429
	0.027	0.353	0.069	0.071	8	0.696	0.482
	0.038	0.162	0.084	0.042	5	0.357	0.314
	0.039	0.165	0.086	0.043	5	0.364	0.320
	0.036	0.140	0.088	0.040	5	0.378	0.329
	0.034	0.154	0.058	0.034	-	0.219	0.275
	0.029	0.142	0.075	0.032	7	0.372	0.389
	0.074	0.286	0.059	0.114	49	1.315	1.727
	0.088	0.079	2.513	0.283	-	1.048	-
	0.040	0.045	4.632	0.346	-	1.387	-

NUTRITIVE VALUES OF FOOD - VITAMINS (PER 100 GRAMS)

FOOD	Common Portion	Weight (in grams)	A (mg)	C (mg)
halibut	1 fillet	159	179	-
herring, cooked	1 fillet	143	102	0.7
mackerel, cooked	1 fillet	88	180	0.4
ocean perch	1 fillet	50	46	-
salmon, pink, canned	3 oz	85	55	0.0
trout, rainbow, cooked	1 fillet	62	75	3.7
tuna, canned in water	3 oz	85	NA	
POULTRY				
chicken, broilers or fryers, fresh only, roasted	1 c	140	53	
chicken, dark, with skin, roasted	1 c	140	72	0
chicken, light, without skin, roasted	1 c	140	29	0
turkey, fryer, roasters, flesh only roasted	1 c	140	0	
turkey, light, without skin, roasted	1 c	140	0	0
turkey, dark without skin, roasted	1 c	140	0	0

NUTRITIVE VALUES OF FOOD - VITAMINS (PER 100 GRAMS)

	Thiamine (mg)	Riboflavin (mg)	Niacin (mg)	B-6 (mg)	Folacin (mg)	B-12 (mg)	Pantothenic (mg)
	0.069	0.091	7.123	0.397	-	1.366	-
	0.112	0.299	4.124	0.348	-	13.141	-
	0.159	0.412	6.850	0.460	-	19.000	-
	-	0.134	2.436	-	-	1.154	-
	0.023	0.186	6.536	-	-	17 RE	-
	0.085	0.225	-	-	-	22 RE	-
				0.378	4.7		
	0.069	0.178	9.173	0.47	6	0.33	1.104
	0.073	0.227	6.548	0.36	8	0.32	1.210
	0.065	0.116	12.421	0.60	4	0.34	0.972
	0.046	0.188	5.326	0.48	8	0.39	1.012
	0.041	0.136	6.936	0.57	6	0.39	0.715
	0.051	0.248	3.471	0.38	10	0.39	1.353

CHART D-2

GOOD SOURCES OF VITAMIN E

FOOD	Portion	Amount in I.U. (International Units)
whole wheat bread	1 slice	0.3
whole wheat flour	1 cup	3.12
brown rice	1 cup	3
corn oil	1 Tablespoon	11.3
olive oil	1 Tablespoon	1.7
peanut oil	1 Tablespoon	3.4
sunflower oil	1 Tablespoon	5.2
sesame oil	1 Tablespoon	4
soybean oil	1 Tablespoon	12.7
sunflower oil	1 Tablespoon	1.3
wheat germ oil	1 Tablespoon	34.6
apple	1 medium	1
banana	1	0.6
mango	1	3
almonds	1 cup	21.3
brazil nuts	1 cup	9.1
hazel nuts	1 cup	28
peanuts	1 cup	9.36
pecans	1 cup	1.5
walnuts	1 cup	1.5
cabbage	1 cup	0.2
cauliflower	1 cup	0.15
celery	1 cup	0.57
cucumber	1 cup	8.4
kale	1 cup	8
mushrooms	1 cup	0.58
onions, mature	1 cup	0.442
peas, green	1 cup	3.1
spinach	1 cup	1.25
tomato	1 medium	0.54
turnip greens	1 cup	3.4

CHART D-3

VITAMIN K

- present in cabbage, cauliflower, soybeans, spinach, wholegrains, wheatgerm, wheatbran, potatoes, tomatoes, green leafy vegetables, spinach, kale, alfalfa, corn, mushrooms, oats, peas, strawberries

CHART D-4

GOOD SOURCES OF BIOTIN

FOOD	Portion	Amount in Micrograms
buckwheat flour	1 cup	2.9
corn flour	1 cup	1.6
soy flour	1 cup	49
wholewheat flour	1 cup	6
brown rice	1 cup	18
haddock	1 lb.	1.36
halibut	1 lb.	9.06
almonds	1 cup	25
peanuts	1 cup	49
walnuts	1 cup	37
apple	1	1.8
banana	1	6
cantaloupe	1/2	6
currants, black	1 cup	2.5
elderberries	1 cup	3
grapes, slip skin	1 cup	3
orange	1	1.8
peach	1	2
raisins	1 cup	7
raspberries	1 cup	2.28
strawberries	1 cup	1.6
watermelon	1 cup	4

GOOD SOURCES OF BIOTIN

FOOD	Portion	Amount in Micrograms
asparagus	1 cup	0.675
beet greens	1 cup	3
carrots	1 cup	4.5
cauliflower	1 cup	1.5
corn	1 cup	1.95
leeks	3-4	1.4
mushrooms	1 cup	11.2
onions, mature	1 cup	1.53
spinach	1 cup	3.5
tomato	1 medium	2

RECOMMENDED INTAKE 150-200 MICROGRAMS/DAY

APPENDIX E

FIBER CONTENT OF FOOD (PER 100 GRAMS)

FOOD	weight of common portion	amount grams	Fiber
GRAINS AND FLOUR			
amaranth	1/2 cup	98	3.77
arrowroot	1/3 cup	43	-
barley, pearled, cooked	1/2 cup	79	0.23
buckwheat groats, roasted, cooked	1/2 cup	99	0.52
buckwheat flour, whole groat	1/2 cup	60	
bulgur, cooked	1/2 cup	91	0.35
cornmeal, whole-grain	1/4 cup	30	1.84
couscous, cooked	1/2 cup	90	0.14
millet, cooked	1/2 cup	120	0.36
oats, rolled or oatmeal, cooked	1 cup	234	0.2
quinoa	1/2 cup	85	-
rice, brown, long-grain, cooked	1/2 cup	98	0.34
rice flour, brown	1/2 cup	79	1.29
rye flour, dark	1/2 cup	64	-
triticale, flour,	1/2 cup	65	1.50
wheat flour, wholegrain	1/2 cup	60	2.10
wheat, sprouted	1/3 cup	36	-
wild rice, cooked	1/2 cup	82	0.33
LEGUMES			
adzuki beans, cooked, boiled	1/2 cup	115	2.02
black beans, cooked, boiled	1/2 cup	86	2.03
kidney beans, cooked, boiled	1/2 cup	88	2.81
navy beans, cooked, boiled	1/2 cup	91	3.14
pinto beans, cooked, boiled	1/2 cup	85	3.02
white beans, cooked, boiled	1/2 cup	90	2.49
chickpeas, cooked, boiled	1/2 cup	82	2.50
lentils, cooked, boiled	1/2 cup	99	2.76

FIBER CONTENT OF FOOD (PER 100 GRAMS)

FOOD	weight of common portion	amount grams	Fiber
lima beans, cooked, boiled	1/2 cup	94	3.09
mungbeans, cooked, boiled	1/2 cup	101	0.46
split peas, cooked, boiled	1/2 cup	98	1.97
peanuts, all types, raw	1 oz.	28	4.85
soybeans, cooked, boiled	1/2 cup	86	2.03
SOY PRODUCTS			
miso	1/2 cup	138	2.47
tamari	1 tsp	18	0.0
tempeh	1/2 cup	83	2.99
soymilk	1/2 cup	120	-
tofu, raw, firm	1/4 block	81	0.15
NUTS AND SEEDS			
almonds, dried, unblanched	1 oz.	28.4	2.71
brazil nuts, dried, unblanched	1 oz.	28.4	2.29
cashew nuts, dry, roasted	1 oz.	28.4	0.70
filbert nuts or hazelnuts, dried, unblanched	1 oz.	28.4	3.80
flax seed	1 oz.	28.0	8.8
pecans, dried	1 oz.	28.4	1.60
pinenuts, dried	1 oz.	28.4	1.88
pistachio nuts, dried	1 oz.	28.4	0.80
walnuts, dried	1 oz.	28.4	6.46
pumpkin/squash seeds, dried	1 oz.	28.4	2.22
sesame seeds, whole, dried	1 Tbsp.	9	4.60
sunflower seed kernals, dried	1 oz.	28.4	4.16
FRUITS			
apples, raw with skin	1 fruit	138	0.77
apricots, raw	3 fruits	106	0.60
[illegible]cadoes, all types, raw	1 fruit	201	2.11
[illegible]as, raw	1 fruit	114	0.50
[illegible]berries	1/2 cup	72	4.10

FIBER CONTENT OF FOOD (PER 100 GRAMS)

FOOD	weight of common portion	amount grams	Fiber
blueberries	1 cup	145	1.30
carambola, raw	1 fruit	127	0.92
cherries, raw, sweet	10 fruit	68	0.40
cranberries, raw	1 cup	95	1.20
dates, domestic, natural dry	10 fruit	83	2.20
figs, raw	1 fruit	50	1.20
figs, dried, uncooked	10 fruit	187	4.80
grapefruit, raw, pink, red, white, all areas	1/2 fruit	120	0.20
grapes (American type) raw	10 fruit	24	0.76
guavas, raw, commercial	1 fruit	90	5.60
kiwi fruit, raw	1 fruit	76	1.10
lemons, raw, without peel	1 fruit	58	0.40
limes, raw	1 fruit	67	0.50
mangos, raw	1 fruit	207	0.84
melons, cantaloupe, raw	1/2 fruit	267	0.36
casaba, raw	1/10 fruit	164	0.50
honeydew, raw	1/10 fruit	129	0.60
nectarines, raw	1 fruit	136	0.40
oranges, raw, all varieties	1 fruit	131	0.43
papayas, raw	1 fruit	304	0.77
peaches, raw	1 fruit	87	0.64
pears, raw	1 fruit	166	1.40
persimmons, raw	1 fruit	168	1.48
pineapple, raw	1 slice	84	0.54
plums, raw	1 fruit	66	0.60
pomegrantes	1 fruit	154	0.20
raisins, seedless	1 cup, not packed	145	1.43
raspberries, raw	1 cup	123	3.00
strawberries, raw	1 cup	149	0.53
tangarines	1 cup	84	0.33
watermelon	1/16 fruit	482	0.30

FIBER CONTENT OF FOOD (PER 100 GRAMS)

FOOD	weight of common portion	amount grams	Fiber
VEGETABLES AND SPROUTS:			
alfalfa seeds, sprouted, raw	1 cup	33	1.64
artichokes, raw	1 artichoke	128	1.06
asparagus, raw	1/2 cup	67	0.83
beans, lima, cooked, boiled, drained	1/2 cup	123	2.09
mung beans, sprouted, raw	1/2 cup	52	0.81
beans, snap, cooked	1/2 cup	62	1.43
beets, raw	1/2 cup	68	0.80
beets, cooked	1/2 cup	85	0.85
beet greens, raw	1/2 cup	19	1.30
beet greens, cooked	1/2 cup	72	1.05
broad beans, cooked	-	-	1.90
broccoli, raw	1/2 cup	44	1.11
brussel sprouts, raw	1 sprout	19	1.51
brussel sprouts, cooked	1 sprout	21	1.37
cabbage, raw	1/2 cup	35	0.80
cabbage, cooked	1/2 cup	75	0.60
cabbage, red, raw	1/2 cup	35	1.00
carrots, raw	1/2 cup	55	1.04
carrots, cooked	1/2 cup	78	1.47
cauliflower,raw	1/2 cup	50	0.85
cauliflower, cooked	1/2 cup	62	0.82
celery, raw	1 stalk	40	0.69
swiss chard, raw	1/2 cup	18	0.80
collards, raw	1/2 cup	93	0.57
sweet corn, raw	1/2 cup cut	77	0.70
sweet corn, cooked	1/2 cup cut	82	0.60
cucumber, raw	1/2 cup	52	0.60
[illegible] greens, raw	1/2 cup	28	1.60
[illegible] greens, cooked	1/2 cup	52	1.30
[illegible] ooked	1/2 cup	48	0.97
[illegible] /	1/2 cup	25	0.90
[illegible]	1 clove	3	1.50

FIBER CONTENT OF FOOD (PER 100 GRAMS)

FOOD	weight of common portion	amount grams	Fiber
ginger root, raw	5 slices	11	1.03
kale, raw	1/2 cup	34	1.50
kale, cooked	1/2 cup	65	0.80
kohlrabi, raw	1/2 cup	70	1.00
leeks, raw	1/4 cup	26	1.51
lentils, sprouted, raw	1/2 cup	38	3.05
lettuce, romaine	1/2 cup	28	0.70
mushrooms, raw	1/2 cup	35	0.75
mustard greens, raw	1/2 cup	28	1.10
okra, cooked	1/2 cup	80	0.70
onions, raw	1 Tbsp.	10	0.44
parsley, raw	10 sprigs	10	1.20
parsnips, raw	1/2 cup	67	2.00
peas, edible - podded, raw	1/2 cup	72	2.50
peas, green, raw	1/2 cup	78	2.21
peas, mature, sprouted, raw	1/2 cup	60	2.78
peppers, sweet, raw	1 pepper	74	1.20
potato, baked, flesh & skin	1 potato	202	0.66
pumpkin, cooked	1/2 cup	122	0.83
radish seeds, sprouted, raw	1/2 cup	19	-
rutabagas, cooked	1/2 cup	85	1.04
soybeans, sprouted, raw	1/2 cup	35	2.30
soybeans, green, cooked	1/2 cup	90	1.85
spinach, raw	1/2 cup	28	0.89
summer squash, raw	1/2 cup	65	0.60
summer squash, cooked	1/2 cup	90	0.60
winter squash, all varieties, baked	1/2 cup	102	0.71
sweet potato, baked in skin	1 potato	114	0.80
tomatoes, red, ripe, raw	1 tomato	123	0.47
turnips, raw	1/2 cup	65	0.90
turnip greens, raw	1/2 cup	28	0.80
watercress, raw	1/2 cup	17	0.70
yams, baked	1/2 cup	75	-

APPENDIX F

PROTEIN CONTENT OF FOOD *(with Essential Amino Acids Values)*

Total Protein *(in grams)* = Total protein in grams/100 grams of edible portion, including both essential and non-essential amino acids.

Total E.A.A. *(Essential Amino Acids)* in grams/100 grams of edible portion:

First value listed = Total essential amino acids for adults

Second value listed = Total essential amino acids plus arginine and histidine, essential for children

FOOD	Total Protein (grams)	Total E.A.A. adult/child (gm)	Tryptophan (gm)
GRAINS AND FLOUR:			
amaranth	14.45 g	4.394/5.843	0.181
arrowroot flour	0.30	0.083/0.099	0.004
barley, pearled, cooked	2.26	0.717/0.881	0.038
buckwheat groats, roasted, cooked	3.38	1.039/1.368	0.049
buckwheat flour, whole groat	12.62	3.876/5.105	0.183
bulghur, cooked	3.08	0.876/1.091	0.048
cornmeal, whole grain	8.12	2.857/3.51	0.057
couscous, cooked	3.79	1.033/1.25	0.049
millet, cooked	3.51	2.318/2.515	0.038
oats, rolled or oatmeal, cooked	2.6	0.861/1.105	0.036
quinoa	13.10	3.839/5.071	-
rice, brown, long-grain, cooked	2.58	0.892/1.154	0.033
rice flour, brown	7.23	2.497/3.229	0.092
rye flour, dark	14.03	4.264/5.212	0.159
triticale, flour, whole-grain	13.18	3.805/4.797	0.158
wheat flour, whole-grain	13.70	3.895/4.854	0.212
wheat, sprouted	7.49	2.235/2.856	0.115
wild rice, cooked	3.99	1.335/1.747	0.049
…ked, boiled	7.52	3.401/4.085	0.072
…ed, boiled	8.86	3.261/4.057	0.105
…ked, boiled	8.67	3.192/3.971	0.103

…TA NOT AVAILABLE

PROTEIN CONTENT OF FOOD *(with Essential Amino Acids Values)*

Threonine (gm)	Isoleucine (gm)	Leucine (gm)	Lysine (gm)	Methionine (gm)	Phenylalanine (gm)	Valine (gm)	Arginine (gm)	Histidine (gm)
0.558	0.582	0.879	0.747	0.226	0.542	0.679	1.060	0.389
0.012	0.012	0.010	0.013	0.006	0.012	0.014	0.012	0.004
0.077	0.083	0.154	0.084	0.043	0.127	0.111	0.113	0.051
0.129	0.127	0.212	0.172	0.044	0.133	0.173	0.250	0.079
0.482	0.474	0.792	0.640	0.164	0.495	0.646	0.935	0.294
0.089	0.114	0.208	0.085	0.048	0.145	0.139	0.144	0.071
0.305	0.291	0.996	0.228	0.170	0.399	0.411	0.405	0.248
0.100	0.147	0.259	0.073	0.059	0.184	0.162	0.140	0.077
0.113	0.148	0.446	0.067	0.070	0.185	0.184	0.122	0.075
0.088	0.106	0.196	0.107	0.048	0.137	0.143	0.182	0.062
0.459	0.472	0.786	0.734	0.262	0.537	0.589	0.918	0.314
0.095	0.109	0.214	0.099	0.058	0.133	0.151	0.196	0.066
0.265	0.306	0.598	0.276	0.163	0.373	0.424	0.548	0.184
0.486	0.541	0.970	0.486	0.209	0.710	0.703	0.635	0.313
0.409	0.484	0.920	0.369	0.206	0.644	0.615	0.678	0.314
0.395	0.508	0.926	0.378	0.212	0.646	0.618	0.642	0.317
0.254	0.287	0.507	0.245	0.116	0.350	0.361	0.425	0.196
0.127	0.167	0.276	0.170	0.119	0.195	0.232	0.308	0.104
0.255	0.300	0.632	0.567	0.79	0.398	0.387	0.486	0.198
0.373	0.391	0.708	0.608	0.133	0.479	0.464	0.549	[illegible]
0.365	0.383	0.693	0.595	0.130	0.469	0.454	0.537	

PROTEIN CONTENT OF FOOD (with Essential Amino Acids Values)

FOOD	Total Protein (grams)	Total E.A.A. adult/child (gm)	Tryptophan (gm)
navy beans, cooked, boiled	8.70	3.201/3.982	0.103
pinto beans, cooked, boiled	8.21	3.024/3.762	0.097
white beans, cooked, boiled	9.73	3.578/4.451	0.115
chickpeas, cooked, boiled	8.86	2.981/4.06	0.085
lentils, cooked, boiled	9.02	3.048/3.999	0.081
lima beans, cooked, boiled	7.80	3.053/3.769	0.092
mung beans, cooked, boiled	7.02	2.51/3.207	0.076
split peas, cooked, boiled	8.34	2.796/3.743	0.093
peanuts, all types, raw	25.80	7.374/11.111	0.250
soybeans, cooked, boiled	16.64	6.159/7.899	0.242
SOY PRODUCTS:			
miso	11.81	4.869/5.945	0.143
tamari soy sauce	10.51	NA	NA
tempeh	18.95	7.071/8.886	0.282
soymilk	2.75	1.337/1.622	0.043
tofu, raw, firm	15.78	5.676/7.185	0.246
NUTS AND SEEDS:			
almonds, dried, unblanched	19.95	6.549/9.602	0.358
brasil nuts, dried, unblanched	14.34	5.72/8.512	0.260
cashew nuts, dry roasted	15.31	5.767/7.907	0.237
filberts or hazelnuts, dried, unblanched	13.04	4.241/6.723	0.216
pecans, dried	7.75	2.567/3.899	0.199
pine nuts, dried	24.00	7.218/12.461	0.303
pistachio nuts, dried	20.58	7.91/10.632	0.283
walnuts, dried	24.35	7.321/11.662	0.322
pump[illegible]h seeds, dried	24.54	10.255/14.969	0.431
[illegible]whole, dried	17.73	6.33/9.482	0.388
[illegible]ernels, dried	22.78	7.989/11.024	0.348

PROTEIN CONTENT OF FOOD (with Essential Amino Acids Values)

Threonine (gm)	Isoleucine (gm)	Leucine (gm)	Lysine (gm)	Methionine (gm)	Phenylalanine (gm)	Valine (gm)	Arginine (gm)	Histidine (gm)
0.366	0.384	0.695	0.597	0.131	0.470	0.455	0.539	0.242
0.346	0.363	0.656	0.564	0.124	0.444	0.430	0.509	0.229
0.409	0.429	0.776	0.668	0.146	0.526	0.509	0.602	0.271
0.329	0.380	0.631	0.593	0.116	0.475	0.372	0.835	0.244
0.323	0.390	0.654	0.630	0.077	0.445	0.448	0.697	0.254
0.337	0.411	0.673	0.523	0.099	0.449	0.469	0.478	0.238
0.230	0.297	0.544	0.490	0.084	0.425	0.364	0.492	0.205
0.296	0.344	0.598	0.602	0.085	0.384	0.394	0.744	0.203
0.883	0.907	1.672	0.926	0.317	1.337	1.082	3.085	0.652
0.723	0.807	1.355	1.108	0.224	0.869	0.831	1.291	0.449
0.639	0.811	1.129	0.660	0.149	0.596	0.742	0.747	0.329
NA	NA	NA	NA	NA	NA	NA	NA	NA
0.770	1.002	1.636	1.125	0.265	1.012	0.979	1.317	0.498
0.113	0.144	0.241	0.179	0.040	0.151	0.141	0.214	0.071
0.644	0.782	1.199	1.039	0.202	0.768	0.796	1.050	0.459
0.739	0.866	1.552	0.666	0.227	1.113	1.028	2.495	0.558
0.460	0.601	1.187	0.541	1.014	0.746	0.911	2.390	0.402
0.592	0.731	1.285	0.817	0.274	0.791	1.040	1.741	0.399
0.448	0.568	1.100	0.399	0.162	0.686	0.662	2.155	0.327
0.253	0.322	0.520	0.292	0.186	0.409	0.386	1.105	0.227
0.761	0.933	1.730	0.901	0.430	0.919	1.241	4.668	0.575
0.722	0.975	1.677	1.278	0.381	1.184	1.410	2.186	0.536
0.730	0.978	1.704	0.721	0.473	1.107	1.286	3.661	0.680
0.903	1.264	2.079	1.833	0.551	1.222	1.972	4.033	0.681
0.736	0.763	1.358	0.569	0.586	0.940	0.990	2.630	0.522
0.928	1.139	1.659	0.937	0.494	1.169	1.315	2.403	0.632

PROTEIN CONTENT OF FOOD (with Essential Amino Acids Values)

FOOD	Total Protein (grams)	Total E.A.A. adult/child (gm)	Tryptophan (gm)
FRUITS:			
apples, raw, with skin	0.19	0.057/0.066	0.002
apricots, raw	1.40	0.382/0.454	0.015
avocados, raw, all varieties	1.98	0.577/0.665	0.021
bananas, raw	1.03	0.294/0.422	0.012
blackberries, raw	0.72	-	NA
blueberries,	0.67	0.157/0.201	0.003
carambola, raw	0.54	0.186/0.201	0.004
cherries, sweet, raw	1.20	-	NA
cranberries, raw	0.39	-	NA
dates, domestic, natural & dry	1.97	0.441/0.537	0.050
figs, raw	0.75	0.168/0.196	0.006
figs, dried, uncooked	3.05	0.688/0.801	0.026
grapefruit, raw, pink , red, white, all areas	0.63	0.02	0.002
grapes, (American type) raw	0.63	0.103/0.172	0.003
guavas, common, raw	0.82	0.181/0.209	0.007
kiwifruit, raw	0.99	-	NA
lemons	1.10	-	NA
limes	0.70	0.019	0.003
mangoes	0.51	0.165/0.196	0.008
melons, cantaloupe, raw	0.88	-	NA
casaba, raw	0.90	-	NA
honeydew, raw	0.46	-	NA
nectarines, raw	0.94	-	NA
oranges, raw, all varieties	0.94	0.210/0.293	0.009
papayas, raw	0.61	0.089/0.104	0.008
peaches, raw	0.70	0.189/0.220	0.002
pea[illegible]	0.39	0.084/0.095	-
[illegible]	0.58	0.201/0.238	0.010
[illegible]	0.39	0.113/0.140	0.005
[illegible]	0.79	0.112/0.138	-

PROTEIN CONTENT OF FOOD (with Essential Amino Acids Values)

Threonine (gm)	Isoleucine (gm)	Leucine (gm)	Lysine (gm)	Methionine (gm)	Phenylalanine (gm)	Valine (gm)	Arginine (gm)	Histidine (gm)
0.007	0.008	0.012	0.012	0.002	0.005	0.009	0.006	0.003
0.047	0.041	0.077	0.097	0.006	0.052	0.047	0.045	0.027
0.066	0.071	0.123	0.094	0.037	0.068	0.097	0.059	0.029
0.034	0.033	0.071	0.048	0.011	0.038	0.047	0.047	0.081
NA	NA	NA	NA	NA	NA	NA	NA	NA
0.018	0.021	0.040	0.012	0.011	0.024	0.028	0.034	0.010
0.023	0.023	0.040	0.040	0.011	0.019	0.026	0.011	0.004
NA	NA	NA	NA	NA	NA	NA	NA	NA
NA	NA	NA	NA	NA	NA	NA	NA	NA
0.052	0.047	0.088	0.060	0.022	0.056	0.066	0.066	0.030
0.024	0.023	0.033	0.030	0.006	0.018	0.028	0.017	0.011
0.100	0.093	0.133	0.122	0.025	0.074	0.115	0.070	0.043
			0.016	0.002				
0.017	0.005	0.013	0.014	0.021	0.013	0.017	0.046	0.023
0.031	0.030	0.055	0.023	0.005	0.002	0.028	0.021	0.007
NA	NA	NA	NA	NA	NA	NA	NA	NA
NA	NA	NA	NA	NA	NA	NA	NA	NA
			0.014	0.002				
0.019	0.018	0.031	0.041	0.005	0.017	0.026	0.019	0.012
NA	NA	NA	NA	NA	NA	NA	NA	NA
NA	NA	NA	NA	NA	NA	NA	NA	NA
NA	NA	NA	NA	NA	NA	NA	NA	NA
NA	NA	NA	NA	NA	NA	NA	NA	NA
0.015	0.025	0.023	0.047	0.020	0.031	0.040	0.065	0.018
0.011	0.008	0.016	0.025	0.002	0.009	0.010	0.010	0.005
0.027	0.020	0.040	0.023	0.017	0.022	0.038	0.018	0.013
0.010	0.011	0.020	0.014	0.005	0.010	0.014	0.007	0.004
0.030	0.025	0.042	0.033	0.005	0.026	0.030	0.025	0.012
0.012	0.013	0.019	0.025	0.011	0.012	0.016	0.018	0.009
0.016	0.016	0.021	0.017	0.006	0.017	0.019	0.013	0.0[illegible]

PROTEIN CONTENT OF FOOD (with Essential Amino Acids Values)

FOOD	Total Protein (grams)	Total E.A.A. adult/child (gm)	Tryptophan (gm)
pomegranates, raw	0.95		NA
raisins, seedless	3.39		NA
raspberries, raw	0.91		NA
strawberries	0.61	0.133/0.171	0.007
tangerines, raw	0.63	0.142/0.198	0.006
watermelon, raw	0.62	0.17/0.235	0.007
VEGETABLES AND SPROUTS:			
alfalfa seeds, sprouted, raw	3.99	0.903	-
artichokes, raw	2.66		NA
asparagus, raw	3.06	0.724/0.914	0.030
beans, lima, cooked, boiled, drained	6.81	2.63/3.317	0.089
mung beans, mature seeds, sprouted, raw	3.04	0.869/1.136	0.037
beans, snap, cooked, boiled, drained	1.89	0.563/0.674	0.020
beets, raw	1.48	0.332/0.390	0.017
beets, cooked, boiled, drained	1.06	0.237/0.279	0.012
beet greens, raw	1.82	0.372/0.452	0.029
beet greens, cooked, boiled, drained	2.57	0.636/0.748	0.040
broad beans, cooked, boiled, drained	4.80	1.591/2.103	0.048
broccoli, raw	2.98	0.747/0.942	0.029
brussel sprouts, raw	3.38	0.88/1.159	0.037
brussel sprouts, cooked, boiled, drained	2.55	0.664/0.874	0.028
cabbage, raw	1.21	0.338/0.432	0.012
cabbage, cooked, boiled, drained	0.96	0.267/0.340	0.010
cabbage, red, raw	1.39	0.386/0.493	0.014
carrots, raw	1.03	0.256/0.315	0.011
carrots, cooked, boiled, drained	1.09	0.271/0.333	0.012
cauli[illegible]	1.99	0.596/0.732	0.026
[illegible]d, boiled, drained	1.87	0.56/0.688	0.025
[illegible]	0.66	0.155/0.186	0.009
[illegible]	1.80	0.715/0.868	0.017

PROTEIN CONTENT OF FOOD (with Essential Amino Acids Values)

Threonine (gm)	Isoleucine (gm)	Leucine (gm)	Lysine (gm)	Methionine (gm)	Phenylalanine (gm)	Valine (gm)	Arginine (gm)	Histidine (gm)
NA	NA	NA	NA	NA	NA	NA	NA	NA
NA	NA	NA	NA	NA	NA	NA	NA	NA
NA	NA	NA	NA	NA	NA	NA	NA	NA
0.019	0.014	0.031	0.025	0.001	0.018	0.018	0.026	0.012
0.010	0.017	0.016	0.032	0.013	0.021	0.027	0.044	0.012
0.027	0.019	0.018	0.062	0.006	0.015	0.016	0.059	0.006
0.134	0.143	0.267	0.214			0.145		
NA	NA	NA	NA	NA	NA	NA	NA	NA
0.085	0.112	0.133	0.145	0.029	0.072	0.118	0.143	0.047
0.289	0.438	0.535	0.450	0.068	0.336	0.425	0.456	0.231
0.078	0.132	0.175	0.166	0.034	0.117	0.130	0.197	0.070
0.082	0.069	0.116	0.091	0.023	0.069	0.093	0.076	0.035
0.044	0.044	0.063	0.053	0.017	0.042	0.052	0.038	0.020
0.031	0.032	0.045	0.038	0.012	0.030	0.037	0.028	0.014
0.054	0.038	0.081	0.053	0.015	0.048	0.054	0.052	0.028
0.076	0.053	0.115	0.075	0.021	0.068	0.076	0.073	0.039
0.178	0.215	0.370	0.313	0.037	0.195	0.235	0.397	0.115
0.091	0.109	0.131	0.141	0.034	0.084	0.128	0.145	0.050
0.120	0.132	0.152	0.154	0.032	0.098	0.155	0.203	0.076
0.091	0.100	0.114	0.116	0.024	0.074	0.117	0.153	0.057
0.042	0.061	0.063	0.057	0.012	0.039	0.052	0.069	0.025
0.033	0.048	0.049	0.045	0.010	0.031	0.041	0.054	0.019
0.048	0.070	0.072	0.065	0.014	0.044	0.059	0.079	0.028
0.038	0.041	0.043	0.040	0.007	0.032	0.044	0.043	0.016
0.040	0.043	0.046	0.043	0.007	0.034	0.046	0.045	0.017
0.072	0.076	0.116	0.107	0.028	0.071	0.100	0.096	0.040
0.068	0.071	0.109	0.100	0.026	0.067	0.094	0.090	0.038
0.019	0.020	0.031	0.026	0.005	0.019	0.026	0.020	0.011
0.083	0.147	0.130	0.099	0.019	0.110	0.110	0.117	0.036

PROTEIN CONTENT OF FOOD (with Essential Amino Acids Values)

FOOD	Total Protein (grams)	Total E.A.A. adult/child (gm)	Tryptophan (gm)
collards, raw	1.57	0.465/0.575	0.020
sweet corn, raw	3.22	1.168/1.388	0.023
sweet corn, cooked, boiled, drained	3.32	0.556/0.782	0.023
cucumber, raw	0.54	0.117/0.159	0.004
dandelion greens, raw	2.70		NA
dandelion greens, cooked	2.00		NA
eggplant, cooked	0.83	0.252/0.317	0.008
endive, raw	1.25	0.418/0.503	0.005
garlic, raw	6.36	1.571/2.318	0.066
ginger root, raw	1.74	0.361/0.434	0.012
kale, raw	3.30	1.194/1.447	0.040
kale, cooked	1.90	0.466/0.612	0.023
kohlrabi, raw	1.70	0.362/0.486	0.010
leeks, raw	1.50	0.430/0.533	0.012
lentils, sprouted, raw	8.96	2.94/3.808	-
lettuce, romaine	1.62	0.685/0.801	0.012
mushrooms, raw	2.09	0.78/0.939	0.047
mustard greens, raw	2.70	0.608/0.853	0.030
okra, cooked	1.87	0.481/0.588	0.016
onions, raw	1.18	0.251/0.428	0.017
parsley, raw	2.20	0.270	0.036
parsnips, raw	1.20		NA
peas, edible, podded, raw	2.80	1.242/1.393	0.027
peas, green, raw	5.41	1.592/2.127	0.037
peas, mature, sprouted, raw	8.80	1.646/2.297	-
peppers, sweet, raw	0.85	0.223/0.298	0.011
potatoes, baked, flesh & skin	2.30	0.759/0.915	0.036
pumpkin, cooked, boiled, drained	0.72	0.182/0.232	0.009
radishes, raw	0.60	0.197/0.250	0.004
radish seeds, sprouted, raw	3.81		NA
rutabagas, cooked	1.10	0.253/0.416	0.012

PROTEIN CONTENT OF FOOD (with Essential Amino Acids Values)

Threonine (gm)	Isoleucine (gm)	Leucine (gm)	Lysine (gm)	Methionine (gm)	Phenylalanine (gm)	Valine (gm)	Arginine (gm)	Histidine (gm)
0.055	0.064	0.097	0.075	0.021	0.056	0.077	0.080	0.030
0.129	0.129	0.348	0.137	0.067	0.150	0.185	0.131	0.089
0.133	0.133	0.358	0.141	0.069	0.155	0.191	0.135	0.091
0.015	0.017	0.023	0.022	0.004	0.015	0.017	0.034	0.008
NA	NA	NA	NA	NA	NA	NA	NA	NA
NA	NA	NA	NA	NA	NA	NA	NA	NA
0.030	0.036	0.052	0.039	0.009	0.035	0.043	0.046	0.019
0.050	0.072	0.098	0.063	0.014	0.053	0.063	0.062	0.023
0.157	0.217	0.308	0.273	0.076	0.183	0.291	0.634	0.113
0.036	0.051	0.074	0.057	0.013	0.045	0.073	0.043	0.030
0.147	0.197	0.231	0.197	0.032	0.169	0.181	0.184	0.069
0.085	0.114	0.133	0.114	0.018	0.097	0.104	0.106	0.040
0.049	0.078	0.067	0.056	0.013	0.039	0.050	0.105	0.019
0.063	0.052	0.096	0.078	0.018	0.055	0.056	0.078	0.025
0.328	0.326	0.628	0.712	0.105	0.442	0.399	0.611	0.257
0.074	0.105	0.098	0.105	0.020	0.068	0.087	0.088	0.028
0.094	0.083	0.128	0.211	0.040	0.081	0.096	0.103	0.056
0.072	0.098	0.083	0.123	0.025	0.072	0.105	0.197	0.048
0.061	0.065	0.098	0.075	0.020	0.061	0.085	0.078	0.029
0.028	0.042	0.041	0.056	0.010	0.030	0.027	0.158	0.019
			0.219	0.015				
NA	NA	NA	NA	NA	NA	NA	NA	NA
0.099	0.161	0.228	0.202	0.011	0.090	0.273	0.134	0.017
0.203	0.195	0.323	0.317	0.082	0.200	0.235	0.428	0.107
0.186	0.171	0.365	0.384	0.069	0.251	0.220	0.484	0.167
0.031	0.027	0.044	0.038	0.010	0.026	0.036	0.041	0.017
0.084	0.093	0.138	0.140	0.036	0.102	0.130	0.106	0.050
0.021	0.023	0.034	0.039	0.008	0.023	0.025	0.039	0.011
0.029	0.030	0.037	0.035	0.007	0.023	0.032	0.040	0.013
NA	NA	NA	NA	NA	NA	NA	NA	NA
0.042	0.046	0.035	0.036	0.009	0.029	0.044	0.136	0.027

PROTEIN CONTENT OF FOOD (with Essential Amino Acids Values)

FOOD	Total Protein (grams)	Total E.A.A. adult/child (gm)	Tryptophan (gm)
soybeans, mature seed, sprouted, raw	13.09	3.095/3.686	0.181
soybeans, green, cooked	12.35	4.065/5.391	0.150
spinach, raw	2.86	1.048/1.274	0.039
summer squash, raw, all varieties	1.18	0.326/0.401	0.011
summer squash, all varieties, cooked	0.91	0.252/0.310	0.008
winter sqush, all varieities, baked	0.89	0.242/0.308	0.013
sweet potatoes, cooked, baked in skin	1.72	0.661/0.773	0.021
tomatoes, red, ripe, raw	0.89	0.170/0.205	0.007
turnips, raw	0.90	0.197/0.235	0.009
turnip greens, raw	1.50	0.649/0.779	0.026
watercress, raw	2.30	0.827/1.017	0.030
yam, baked	1.49	0.415/0.572	0.012
SPROUTS:			
alfalfa seeds, sprouted, raw	3.99	0.903	-
kidney beans, sprouted, raw	4.20	1.419/1.765	0.044
lentils, sprouted, raw	8.96	2.94/3.808	-
mungbeans, sprouted, raw	3.04	0.869/1.136	0.037
peas, sprouted, raw	8.80	1.646/2.297	-
radish seed, sprouted, raw	3.81		NA
soybeans, mature seed, sprouted, raw	13.09	3.095/3.686	0.181
wheat, sprouted, raw	7.49	2.235/2.856	0.115

PROTEIN CONTENT OF FOOD (with Essential Amino Acids Values)

Threonine (gm)	Isoleucine (gm)	Leucine (gm)	Lysine (gm)	Methionine (gm)	Phenylalanine (gm)	Valine (gm)	Arginine (gm)	Histidine (gm)
0.458	0.394	0.664	0.552	0.088	0.316	0.442	0.379	0.212
0.492	0.543	0.883	0.739	0.150	0.559	0.549	0.994	0.332
0.122	0.147	0.223	0.174	0.053	0.129	0.161	0.162	0.064
0.028	0.042	0.069	0.065	0.017	0.041	0.053	0.050	0.025
0.022	0.033	0.053	0.050	0.013	0.032	0.041	0.038	0.020
0.027	0.035	0.050	0.033	0.011	0.035	0.038	0.049	0.017
0.086	0.086	0.126	0.085	0.042	0.103	0.112	0.080	0.032
0.022	0.021	0.033	0.033	0.008	0.023	0.023	0.022	0.013
0.025	0.036	0.033	0.036	0.011	0.017	0.030	0.024	0.014
0.082	0.078	0.137	0.098	0.034	0.092	0.102	0.094	0.036
0.133	0.093	0.166	0.134	0.020	0.114	0.137	0.150	0.040
0.052	0.050	0.094	0.058	0.020	0.069	0.060	0.124	0.033
0.134	0.143	0.267	0.214			0.145		
0.176	0.186	0.302	0.239	0.044	0.212	0.216	0.228	0.118
0.328	0.326	0.628	0.712	0.105	0.442	0.399	0.611	0.257
0.078	0.132	0.175	0.166	0.034	0.117	0.130	0.197	0.070
0.186	0.171	0.365	0.384	0.069	0.251	0.220	0.484	0.167
NA	NA	NA	NA	NA	NA	NA	NA	NA
0.458	0.394	0.664	0.552	0.088	0.316	0.442	0.379	0.212
0.254	0.287	0.507	0.245	0.116	0.350	0.361	0.425	0.196

REFERENCES

CHAPTER 1 – *Intuitive Eating*

1. Ehret, Arnold. *Mucousless Diet Healing System*. Beaumont, CA: Ehret Literature Publishing Co., 1972.
2. Herrin, Angelia, "1988 Surgeon General's Report – 68% of All Deaths in U.S. are Diet Related," *Buffalo Evening News*, 1991, A-8.
3. Shealy, Norman M.D., Ph.D. and Caroline M. Myss M.A. *The Creation of Health.* Walpole, NH: Stillpoint Publishing, 1988, pp. 333-343.
4. Ibid, p. 11.
5. Schleifer, S.J., Keller, S.E., Camerino, M., Thornton, J.C., and Stein, M. "Suppression of Lymphocyte Stimulation Following Bereavement." *Journal of the American Medical Association*, 250(3), 1983, 374-377.
6. Shealy, pp. 333-343.

CHAPTER 2 – *Environmental Causes of Disease*

1. Lakhovsky, George. *LaCabale Historire d'une De-couverte* (L'oscillation Cellulaire). Paris: G. Doiw, 1934.
2. Gerber, Richard M.D. *Vibrational Medicine*. Santa Fe, NM: Bear and Company, 1988.
3. Ibid., pp. 122-123.
4. Becker, Robert O. M.D. and Gary Selden. *The Body Electric*. New York: William Morrow and Company, 1985.

5. Brodeur, Paul. "Zapping of America." *People Magazine.* December 1989.
6. Becker, Robert O. *Cross Currents: The Perils of Electropollution.* Los Angeles, CA: Jeremy P. Tarcher, 1990.
7. Dadd, Deborah Lynn. *The Non-Toxic Home.* Los Angeles, CA: Jeremy P. Tarcher, 1986.
8. "Is Your Water Safe?" *U.S. News & World Report,* July 29, 1991.
9. Ibid.
10. *In Health Magazine,* Sept.-Oct. 1991.
11. Ibid.
12. Voisin, Andre. *Soil, Grass, and Cancer.* South West Territory: London Crosby Lockwood & Son, L.T.D., 1959.
13. Ibid.
14. Gerson, Max M.D. *A Cancer Therapy – Results of Fifty Cases.* Del Mar, CA: Totality Books, 1958.
15. Robbins, John. *Diet for a New America.* Walpole, NH: Stillpoint Publishing, 1989, pp. 301-305.
16. Ibid.
17. Ibid., p. 343.
18. Buist, Robert Ph.D. *Food Chemical Sensitivity.* Garden City Park, NY: Avery Publishing Group, Inc., 1988, pp. 99-105.
19. Ibid.
20. Ibid.
21. Ibid., p. 66.
22. Ibid.
23. Robbins, p. 331.
24. Ibid.
25. Ibid., p. 330.
26. Ibid.
27. Buist, pp. 99-105.
28. Power, Kathleen M. "Food Irradiation: A Report to the Chiropractic Profession." *Today's Chiropractic Newsletter,* March 4, 1987.

CHAPTER 3 – *Nutrition Against Disease*

1. Tilden, John H. M.D. *Toxemia Explained.* Yorktown, TX: Life Science.
2. Cheraskin, E. M.D., W.M. Ringsdorf Jr. D.M.D., and J.W. Clark D.D.S. *Diet and Disease.* New Canaan, CT: Keats Publishing, Inc., 1968.

CHAPTER 4 – *Your Nutritional Primer*

1. Garten, Max, N.D. *Civilized Diseases And Their Circumvention.* San Jose, CA: Maxmillion World Publishers, pp. 37-38.
2. Gerson, Max, M.D. *A Cancer Therapy.* Del Mar, CA: Totality Books, 1958, p. 80.
3. Bionomics Health Research Institute of Tucson, AZ. (9702 Paseo Corona). *Overnutrition – All About Protein.* 1983, p. 10.
4. Ibid., p. 12.
5. Garten, p. 49.
6. Guyton, Arthur C., M.D. *Textbook of Medical Physiology.* Philadelphia, PA: W.B. Saunders, 1976, p. 970.
7. Bionomics Health Research Institute, p. 23.
8. Garten, p. 53.
9. McDougall, Dr. John and Mary McDougall. *The McDougall Plan.* Hampton, N.J.: New Century Publishing, Inc., 1983, pp. 95-106.
10. Robbins, John. *Diet For A New America.* Walpole, N.H.: Stillpoint Publishers, 1989, p. 195.
11. Correl, Dr. Alexis. *Man the Unknown.* New York: Harper and Row, 1935.
12. Bionomics Health Research Institute, p. 47.
13. Robbins, p. 195.
14. Pfeiffer, Carl, C., Ph.D., M.D. *Mental and Elemental Nutrients,* New Canaan, CT: Keats Publishing, Inc., 1975, p. 116-121.
15. Ibid., p. 125.

CHAPTER 5 – *Enzymes and Health*

1. Howell, Edward. *Food Enzymes For Health and Longevity.* P.O. Box 64, Woodstock Valley, CT 06282: Omangod Press. New copyright, 1980, by National Enzyme Company, Forsyth, MO.

   All the following references are reproduced here as they appear in Dr. Howell's original work.
2. Chemical Reviews, 13: 501-12 (1933)
3. *Food Enzymes For Health and Longevity.* by Dr. Edward Howell - Introduction by Viktoras Kulvinskas, Pub. Omangod Press 1986
4. *Enzymes and Hormones* by Elizabeth D. McCarter, B.S., M.Ed. D.Sc. and Robert McCarter, B.S., M.S., Ph.D. Publishers – Bionomics Health Research Institute of Tucson 1983
5. See note 2 above.
6. Biochemistry Zeit, 208: 415-27 (1929)
7. Journal of Experimental Medicine, 55: 505-9 (1932)
8. Enzymologia 1: 145-50 (1936)

9. Compt Rend. sociological biology, 112: 549-50 (1933)
10. Zeit, physiological chemistry, 221: 13-32 (1933)
11. Journal of clinical investigations, 13: 517-32 (1934)
12. American Journal of Digest. Dis. & Nut., 2: 230-5 (1935)
13. Proc Soc(iological) (Exp)periments (Bio)logy & (Med)icine, 28: 948-51 (1930-1)
14. *Enzyme Therapy*. Max Wolf, M.D. and Karl Ransbager, Ph.D. (Regent House, Los Angeles, CA, 1972)
15. Arch. F. Tierer v. Tierz 4: 507-25 (1931)
16. Klin. Woch, 9: 2295-6 (1930)
17. Therap. Arch. U.S.S.R., 12: 140-4 (1934)
18. See note 2 above
19. Sei-i-kai Mod. Journal, 54: 1531-8 (1935)
20. Arch. Verdanugskrankh, 49: 168-200 (1931)
21. Biochem. Zeit., 240: 328-56 (1931)
22. Amer. Journ. Digest. Dis., 5: 184-9 (1938)
23. Journal of Exptl. Zool., 76: 325-52 (1937)
24. *The McDougall Plan*, by John A. McDougall, M.D. & Mary A. McDougall (New Century Publishers, Inc., NJ 1983)
25. Bibliotek for Larger, 123: 437-70 (1931)
26. Nagoya Journal of Medical Science 3: 51-73 (1928)
27. Biochem zeit. 275: 216-33 (1935)
28. "The Influence of Food Cooking on the Blood Formula of Man" by Paul Kouchakoff, M.D. (Institute of Clinical Chemistry, Lausanne, Switzerland, 1930)
29. Same as note 28 above
30. "Survival into the 21st Century" by Viktoras Kulvinskas, (Omangod Press, Fairfield, Iowa, 1975)
31. Ibid.
32. Biochem. zeit. 288: 149-54 (1936)
33. Amer. Jour. Dig. Dis. & Nut. (Jan. 1934-5)
34. Same as note 2 above.
35. Journal of Nutrition, 13: 15-28 (1937)

CHAPTER 6 – *Eating For Life: From Degeneration to Regeneration*

1. Kulvinskas, Viktoras, M.S. *Survival Into The 21st Century*. Wethersfield, CT: Omangod Press, 1975, pp. 48-50.
2. Ibid.
3. Cousens, Gabriel, M.D. *Conscious Eating*. Santa Rosa, CA: Vision Books International, 1992, p. 360.
4. Quillin, Patrick, Ph.D., R.D. *Healing Nutrients*. Vintage Books, Division of Random House, 1987, p. 198.

5. Ibid., pp. 130-135.
6. Wagner, Eugene S., Ph.D. *The Vital Spark of Life*. Indiana University School of Medicine, p. 13.
7. "Alternatives Newsletter". Mountain Home Publishing, Vol. 2, No. 8, Feb. 1988.
8. Ibid.
9. Ibid.
10. Ibid.
11. Walford, Roy L. M.D. *The 120-Year Diet*. New York, NY: Pocket Books, Simon & Schuster, 1986.
12. Ibid., p. 56.
13. Ibid., p. 98.
14. Graham, Sylvester, M.D. *Science of Human Life*. New York: Fowler & Wells, 1883.
15. Ibid.
16. Walford, p. 72.

CHAPTER 7 – *Detoxification: The First Step In Your Transition*

1. Lindlahr, Henry, M.D. *Philosophy of Natural Therapeutics*. Chicago: Lindlar Publishing, 1922.
2. Kordich, Jay. *The Juiceman's Power of Juicing*. New York: William Morrow & Company, Inc., 1992.
3. Bragg, Paul, N.D. *The Miracle of Fasting*. Santa Ana, CA: Health Science, 1975.
4. Kloss, Jethro. *Back To Eden*. Santa Barbara, CA: Woodbridge Press, 1972.

CHAPTER 8 – *The Transitional Diet, Stage I*

1. Cousens, Gabriel, M.D. *Conscious Eating*. Santa Rosa, CA: Vision Books International, 1992, p. 366.
2. Quillin, Patrick, Ph.D., R.D. *Healing Nutrients*. New York, NY: Vintage Books, Division of Random House, 1987, P. 158.
3. Ibid., p. 243.
4. Ibid., p. 158.
5. Cousens, p. 202.
6. Ballentine, Rudolph, M.D. *Transition to Vegetarianism*. Honesdale, PA: Himalayan International Inst., 1987, p. 68.
7. Cousens, p. 189.
8. Ibid., p. 189.
9. Ibid., p. 185.
10. Ibid., p. 187.
11. Kulvinskas, Viktoras. *Love Your Body*. Wethersfield, CT: Omangod Press.
12. Kulvinskas, Viktoras. *Survival Into The 21st Century*. Wethersfield, CT: Omangod Press, 1975.

CHAPTER 9 – *The Health Benefits of Juicing*

1. Murray, Michael T., N.D. *The Complete Book of Juicing*. Rocklin, CA: Prima Publishing, 1992, p. 38.
2. *Wellness Letter*, University of California, Berkeley. December 1990; Vol. 7, No. 3.

INDEX

RETAIL ORDER FORM

NAME: ______________________

SHIPPING ADDRESS: ______________________

CITY: __________ STATE: __________ ZIP CODE: __________

QTY.	DESCRIPTION	COST		TOTALS
		US Mail	UPS	
	NATURAL HEALING WITH HERBS, 408 pages by Humbart "Smokey" Santillo, N.D.	$16.50	$19.00	
	HERBS, NUTRITION AND HEALING, 300 Minutes 4 Cassette Herbal Seminar Series by Humbart "Smokey" Santillo, N.D.	$46.75	$48.75	
	FOOD ENZYMES: The Missing Link to Radiant Health, 80 pages by Humbart "Smokey" Santillo, N.D.	$ 6.75	$ 8.75	
	FOOD ENZYMES: The Missing Link to Radiant Health, 150 Minures 3 Audio Cassette Recording of Food Enzymes and a Copy of the Book	$47.25	$49.25	
	ENERGETICS OF JUICING: The Key to Longevity, Health & Energy, 120 minures, 2 Cassette Seminar by Humbart "Smokey" Santillo, N.D. and a 48-Page Book	$31.75	$33.75	
	INTUITIVE EATING: EveryBody's Natural Guide To Total Health And Lifegiving Vitality Through Food, 450 pages by Humbart "Smokey" Santillo, N.D.	$18.50	$20.25	
		TOTAL ENCLOSED US FUNDS ONLY		

☐ **CHECK *or***
☐ **MONEY ORDER**

FOR SHIPPING OUTSIDE U.S. PLEASE ADD 25% FOR U.S. MAIL DELIVERY

Mail to: HOHM PRESS • P.O. Box 2501 • Prescott, Arizona U.S.A. 86302

PRICES SUBJECT TO CHANGE OVER TIME

RETAIL ORDER FORM

NAME:

SHIPPING ADDRESS:

CITY: STATE: ZIP CODE:

QTY.	DESCRIPTION	COST		TOTALS
		US Mail	UPS	
	NATURAL HEALING WITH HERBS, 408 pages by Humbart "Smokey" Santillo, N.D.	$16.50	$19.00	
	HERBS, NUTRITION AND HEALING, 300 Minutes 4 Cassette Herbal Seminar Series by Humbart "Smokey" Santillo, N.D.	$46.75	$48.75	
	FOOD ENZYMES: The Missing Link to Radiant Health, 80 pages by Humbart "Smokey" Santillo, N.D.	$ 6.75	$ 8.75	
	FOOD ENZYMES: The Missing Link to Radiant Health, 150 Minures 3 Audio Cassette Recording of Food Enzymes and a Copy of the Book	$47.25	$49.25	
	ENERGETICS OF JUICING: The Key to Longevity, Health & Energy, 120 minures, 2 Cassette Seminar by Humbart "Smokey" Santillo, N.D. and a 48-Page Book	$31.75	$33.75	
	INTUITIVE EATING: EveryBody's Natural Guide To Total Health And Lifegiving Vitality Through Food by Humbart "Smokey" Santillo, N.D.	$18.50	$20.25	
		TOTAL ENCLOSED US FUNDS ONLY		

❏ CHECK *or*
❏ MONEY ORDER

FOR SHIPPING OUTSIDE U.S. PLEASE ADD 25% FOR U.S. MAIL DELIVERY

Mail to: HOHM PRESS • P.O. Box 2501 • Prescott, Arizona U.S.A. 86302

PRICES SUBJECT TO CHANGE OVER TIME

HERBAL SEMINAR TAPES

These tapes are a live recording of an Herbal Seminar presented to laypersons, doctors, and other professionals by Humbart "Smokey" Santillo, N.D. The presentation begins with the basics of herbology and extends into a comprehensive coverage of therapies used in clinics throughout the world. It correlates historical herbology with the most recent in American and Chinese herbal philosophies. Following is a description of the content of each tape:

TAPE #1:

Side A—This side explains the role that the mind plays in healing—how ideas and thoughts affect the body and how, when negative, they result in dis-ease (disease). An interesting discussion explains how parts of the brain relay thought energy throughout the body, causing tension, stress, and other psychosomatic disorders. Once you understand this material, you are in a position to improve your mental attitude and avoid the negative effects of stress. The physical cause of disease is explained on this side along with other related subjects such as acid-alkaline balance, cleansing diets, detoxification, enervation (lowered nerve energy), and toxemia. These subjects lead into a complete discussion of acute and chronic diseases.

Side B—The three functions of herbs: eliminating, maintaining (balance), and building, are presented. These functions are coordinated with the healing purposes of herbs, such as demulcents, laxatives, expectorants, etc. Also discussed here, and continuing to Tape #2, are eight major therapies used to treat disease.

TAPE #2:

Side A—This tape explains treatments such as stimulation therapy, tranquilization therapy, blood purification and tonification therapies.

Side B—This side continues with more therapies such as sweating, emesis, diuresis, and purging. Herbs are listed under each therapy with a full discussion of herbal properties and their definitions.

TAPE #3:

Side A—This tape gives a complete explanation of how to prepare and use herbal infusions, decoctions, boluses, douches, electuaries, pills, enemas, tinctures, and oils.

Side B—A continuation of the previous side with discussions of how to prepare and use poultices, plasters, castor oil packs (for treatment of tumors), capsules, salves, and concentrates.

TAPE #4:

Side A—In Chinese medicine, diseases are categorized as being either hot or cold. This concept is explored along with suggested ways for determining which illnesses fall into these categories. Dietary suggestions are presented, including cleansing and transition diets. Primary and secondary symptoms are discussed, along with how to determine one's major weaknesses and strengths. This gives the herbalist a basis to determine which part of the body to treat.

Side B—This side includes a thorough explanation of how to treat colds, fevers, and flus using cold sheet treatments, hydrotherapy, and the herbs fenugreek, catnip, fennel, comfrey, and thyme. Most important on this tape is an explanation of how to build proper herbal formulas for both acute and chronic illnesses. The final part of this presentation deals with how each disease goes through five stages of development from the onset to the cure. Symptoms are discussed to help a therapist recognize the stages of the disease and choose the proper herbs for treatment.

* * *

These tapes include concentrated, easy-to-understand information which can be of assistance to anyone who has the interest. This information is invaluable for laypersons, doctors, or students who want to enhance their own health or wish to help others.

INTUITIVE EATING:

EveryBody's Natural Guide To Total Health And Lifegiving Vitality Through Food

by Humbart "Smokey" Santillo, N.D.

"Imagine being so attuned to your body that you knew exactly what it needed—when to add protein to your diet; what vegetables and fruits would immediately remedy any imbalance; what foods would help you through a period of emotional turmoil. This is no fantasy, however. It is a very real possibility. One that I have lived, and shared with thousands of clients. This is INTUITIVE EATING."

—*"Smokey" Santillo, from Chapter 1*

The natural voice of the body has been drowned out by the shouts of addictions, overconsumption, and devitalized and preserved foods. Millions battle the scale daily, experimenting with diets and nutritional programs, only to find their victories short-lived at best, confusing and demoralizing at worst. Intuitive Eating is an alternative.

Intuitive Eating is a handbook for developing a personalized relationship to food and nutrition characterized by self-awareness and environmental sensitivity. The author lays a firm foundation in the basics of nutrition and then guides the reader through a gentle, three-stage transitional diet with practical directions in the use of fresh juices and enzymes.

Meal plans and sample recipes, including health snacks and desserts, make the transition easy and enjoyable. Extensive charts provide an invaluable reference on the nutritional contents (protein values, vitamins, minerals, fat content, etc.) of most common foods.

Preface by Victor Kulvinskas, author of *Survival Into The 21st Century.*
Introduction by Jay Kordich, author of *The Juiceman's Power of Juicing.*

INTUITIVE EATING: *EveryBody's Natural Guide To Total Health And Lifegiving Vitality Through Food*
by Humbart "Smokey" Santillo, N.D., $16.95 US Funds
• 0-934252-27-0 Health/Nutrition, 420 pages/Trade Paper

TO ORDER BOOK, PLEASE SEE ACCOMPANYING ORDER FORM

NATURAL HEALING WITH HERBS
CORRESPONDENCE COURSE INFORMATION

This correspondence course has been written by the author for both the layperson and the physician. It is a course that will help prepare an individual to conduct his or her own herbal practice. The instruction presented in the course is unique in that it is coordinated with the material in the book *Natural Healing With Herbs*, which helps to make it simple for all to understand. Therapies utilizing nutritional foods, and both Chinese and American herbs (including their philosophies), are thoroughly discussed to furnish an understanding of both Eastern and Western medicine.

The course is divided into separate sections with questions and answers at the end of each section. Upon completion of the course, a final examination will be provided for the student to take and then mail back to the author for correction. The student, upon satisfactorily completing the course, will receive his or her Master Herbalist Degree. There is no time schedule on completing the course; some students may take six months, others may take one year or more. The student may proceed at his or her own pace.

The course is available for only $375.00 and an additional $16.50 if you have not purchased the book, *Natural Healing With Herbs*. It is essential that the student purchase the entire course plus the book, *Natural Healing With Herbs* at the same time. (If two or more courses are ordered at the same time, you pay only $350.00 each.) Students who prefer may make two payments. The first payment is $275.00 and includes only the first part of the course. A preliminary lesson preview is available for $7.00. The second part of the course will be mailed to the student upon receipt of the second payment of $100.00, which will be due within 30 days of the mailing date of the first part. (This includes shipping and handling charges.) A special price is offered to retail health food store owners or managers. Please write to the address below for more information. Make all checks or money orders (in U.S. funds only), payable to Humbart Santillo. Allow 3 - 4 weeks for delivery for courses paid by money order and 7 - 8 weeks for delivery for courses paid by check.

To assist the student, additional tapes are available, including some recorded live at herbal seminars given internationally by the author. These tapes contain further instruction on the proper use of herbs, diet, and the role the mind plays in healing.

Hundreds of people have been satisfied with this information. If within a two week trial period you find you are not satisfied with the material you have received, return the course for your refund minus $25.00 processing fee. This is a wonderful opportunity for the true seeker of herbal knowledge to receive proper, factual instruction.

To order courses or for more information, please write (no phone calls will be accepted): **Herbal Correspondence Course**, P.O. Box 468, East Amherst, New York 14051.

This course of study includes the following subjects:

Anatomy and Physiology

- Body Systems
- Pathology and Herbal Remedies

The Cause of Disease

- The Cell
- Elimination
- Acute and Chronic Diseases

The Properties of Herbs

The Chemical Constituents of Plants

Herbal Preparations

Herbal Formulations

Methods of Application

Diagnosis

- Pulse Diagnosis
- Questioning
- Yin Yang Theory
- Five Element Theory

The Ten Herbal Therapies

Physio-Medical Approach to Healing

Treatment of Inflammation and Pain

Monitoring the Healing Process

- Using the Temperature, Pulse, Blood Pressure, Urine and Saliva

Herbs for Pregnancy and Female Diseases

Herbs for Male Diseases

Chinese Herbs

Vitamins and Minerals in Plants

Food as Medicine